Prevention vs. Treatment

Prevention vs. Treatment

What's the Right Balance?

EDITED by HALLEY S. FAUST and

PAUL T. MENZEL

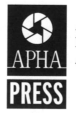

American
Public Health
Association

www.aphabookstore.org

OXFORD
UNIVERSITY PRESS

OXFORD
UNIVERSITY PRESS

Oxford University Press, Inc., publishes works that further
Oxford University's objective of excellence
in research, scholarship, and education.

Oxford   New York
Auckland   Cape Town   Dar es Salaam   Hong Kong   Karachi
Kuala Lumpur   Madrid   Melbourne   Mexico City   Nairobi
New Delhi   Shanghai   Taipei   Toronto

With offices in
Argentina   Austria   Brazil   Chile   Czech Republic   France   Greece
Guatemala   Hungary   Italy   Japan   Poland   Portugal   Singapore
South Korea   Switzerland   Thailand   Turkey   Ukraine   Vietnam

Published by Oxford University Press, Inc.
198 Madison Avenue, New York, New York 10016
www.oup.com

Oxford is a registered trademark of Oxford University Press

Library of Congress Cataloging-in-Publication Data

Prevention vs. treatment : what's the right balance? / edited by Halley S. Faust and Paul T. Menzel.
    p. ; cm.
Includes bibliographical references and index.
ISBN 978-0-19-983737-3
1. Medicine, Preventive—United States. 2. Preventive health services—United States.
3. Evidence-based medicine—United States. I. Faust, Halley S. II. Menzel, Paul T., 1942-
[DNLM: 1. Preventive Health Services—United States. 2. Evidence-Based Medicine—United States.
3. Health Promotion—United States. 4. Primary Prevention—United States.
5. Religion and Medicine—United States. 6. Therapeutics—United States. WA 108]
RA425.P725 2012
614.4'40973—dc22   2011010087

To Ruth Anne, Halley's double chai *patient love; his wonderful sons and daughter-in-law, Josh, Aaron, and Rachel; and his beautiful grandchildren, Natalie Sam and Maya Bella.*

In memory of Susan Louise Blank (1942–2007), Paul's late wife, who gained six wonderful years of life from state-of-the-art medical treatment; of his mother, Annemarie Mueller Menzel (1913–2010), a model of how a deeply good heart and a stress-free disposition can seemingly lengthen life; and of his sister, Rhea Menzel Whitehead (1936-2011), whom acute care could not rescue.

CONTENTS

ACKNOWLEDGMENTS

Many people and organizations have been instrumental in inspiring the editors to take on this project. We are grateful to the American College of Preventive Medicine for initiating at its annual meeting in 2004 the seminar on the ethics of prevention that eventually gave birth to this volume. We also thank Kenneth Warner, immediate past Dean of the University of Michigan School of Public Health; the Altarum Institute of Ann Arbor, particularly Charles Roehrig and George Miller; and Thomas Murray, Michael Gusmano, and others at the Hastings Center who have encouraged us in this project.

We especially thank our contributing authors. They responded enthusiastically to our invitations, were instrumental in the thinking, strategy, and development of the volume, and have patiently worked with us through two years of the book's assembly. Most of them developed their papers specifically for this book; we are grateful for their industriousness, scholarly care, good nature in light of our editing and suggestions, and timeliness in meeting deadlines.

Finally, we thank Oxford University Press, especially Peter Ohlin, Lucy Randall, Karen Kwak, Veena Deepak, and two anonymous reviewers of the manuscript. The American Public Health Association, especially through the efforts of Nina Tristani, has lent an unusually important hand to the project by working with Oxford University Press as co-publisher.

Halley Faust thanks foremost Paul Menzel, without whom this project would not have seen the light of day; Halley is grateful to have Paul as a colleague and friend. Halley also thanks Kevin Patrick, Steve Woolf, Doug Kamerow, Caroline Burnett, Mike Parkinson, Mark Johnson, Mark Cherry, and Stephen Angle. He appreciates and thanks his philosophy teachers and mentors at Wesleyan who helped him develop his foundation in ethics and philosophy of science: Lori Gruen, Joe Rouse, Kelly Sorensen, and Eric Schliesser, and former Senior Associate Provost, Billy Weitzer. In addition, Halley thanks his colleagues at the

American College of Preventive Medicine, his fellow clinical ethics fellows and mentors from the University of Toronto Joint Centre for Bioethics, especially former directors Peter Singer and Ross Upshur, and his current colleagues at the University of New Mexico's Department of Family and Community Medicine. He is indebted to all those who worked with him in the health care industry over the past 35 years, giving him opportunities, and prodding his thinking and understanding of the behavior of patients, physicians, health care professionals, and policy makers, especially Bill Thar, Bob Scranton, Larry Brilliant, John Atwater, Hugh Tilson, Keith Stevenson, Tom James, Larry Kries, Phil Bredesen, Richard Cooper, Jay Ripps, Dave Reed, Mark Buchanan, Skip Creasey, Hazel Keimowitz, Mike Barry, Paul Bonta, and Marki Ware. Finally, Halley thanks his wife, Ruth Anne, for her encouragement and moral support during the many times he said, "Have to work on the book."

Paul Menzel is grateful above all for the fact that an accomplished and philosophically astute preventive medicine physician proposed to him this project; subsequently, Halley's patience, persistence, and insight always made the work a pleasure. Paul's preparation on this topic was laid in the three previous decades, when he benefitted from the specific encouragement of Baruch Brody, Daniel Callahan, Ruth Faden, and Peter Singer, among others, and from collaborative writing with Erik Nord, Peter Ubel, Jeff Richardson, Marthe Gold, Paul Dolan, and Jan Abel Olsen. Pacific Lutheran University always provided him with an ideal setting for undergraduate teaching, cross-disciplinary stimulation, and valued scholarship. In recent years he has especially appreciated the support of Bonnie Steinbock and their many fertile conversations.

CONTRIBUTORS

Roy Branson, PhD, is Professor of Religion and Associate Dean of the School of Religion at Loma Linda University, where he directs the University's Center for Christian Bioethics. Branson took his doctorate in Religious Ethics from Harvard University before joining the faculty of the Seventh-day Adventist Seminary to establish their ethics program. After moving to the Kennedy Institute of Ethics at Georgetown University, he co-edited *Ethics and Health Policy* with Robert Veatch. He has written on ethics and religious apocalyptic for the *Kennedy Institute of Ethics Journal* and in chapters of several volumes published within the Seventh-day Adventist community. He has served as President of the Adventist Society for Religious Studies and started the Interreligious Coalition on Smoking or Health, the first faith-based lobby (Catholic–Protestant–Jewish–Muslim) for public policies regulating tobacco use.

Ho Mun Chan, PhD, MSc, is Associate Professor of Philosophy in the Department of Public and Social Administration, City University of Hong Kong. His BA and MPhil are from the University of Hong Kong in philosophy, his MSc from the University of Sussex in knowledge-based systems, and his PhD in philosophy from the University of Minnesota. His publications have focused on comparative social and political philosophy, applied and comparative ethics, and the philosophy of science and technology. In health care ethics he has published on health care justice, resource allocation, organ transplantation, surrogate motherhood, informed consent, advance directives, long-term care, euthanasia, and end-of-life decision making. He is currently a member of the Clinical Ethics Committee of the Hospital Authority in Hong Kong and chairs its Working Group on Advance Directives.

Norman Daniels, PhD, is Mary B Saltonstall Professor and Professor of Ethics and Population Health in the Department of Global Health and Population at

Harvard School of Public Health. He was formerly chair of the Philosophy Department at Tufts University, where he taught until 2002; his most recent books include *Just Health: Meeting Health Needs Fairly* (Cambridge 2008); *Setting Limits Fairly: Learning to Share Resources for Health,* 2nd edition (Oxford 2008); *From Chance to Choice: Genetics and Justice* (2000); and *Is Inequality Bad for Our Health?* (2000). His research is on justice and health policy, including priority setting in health systems, fairness and health systems reform, health inequalities, and intergenerational justice. He directs the Ethics concentration of the Health Policy PhD, recently won the Everett Mendelsohn Award for mentoring graduate students, and teaches courses on ethics and health inequalities and justice and resource allocation.

Halley S. Faust, MD, MPH, MA, is Clinical Associate Professor of Family and Community Medicine at the University of New Mexico, and for 15 years has been managing member of Jerome Capital, LLC, a venture capital firm involved mostly in high technology medical ventures. He is also President-Elect of the American College of Preventive Medicine (ACPM), Chairperson of the Committee on Ethics of the ACPM, and former chairperson of ACPM's Policy and Finance Committees. He has taught epidemiology, health policy, and bioethics at several universities and has been on the bioethics committees and institutional review boards of two medical centers. Earlier in his career he spent 8 years as a senior manager at Aetna Life Insurance Company and Health America Corporation, and 6 years as the medical director of a public health department. His MA is in philosophy from Wesleyan University, CT and his MPH is in health planning and administration from the University of Michigan. He is board certified in general preventive medicine and medical management, and was a clinical ethics fellow at the University of Toronto's Joint Centre for Bioethics. He is a fellow of the American College of Preventive Medicine and the American College of Physician Executives.

Shimon Glick, MD, is Professor (emeritus) of Medicine at Ben Gurion University in Beer Sheva, Israel, and Editor of the journal *ASSIA-Jewish Medical Ethics.* He received his MD from the Downstate Medical Center, Brooklyn, NY, training in internal medicine and endocrinology. After positions as Chief of Medical Services at the Coney Island Hospital in Brooklyn and Clinical Professor of Medicine at the Downstate Medical Center, he emigrated in 1974 to Israel to become founding Chairman of the Division of Medicine at the Ben Gurion University Faculty of Health Sciences. He subsequently served there as Dean, head of the Moshe Prywes Center for Medical Education, and acting head of the Lord Rabbi Jakobovits Center for Jewish Medical Ethics. For over a decade he served as ombudsman for Israel's National Health Service. He is the father of 6, grandfather of 46, and greatgrandfather of 30.

Paul Hughes-Cromwick, MA, is Senior Analyst at Altarum Institute (Ann Arbor), where he leads outreach and marketing for the Altarum Center for Sustainable Health Spending. He took his MA in economics from Clark University, after a BS from Notre Dame in mathematics and philosophy. He was Chairman of the Board of Care Choices HMO (Farmington, MI) until its sale and currently sits on the Board of Directors of St. Joseph Mercy Oakland Hospital, Pontiac, MI. Co-author of "Quantifying National Spending on Wellness and Prevention" in *Beyond Health Insurance: Public Policy to Improve Health*, he serves as project manager of the National Heart, Lung, and Blood Institute funded study, *Systems Science Methods for Addressing the Cardiovascular Disease Prevention-Treatment Trade-Off.*

Alan Jotkowitz, MD, is Director of the Jakobovits Center for Jewish Medical Ethics, Faculty of Health Sciences, Ben Gurion University of the Negev, Israel. He is also Senior Lecturer in Medicine and a Senior Physician, Department of Medicine, Soroka University Medical Center, Beer-Sheva, Israel. He is the author of numerous articles in the *American Journal of Bioethics*, the *Journal of Medical Ethics*, and the *Journal of Jewish Medical Ethics*.

Nuala Kenny, OC, BA, MD, FRCP(C), is Emeritus Professor of Bioethics at Dalhousie University in Halifax, Nova Scotia and the Ethics and Health Policy Advisor to the Catholic Health Alliance of Canada. She is a member of the Sisters of Charity of Halifax. After a distinguished career in pediatrics and medical education, she founded the Department of Bioethics at Dalhousie in 1995. In 1999 she was seconded as Deputy Minister of Health for the Province of Nova Scotia. Past President of both the Canadian Paediatric and Canadian Bioethics Societies and author of over one hundred papers, she has also authored two books, *What Good Is Health Care: Reflections on the Canadian Experience* and *Lost Virtue: Professional Character Development in Medical Education.*

Paul T. Menzel, PhD, is Professor of Philosophy at Pacific Lutheran University. He began his writing on philosophical issues in health economics and health policy with *Medical Costs, Moral Choices: A Philosophy of Health Care Economics for America* (Yale University Press 1983) and *Strong Medicine: The Ethical Rationing of Health Care* (Oxford University Press 1990). In 1999 he began publication of a series of papers with health economists about philosophical questions raised by the methodological structure of cost-effectiveness analysis.

In other essays since he has explored the relationship between justice and liberty in health system structure and health insurance reform.

George Miller, PhD, MSE, is Institute Fellow at Altarum Institute (Ann Arbor), where he applies operations research methods to modelling and analysis of health care issues. He was a lead participant in an Altarum project to estimate national health expenditures by medical condition (published in *Health Affairs*), directed a project to estimate national expenditures on prevention (published in *Advances in Health Economics and Health Services Research*), and is currently principal investigator on a grant from the National Institutes of Health to explore trade-offs between investments in treatment and in prevention. Dr. Miller took his degrees in Industrial and Operations Engineering from the University of Michigan and has served there as Adjunct Assistant Professor.

Diana B. Petitti, MD, MPH, is Professor of Biomedical Informatics at Arizona State University. With her MD from Harvard and MPH from the University of California, Berkeley, she has held positions with the Centers for Disease Control and the University of California, San Francisco School of Medicine. As Director of Research and Evaluation with Kaiser Permanente Southern California, Dr. Petitti was a member of the senior management team that oversaw clinical practice guidelines, technology assessment, and quality measurement and improvement. She has authored more than 200 papers and two books: *Meta-Analysis, Decision Analysis, and Cost-Effectiveness Analysis: Methods for Quantitative Synthesis in Medicine* and, with Ross Brownson, *Applied Epidemiology*. She has served on several national committees addressing issues of evidence-based medicine and its applications, most recently, from 2004 to 2009, as Vice Chair of the United States Preventive Services Task Force.

Thaddeus Mason Pope, JD, PhD, is formerly of Widener Law School, is now Director of the Health Law Institute at Hamline University School of Law. He teaches and writes in health law, bioethics, public health, and torts. Following his JD from Georgetown University he clerked for the U.S. Court of Appeals, Seventh Circuit, and then worked for Arnold and Porter LLP in Los Angeles. Since completing his doctoral dissertation under public health theorist Larry Gostin, he has been deeply engaged in legal, policy, and ethical issues concerning public health law and ethics. In one of his most important publications, "Balancing Public Health against Individual Liberty: The Ethics of Smoking Regulations" (*University of Pittsburgh Law Review* 2000), Pope examines and debunks alleged ethical and policy limits to a growing U.S. emphasis on prevention instead of treatment. He has published widely on public health paternalism.

Charles Roehrig, PhD, MA, is Vice-President of Altarum Institute (Ann Arbor) and Director of their Center for Sustainable Health Spending. He has led the development of the Altarum Health Sector Model (AHSM) to forecast health care expenditures under alternative assumptions about insurance coverage, underlying needs, access to care, and prices paid for care. He has developed estimates of national health expenditures by medical condition (*Health Affairs* February 2009) and by categories of prevention, and is currently researching the impact of disease prevalence on national health expenditures and the trade-off between spending on prevention and treatment of chronic illness. In addition to this applied work, he has published in theoretical econometrics in journals such as *Econometrica* and the *Journal of Econometrics*. Dr. Roehrig took his PhD in economics and his MA in statistics from the University of Michigan.

Louise B. Russell, PhD, is Research Professor in the Institute for Health and Professor in the Department of Economics, Rutgers University, New Brunswick, NJ. An elected member of the Institute of Medicine, Dr. Russell served on IOM's National Cancer Policy Board and on the Committee on Valuing Community-Based, Non-Clinical Prevention Policies and Wellness Strategies. She co-chaired the U.S. Public Health Service Panel on Cost-Effectiveness in Health and Medicine, which published recommendations to improve the quality and comparability of cost effectiveness studies in *Cost-Effectiveness in Health and Medicine* (Oxford University Press, 1996) and three articles in *The Journal of the American Medical Association* (October 1996). She was also a member of the first U.S. Preventive Services Task Force. Her publications include *Educated Guesses. Making Policy About Medical Screening Tests* (University of California 1994) and *Is Prevention Better Than Cure?* (Brookings 1986). She is deputy editor of the journal *Medical Decision Making*.

Ani Turner, BA, is Senior Analyst with Altarum Institute (Ann Arbor) where she leads health workforce analysis and modeling for Altarum's Center for Sustainable Health Spending. As a consultant to government and commercial clients for over two decades, she has researched health care resources, costs, and quality for the Department of Health and Human Services, the Department of Defense, individual States, and private health plans. In her current work she studies the nation's primary care physician workforce for the Council on Graduate Medical Education and updates the federal government's official forecasts of physician supply and demand by specialty.

Aana Marie Vigen, PhD, is Associate Professor of Christian Social Ethics at Loyola University Chicago. A member of the Society of Christian Ethics and the American Association of Bioethics and Humanities, Dr. Vigen serves on the national Genetics Task Force of the Evangelical Lutheran Church in America. She is the author of *Women, Ethics, and Inequality in U.S. Healthcare: "To Count Among the Living"* (Palgrave 2006, 2ⁿᵈ edition 2011), co-editor (with Patricia Beattie Jung) of *God, Science, Sex, Gender, Ethics: An Interdisciplinary Approach to Ethics* (University of Illinois Press 2010), and co-author/editor (with Christian Scharen) of *Ethnography as Christian Theology and Ethics* (Continuum Press 2011).

Robert B. Wallace, MD, is Irene Ensminger Stecher Professor of epidemiology and internal medicine at the University of Iowa. His research activities surround the causes and control of the chronic diseases of older persons. He was a member of the U.S. Preventive Services Task Force and is editor of the current (15th) edition of *Maxcy-Rosenau-Last's Public Health and Preventive Medicine* (McGraw-Hill 2008).

Introduction

HALLEY S. FAUST, MD, MPH, MA, and
PAUL T. MENZEL, PhD ■

In 1977 Benjamin Freedman (1977) wrote, "it is more praiseworthy to save a life than to preserve health" and concluded, "in a closed system providing health services a relative primacy should be given to health care over preventive medicine."

At the time, one of us (Faust) was in the midst of a preventive medicine residency and took great umbrage at Freedman's statement. Many of Faust's values were being challenged just at a time when he was idealistically oriented to encouraging the use of greater resources for prevention. Faust began a written response that he did not complete, but he never forgot his concerns and vowed eventually to write about Freedman's conclusions.

At the same time, the second of us (Menzel) began to answer Freedman's claims in what became a chapter of his *Medical Costs, Moral Choices*. Menzel (1983) generally rejected Freedman's arguments, but he also articulated what he thought were more persuasive, though highly conditional, arguments for treatment's priority. He concluded that the distinction between preventive and rescue medicine has only variable moral weight and ended with a distinctly nonrevolutionary view: we should not so much shrink our commitment to treatment as spend more resources on prevention so that we do not demand more benefit and efficiency from it than we do from treatment.

Two decades later, in 2004, Faust and Menzel met when they led a workshop on the ethics of prevention at the annual meeting of the American College of Preventive Medicine. It is from that collaboration and further discussion that this volume has evolved. The discussion came naturally, stimulated repeatedly by questions about treatment's relationship to prevention presented by the society in which we live. For example:

- Why will we marshal all available resources to save a little girl who's fallen into the well, while we either procrastinate or avoid putting a protective barrier around the well long before she would have fallen in?
- Why is it that health insurance originally was developed to contribute toward catastrophic costs of health care, but was reluctant to include coverage for preventive activities—until government mandates or union bargaining forced coverage for measures such as immunizations and breast and cervical cancer screening?
- Why is it that nutrition and fitness counseling still are rarely covered in health insurance plans?

To avow ideological preference for prevention we use sayings such as Benjamin Franklin's 1736 statement, "An ounce of prevention is worth a pound of cure." We frequently hear comments such as "Preventive medicine—we need more of that." Many physicians in the United States have taken the version of the Hippocratic Oath revised in 1964 by Louis Lasagna (1964), wherein they affirm, "I will prevent disease whenever I can, for prevention is preferable to cure." Yet generally as a society we appear not to follow through with policies to encourage prevention as quickly or as resolutely as we cheer the expansion of treatments as soon as they surface. Physicians similarly usually prioritize treatment over prevention.

The matter is not simply weakness of will in acting on our convictions; in our thinking, too, treatment holds priority. Reallocation from cure to prevention strikes some as "taking from the sick and giving to the healthy," perhaps not a compassionate or fair thing to do.[1] In many of our religious traditions we are urged to care for the current acutely needy as a matter of obligation, while we are urged to help the potentially future needy as something merely desirable and praiseworthy. In specific social philosophies we are urged as a matter of justice to attend to the worst-off first.[2] In health care attending to the worst-off generally means those already suffering from medical ailments, not those

1. Olsen (1993, 263) quotes a Norwegian Health Director as having said that reallocation from cure to prevention implies that "one takes from the sick and gives to the healthy."

2. First articulated in philosophically systematic fashion by John Rawls (1971). Rawls' view, though not only or even primarily its part that accords priority to the worst-off, was made prominent specifically for health care by Norman Daniels, first in *Just Health Care* (1985) and most recently in *Just Health* (2008).

lacking prevention. Were we to carry this to its logical extreme, we might never even get to prevention; the burden of treating all with medical illness and suffering to the maximum extent reasonable could consume all the resources our society was willing to devote to health care.

Realistically we should probably admit that this strong pull to use the great majority of our financial and emotional resources to alleviate immediate suffering before preventing future suffering, whether in thought and attitudes or in behavior, constitutes an actual value and priority of our society. This priority seems stubborn even as economists describe people as *homo economicus* (Pareto 1906), a being that tries to achieve its personal preferences to a maximum extent at minimum cost, knowing what is best for its physical and mental health and acting to attain it. Increasingly, behavioral economists have marshaled empirical evidence that this notion is naive. In their growing field, behavioral economists factor in other cognitive, cultural, and emotional variables that often appear not to represent rational self-interest.

If we thought and acted on the rational, ideal level of *homo economicus*, we would almost certainly give priority to *avoiding* suffering over alleviating and recovering from it. We prefer, after all, to go about our lives in uninterrupted good health from which we do not need to recover. Dependably good health contributes toward our overall well-being, permitting us to work toward fulfilling more completely our life goals and desires.[3] Even if illness can be effectively treated, when we recover we are often unable to return fully to our pre-ailment condition. From any utilitarian perspective it would seem that preventing suffering should be more highly valued than alleviating it.

If preventing disease and maintaining health are rationally preferable to treating disease and rehabilitating from it, two questions about our current situation stand out: (1) What explains why, as a matter of fact, in our Western health care systems—at least in U.S. health care—we concentrate so many more resources on alleviating illness than on preventing it? (2) Can this apparent imbalance be morally justified? These two primary questions provide the focus for this volume. Exploring them requires attention to many different considerations. For this volume we have chosen the empirical considerations of economics in combination with clinical evidence, philosophical moral analysis, and the perspectives of several religious and cultural traditions.

Before providing an orientation to the concerns of the volume's different sections we will first articulate more specific, less impressionistic evidence for the claim that prevention takes second place in competing for resources.

---

3. "Bodily health" is one of the 10 specific capability needs for human functioning according to Martha Nussbaum (2000, 78): "Being able to have good health, including reproductive health; to be adequately nourished; to have adequate shelter."

We will also dispose of some of the most common but inadequate justifications for providing priority to treatment, and define the key terms needed to pursue the central questions of this volume.

EVIDENCE OF PRIORITY OF TREATMENT OVER PREVENTION

Assuming that our values are in part reflected in how we spend our resources of money and time, we can see that our society collectively values treatment-related services over preventive ones. Here are just a few manifestations:

- The work of Miller et al. in this volume (Chapter 2) shows that for every dollar spent in our health care system on prevention services and research, more than 11 dollars are spent on treatment services and research.
- Medicare has paid for renal dialysis since Public Law 92-601 was enacted on October 30, 1972, after only 30 minutes of floor debate and with only one dissenting Senate vote (Lockridge 2004).[4] By contrast, only since 1991 and after years of delays and debates did Medicare and Medicaid cover mammography screening for breast cancer in women. Nattinger and Goodwin (1992) note that "for more than 13 years, one branch of the federal government actively promoted a medical procedure [mammography] that another branch did not reimburse."
- Medicare explicitly permits cost considerations in evaluating certain preventive tests and services, such as screening for colorectal and prostate cancer, as long as those tests and services are recommended with a grade of A or B by the U.S. Preventive Services Task Force (Dhruva et al. 2009).[5] No such explicit permission for considering cost

4. The actual voting and debate discussion was found online at the "History of Dialysis" from the website http://www.kidneycarepartners.org/index.php/dialysis/history.html for Kidney Care Partners, accessed April 10, 2005. That link is no longer operational. See also Schreiner (2000).

5. Except for breast and cervical cancer screening, Medicare precluded preventive services coverage entirely until a 2003 law took effect in 2005. See the 2004 CMS Legislative Summary of H.R. 1, Medicare Prescription Drug, Improvement, and Modernization Act of 2003, Public Law 108-173, http://www.cms.gov/MMAUpdate/downloads/PL108-173summary.pdf, pp 89–90, accessed June 1, 2011. Further coverage was permitted effective January 1, 2009, as an amendment to the law, 42 CFR—PART 410, §410.64, and with the Patient Protection and Affordable Care Act (PPACA) of 2010 (United States Congress 2010), discussed by Faust in Chapter 6 of this volume. Note that even in the PPACA "comparative clinical

applies to treatment services. Since Medicare's inception, while "the consideration of costs in treatment services… [has] not [been] a 'prohibition,'" there has been "a long-standing practice of not considering them in… coverage decision making" (Salive 2009).

- In Medicare authorization, moreover, no requirement exists for specific treatment services to be evaluated by a separate federal body, parallel to that requirement for preventive services. (Historically, third-party claims intermediaries for Medicare have made coverage decisions, though since 1999 the Medicare Coverage Advisory Committee has provided nonbinding advice to Medicare.)
- Postgraduate preventive medicine and public health residency training programs are one of only two types of physician training not funded through Medicare/Medicaid authorization,[6] and frequently they are only minimally funded through Title VII funds. The supply of preventive medicine and public health physicians in the United States has been estimated to be short by 50%: there are an estimated 10,000 currently, and the Institute of Medicine estimated in 2007 that the nation needs another 10,000. Simply to maintain the current level of 10,000, 1,350 residents per year need to be educated; currently fewer than 300 are being trained annually (National Academy of Sciences 2007).
- Public health and preventive medicine physicians receive the lowest mean compensation of physicians in any specialty, fully 10–20% lower than the next lowest medical specialty (Cjeka Search and the American College of Physician Executives 2009, 139).
- Delivery of preventive services is "fragmented and often ineffective and inefficient" (Porter 2009). They are not organized with proper personnel and functionality in primary care physician offices, where they are supposed to be provided. In contrast, surgical and medical intervention services in hospitals have highly developed structures and processes.
- The Patient Protection and Affordable Care Act of 2010 (PL 111-148 or PPACA) specifically includes cost considerations in evaluating

---

effectiveness research" does not mention costs (HR 3590, 609) as compared with "clinical preventive services research," which specifically mentions "cost-effectiveness" as a valid criterion for policy development (HR 3590, 424–425).

6. The other is pediatrics, which gets annual reliable funding through a separate line item for children's hospitals.

prevention, but not when considering the comparative effectiveness of
treatment options (United States Congress 2010).[7]

One of us (H.S.F.), a board certified preventive medicine physician, has
noticed during his years in the health care system that in prosperous times prevention and health promotion programs are instituted at corporations, government, and nonprofits. When economic times are tough, however, employers
and government are loath to eliminate coverage of treatment, whereas prevention programs are often eliminated first. A good recent illustration is that shortly
after passage of the PPACA some in Congress tried to use the appropriations
for the Prevention and Public Health Fund (Section 4002) to offset the increase
in Medicare payments to physicians (Kliff 2010).

In state and local government programs public health funds rarely take precedence over transportation, legal, education, or other funds. Moreover, there is
evidence that in their individual choices, Americans forego prevention in economically rough times more than they do treatment, which is seemingly more
urgent. A survey of the members of the American Academy of Family Physicians
in the midst of the recent economic recession of 2009 noted that "6 out of 10
respondents said they were seeing more health problems as a result of skipped
preventive care, such as screenings, or unfilled prescriptions" (Rubin 2009).

Even in the U.S. legal system, as discussed by Pope in Chapter 10 of this
volume, "Generally, there is no obligation to protect others from harm. Tort law
treats actions differently from omissions. It protects negative rather than positive rights." Admittedly, protection from harm is prominent in some so-called
"product liability" cases, but special contextual reasons may be driving prevention's importance there, and the equivalence in the law is only between not

---

7. Section 4003 of PL 111–148 establishes the Preventive Services Task Force, which "shall
review the scientific evidence related to the effectiveness, appropriateness, and cost-effectiveness of clinical preventive services for the purpose of developing recommendations for the
health care community." The only place "cost-effectiveness" appears again in this Act is when
evaluating hospice (Section 3140) and conducting complaint investigations related to long-
term care facilities (Section 2046). All sections dealing with treatment-related items do not
include the term "cost-effectiveness" though the term "efficient health care services" is used
in evaluating quality improvement activities (Section 933). PL 111–148 replaces the Federal
Coordinating Council for Comparative Effectiveness Research established by Section 804 of
the American Recovery and Reinvestment Act of 2009 (ARRA), with the Patient-Centered
Outcomes Research Institute for clinical effectiveness research that does not include evaluating costs of services or treatments for individual patients, though it does include the ability
of the Institute to look at "the effect on national expenditures associated with a health care
treatment, strategy, or health conditions" (Section 6301). There are specific exclusions for the
use of dollars per quality-adjusted life year (QALY) for thresholds "to determine coverage,
reimbursement, or incentive programs" (Section 1182).

preventing and directly causing *when there is a duty to prevent.* We should not interpret the law as harboring a general equivalence between preventing and alleviating harm, and it is treacherous to emphasize legal obligations to prevent as true counterelements to the typical bias toward providing resources for treatment. Nonetheless, in some parts of the law, the negligent failure to prevent harm is treated as a wrong equal to the wrong of causing harm; in fact, in those cases, the law would say that not preventing harm *is* causing it.

It is also possible that we are currently seeing some movement toward a greater balance between prevention and treatment as people are asked to stand back and express preferences more abstractly about our health care system. In a recent Kaiser Family Foundation survey, 34% wanted to see increased spending on "public health programs to prevent the spread of disease and improve health"; 55% said "keep it about the same" (Kaiser Family Foundation/Harvard School of Public Health 2009).[8] A Robert Wood Johnson Foundation sponsored poll found that "More than three-quarters of American voters support increasing funding for prevention... While a vast majority believes that prevention will in fact save us money, more than 7 in 10 support an investment in prevention regardless of whether it will save money" (Greenberg Quinlan Rosner 2009).

Despite such recent surveys and long-term legal developments, abundant evidence exists that U.S. health care is more strongly predisposed toward treatment. To say "strongly predisposed toward treatment" does not, of course, mean that treatment is always chosen and prevention is never chosen. Priority for treatment does not mean we choose treatment over prevention when treatment is simply ineffective in alleviating harm, much less efficient in doing so,[9] or of high risk even with potentially high benefits. When faced with choosing between prevention or alleviation, with both about *equally* effective/

8. The survey was in the context of the following: "As you know, the federal government has a substantial budget deficit and there are many competing spending priorities facing the next president and Congress. Thinking about the federal budget, do you want to see the next president and Congress increase spending on public health programs to prevent the spread of disease and improve health, decrease spending, or keep it about the same?" Those same surveyed individuals said they would like to see increased spending on Medicare (43.6%), Medicaid (34.1%), and medical care for veterans (64.2%) as well.

9. Though for serious illnesses we often choose to use seemingly inefficient or relatively ineffective resources to attempt to lengthen life and postpone death, even if for very short times. Witness, for example, the use of Avastin or Erbitux in colorectal cancer treatment, which may extend life for 3 to 6 months for $100,000: "The health economic analysis suggests that the marginal cost–utility of bevacizumab plus IFL versus IFL is unlikely to be better than £62,857 per QALY gained [that is, the cost less than £62,857 per QALY] and the marginal cost–utility of bevacizumab plus 5-FU/FA versus 5-FU/FA is unlikely to be better than £88,658 per QALY gained" (Tappenden et al. 2007; more generally, Menzel 2011).

ineffective, efficient/inefficient, or likely to produce the same benefits given the risk, however, Western societies more readily choose alleviating harm over preventing it.

ELIMINATING SOME WEAK JUSTIFICATIONS FOR TREATMENT OVER PREVENTION

More than one author has indicated that the standard for pursuing prevention *should* be higher than the standard for alleviation. In an attention-getting editorial in the *British Medical Journal*, for example, editor Fiona Godlee (2005) claimed that "because it is [en]acted on healthy people, preventive medicine needs even stronger supporting evidence on benefits and harms than therapeutic interventions."

Behind Godlee's claim lay the studies she cited alleging a virtual mania of prevention. The perceived need to keep healthy is pushed to a point at which common-sense health maintenance turns into needless anxiety and excessive diagnosis—to the point at which, subjectively, health becomes imminent illness and risk factors lose their "risk" component and get viewed as illness. A classic example is high blood pressure coming to be seen over time as a disease. The upshot is that people take on the burden of feeling sick when they aren't. Thus Godlee's title: "Preventive medicine makes us miserable."

Admittedly, if prevention is pursued with this much zeal, damage can be done. Perhaps prevention zealotry should require clearer evidence if its true net benefit is to be represented accurately. Those factors, however, should already be included in any good benefit analysis. Beyond these factors why should prevention bear any greater burden of evidence than treatment? And in circumstances more generally, for all the preventive measures not pursued with anything like the excessive zeal that Godlee has in mind, her argument is beside the point.

For different but related reasons, Heidi Malm (2002) claims that prevention should carry a heavier burden of evidence than treatment. "Treatment must be supported by [only] a *preponderance of the available evidence*" whereas prevention requires "*clear and convincing* evidence or, even stronger, evidence showing it to be *beyond a reasonable doubt* that the recommended procedure will be good for the patient, all things considered." Why? According to Malm it is because the doctor initiates the preventive activity (contra treatment, where the patient takes the initiative) and because it is not perceived by the patient to be a necessity; therefore prevention carries a heavier burden of effectiveness proof.

Malm's argument, like Godlee's, is incorrect. First, as opposed to her underlying premise, patients often initiate prevention requests of clinicians. Second, assuming the doctor is working in the best interest of the patient, it is not clear why the doctor's initiating a contact creates a situation requiring a higher burden of proof of effectiveness. Don't patients presume that the doctor is working in their best interest as much in a potentially preventive situation as they do in an acute situation?

Others have used the "prevention paradox" first articulated by Geoffrey Rose (1992, 12) to argue against more aggressive public health measures: "a preventive measure that brings large effects to the community offers little to each participating individual." Illustrations would include advocating a reduction in salt intake to reduce blood pressure, a reduction of trans-fats to reduce cholesterol and adverse heart effects, and increased physical activity to reduce heart disease. To be sure, this "distance" of large community effects from the single individual who might benefit can understandably have an effect on the psychological motivation for prevention, but how does it provide a *reason* for downgrading the importance of prevention?

The distance Rose has noted may be linked to two related problems: (1) public health prevention strategies cannot identify which individual lives will be saved, and (2) later it is difficult to prove that any particular individual's adverse health development has failed to occur *because* of specific previous preventive actions. The latter point applies even in clinical contexts in which preventive medicine is very much administered to identifiable individuals. If a physician assists a patient in changing behaviorally oriented risk factors such as smoking, food intake, or exercise, it is particularly difficult to prove that this assistance is the causal reason that, for example, this patient has not had a heart attack. Without this or some other discernible cause any later good health state is not even an "effect." Without the apparent cause (and therefore an effect) showing itself visibly, it is difficult for the absence of illness to be appropriately attributed to the preventive action even if we have definitive epidemiological evidence that the incidence or gravity of disease events is indeed a result of diminished exposure to known risk factors, or that specific interventions that reduce risk factors are effective. In a multifactorial disease such as cardiovascular disease, the ambiguity is even worse; although the elimination of one or more risk factors can be shown to be effective in large populations, the causal field is so hard to control and contains so many factors that intense efforts of exercise or diet change may not yield any effect for a particular individual.

What demands to be noted, however, is that the very same point applies to most forms of treatment. Adding Erbitux or Avastin for the treatment of colorectal cancer adds *on average* 3–6 months of a quality-adjusted life year

(QALY),[10] which means that for some cancer-afflicted patients *no* marginal QALYs will be added, for others *more* QALYs will be added, and for some patients *marginal* QALYs may even be *lost* because of the side effects of the drug. Double-blind, randomized controlled trials can indicate that on average this or that Erbitux-related effect is likely to occur, but it cannot predict the result for any individual exposed to it. Even after treatment, if a relatively good state of affairs has come about, we often do not know whether that is an effect of the medication or a natural course of the disease *in this particular person.* The obscurity of individual benefits and beneficiaries afflicts not only most prevention, but also much treatment.

These are not the only weak arguments for treatment priority.[11] At this point, suffice it to say that even with such arguments refuted, prevention still struggles to step up to a relationship of equivalence, much less priority. Something more appears to be at play in this competition for resources.

The purpose of this volume is to explore whether deeper and more subtle elements can help to explain and justify our apparent preference for treatment over prevention. Are relatively little known or poorly understood economic considerations part of the explanation? Do sounder moral arguments obtain than those we have briefly assessed above? Do some religious traditions, when well understood, help explain the bias toward treatment? Do any non-U.S. cultural traditions help us better to understand what might be going on in our own culture's bias toward treatment, either by illumination from contrast or reinforcement from similarity? These are the tasks of this volume.

10. A QALY is a constructed unit of health benefit measurement that incorporates life extension and quality-of-life improvement into the same scale, as people are willing to trade them off for each other. If, for example, I am willing to give up 2 of my remaining 10 years of life, when I have a debilitating or painful chronic condition, to gain a cure of my condition (but live only 8 more years), I will have ranked my quality-of-life at 0.8 out of 1.0. Then a procedure that extends my life 10 years but leaves the chronic condition intact will be said to achieve 8.0 QALYs of health benefit.

11. Six others are examined and rejected by Brock and Wikler (2009). Included are arguments based on urgency and the propensity to rescue people already in trouble (so-called "Rule of Rescue"—Jonsen 1986). Brock and Wikler give qualified support, however, to an argument derived from these elements: if urgency and rescue are sufficiently compelling factors to donors and attract funding for treatment that simply cannot be raised for prevention, then a policy of priority for treatment may be morally justified. Perhaps this argument, too, is weak: the very factors on which the funding realities rest, priority for urgency and rescue, have already been rejected as providing a logical justification for priority for treatment. The argument is not strictly circular or question begging, and it does have a practical moral logic in the situation Brock and Wikler hypothesize, but the social reality to which they accede is still morally regrettable. If the society did not accord such mistaken importance to urgency and rescue, more lives yet could be saved by prevention.

DEFINING OUR TERMS

Prevention and Treatment

What do we mean by "preventing harm" and "alleviating harm" in the health care context? The term common to both conditions, "harm," includes suffering, deterioration, loss of function, pain, reduced capacity from normal (either for the individual or species), injury, accident, illness, premature death, etc. In other words, harm is the physical or psychological change from species-specific normal functioning, whether naturally occurring or man induced.[12] In common parlance, harm has occurred (or continues) when a bone is broken, a disease develops, severe stress alters our ability to cope, or a physical or mental trauma occurs. Even in very old age, when a disabling or fatal disease develops, we would say it is a harm to the individual, even if the individual has exceeded all expectations of longevity.[13] Limitation on an individual's ability to function as he or she would reasonably expect to function is a harm.[14]

What a health care provider does to relieve, reduce, or eliminate the harm once it has become manifest in an ailment we call "treatment." It occurs after the harm has shown symptoms (concerns of bodily abnormalities articulated by the patient) or signs (physical examination, laboratory, or radiology findings) discovered during or after a medical encounter. There are many different sorts of treatment, and it is variously referred to as (1) *cure*, a successful elimination of the ailment and usually its cause(s); (2) *acute care*, which attempts to find the cause of the disease and/or relieve symptoms with the hope of moving toward a cure; (3) *rescue medicine*, care to alleviate harm that is framed by the "powerful human proclivity to rescue a single identified endangered life, regardless of cost" (Osborne and Evans 1994); (4) *arresting disease* or severely

---

12. We can argue as to whether the deviation should be measured from normal species-specific functioning or optimal species-specific functioning, and also whether relevant deviation keys off the notion of "normal for this individual" or normal for the species. These are exceptionally difficult issues in the concept of disease and illness, best left to their own literature.

13. If an individual is in severe pain or cannot function to a preferred level, a harm (an exacerbation or advancement of the existing underlying illness) might be *welcome* if it leads to death, as death from the harm is viewed as a relief from suffering. It is not our intention to address this positive sense of "harm" in the volume.

14. Generally we are inclined to restrict this to "reasonable and realistic" expectations, though it is often difficult to specify the content of such limits. Not all cases are problematic, however. If the excessively high expectations are internally generated through, for example, mental illness with motivational deficits, we would probably agree that inability to function as the mentally ill person wishes is not a harm.

retarding its progression, without eliminating or curing it; and (5) *rehabilitation*, helping individuals recover from and become agile again functionally. In this volume we have asked the contributors to use the term *treatment* to encompass any and all of these forms of *alleviating harm*.

We use the term "prevention" to mean *preventing harm*, which in turn occurs when (1) a susceptible person does not yet have an impairment or illness but they might come to have it, and that susceptibility is prevented from coming to fruition for some reasonable time when it might otherwise have occurred; (2) risk factors for disease are reduced (or attempts are made to reduce them); or (3) pre-symptomatic disease is detected early enough that either it can be cured or its impairing effect can be mitigated. We call all three of these conditions *prevention*, as they are all intended to prevent the onset of a disease or detect it in a generally curable stage before it becomes symptomatic to the patient.

The related term "health promotion" may include all of the components of prevention just mentioned, as well as "enhancement"—improvements in health-related well-being from a baseline.[15] Especially in clinical and corporate settings these are often included in "prevention" as well. Though health promotion is not literally the prevention of harm, we allow it to be included in the widest, most generic sense of prevention.

Public health and preventive medicine literature typically refers to three standard forms of prevention. *Primary prevention* prevents disease or disability from even starting (e.g., most public health measures, immunizations, health behavior counseling, and an individual's eating in a nutritionally sound way). *Secondary prevention* interventions detect and arrest disease or disability in early asymptomatic stages (e.g., screening for breast or colorectal cancer). *Tertiary prevention* inhibits already symptomatic illness or injury from progressing.[16] In this volume we have asked the authors to use *prevention* to include the primary and secondary forms, but not tertiary prevention, which we view as a form of treatment.

The fourth type of prevention is called *primordial*, which Last (2001, 143) defines as "the elimination of risk factors, precursors, genetic counseling to avoid genetically determined conditions, etc." (see also Wallace in Chapter 4 of

---

15. For example, enhancing quality of life by engaging in additional physical activity. However, we are not including the "enhancement" often referred to in genetic therapy discussions.

16. According to Last (2001), preventive medicine includes "Actions aimed at eradicating, eliminating, or minimizing the impact of disease and disability, or if none of these is feasible, retarding the progress of disease and disability. . . primary prevention aims to reduce the incidence of disease, secondary prevention aims to reduce the prevalence of disease by shortening its duration, and tertiary prevention aims to reduce the number and/or impact of complications [of disease]."

this volume). Primordial prevention eliminates health threats from a disease or accident causal field. For example, if smoking tobacco were not available agriculturally or commercially, then individuals could not smoke, and smoking is removed as a health threat. Primordial prevention addresses root causes such as smoking, and also social disparities in health—poorer, lesser educated, or rural dwellers, for example, have shorter life expectancies and higher morbidity rates (Braveman, Egerter, and Mockenhaupt 2011). At times it can be difficult to distinguish between primary and primordial prevention, so we collapse the two in most of the discussion in this volume.

Figure 1.1 can be used to illustrate the different types of health care. Illness develops within a causal field impacted by (sometimes) definable health threats, such as smoking, high sodium intake, and lack of physical activity. These health threats, usually called *risk factors*, can be causes of preclinical pathological changes that if identified before they become clinical, might be modified or eliminated, restoring the pre-pathological state A. However, if there is no intervention (or spontaneous cure), the disease may manifest clinically. Clinical manifestation may result in several outcomes, including cure (return to state A) with or without medical intervention, slow reduction in signs and symptoms to a state of minimal disease less healthy than pre-disease functioning, ongoing chronic illness, or slow progression to full disability or death.

Primary prevention intervenes between 0 (absence of all health threats) and A (elimination of health threats). Secondary prevention occurs at B. Treatment occurs at C.

With primary prevention, an illness or injury fails to occur, period. Operationally, in studies of prevention, this does not mean that the illness or injury will *never* occur. What counts as effective prevention avoids the occurrence of a disease or injury within a reasonably foreseeable set of circumstances and during a defined time period. The time period is essential, because eventually we all develop disease, but effective prevention postpones its onset. As Steve Woolf (2008) paraphrases Jim Fries (1980): "the aim of health promotion and disease prevention is not to prevent the inevitable but to 'compress' morbidity, maximizing health until death."

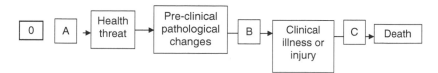

Figure 1.1 The Spectrum of Health and Disease and Where Prevention and Treatment Intervene.

In short, "Where prevention serves to stop the causal chain of events from even starting, treatment ideally 'returns [the] individual to a previous state of health'" (Cutter 2003). Or, as Evans (1988) states, "'What [prevention] treats—if treat be the word—is a set of conditions under which disease may arise."

Priority Relationships

In addition to definitions of treatment and prevention, we also need definitions of the most prominent possible priority relationships between them. First, it is necessary to draw conceptually some distinctions among different kinds of priority.

One kind of claim can be referred to as *effectiveness priority*. In this kind of priority the claim is about either relative effectiveness or cost-effectiveness. For example, treatment might be said to deserve priority because it is more effective (or cost-effective) than prevention in achieving certain health goals. We would not thereby be claiming that *if* prevention and treatment were only *equally* effective or cost-effective in achieving certain defined health goals, treatment still deserved any priority.

Contrast this with what we choose to call *deontological priority*, which claims priority irrespective of the effectiveness or efficiency in achieving goals or results ("teleological" considerations). A claim of priority in this second sense is a claim that a category of care—prevention or treatment, say—ought to obtain resources according to some non-teleological characteristic such as intention, self-consistency in a social context, or in accordance with basic principles of rightness or fairness, even when that care is less effective or efficient.

It is always wise to keep these two different kinds of priority claims distinct. Prevention might be claimed to deserve ("have") priority because it is more effective (or cost-effective) in avoiding a certain disease and achieving a defined segment of health than services that treated the same disease once it has emerged. Or a given treatment might be claimed to have priority over prevention aimed at the same disease even when it was no more (or was less) effective than the preventive effort. The former would be an effectiveness priority claim; the latter would be a claim of deontological priority. Although speaking of "moral priority" may have either a teleological or deontological reference, we will typically use the phrase in the deontological sense.[17]

17. An example of this type of clear concern of priority was recently stated in an article by Leibowitz, Parker and Rotheram-Borus (2011): "Could public support be ethically allocated to provide [pre-exposure prophylaxis] to high-risk, but uninfected [HIV] individuals, while public resources were not available to treat all those currently [HIV] infected?"

We are now in a position to define the different key positions on the moral relationship between treatment and prevention that become the subject of debate.

Equivalence: *No preference should be given to either preventive or treatment services above and beyond what other allocation criteria such as efficiency, effectiveness, and compensatory justice generate.*

Treatment Priority: *Treatment should take priority over prevention when the two are equally effective (or cost-effective) in producing health benefits, and even, up to a point, when treatment is less effective (or cost-effective).*

Prevention Priority: *Prevention should have priority over treatment when it is as effective (or cost-effective) in preserving health as treatment is in restoring health, and it should have priority even, up to a point, when it is less effective or (cost-effective).*

Equivalence does not claim that prevention and treatment are equally likely to achieve a given degree of health-related benefit or cost-effectiveness. Its point instead is to deny that any deontological consideration creates moral priority for treatment that can override an advantage in effectiveness or efficiency for prevention. Similarly, no consideration beyond effectiveness or efficiency should create any advantage for prevention.

Realistically, the predominant moral debate is between Treatment Priority and Equivalence. Prevention Priority is seldom a view that lobbies for contention. Effectiveness priority claims are often made for prevention, but deontological priority claims, while frequently made for treatment, almost never are made for prevention.

Empirical Considerations: Economics and Evidence-Based Medicine

First, of course, we had better have some of our facts straight. We usually work under the impression that in our society's basic approach to health care, prevention is underfunded relative to treatment. It is important to look at the actual evidence for this claim more carefully. For one thing, even if it is generally accurate, there are different possible ways and degrees in which it might be correct, and some particular prevention services may be well supported. For another thing, as Russell notes in Chapter 3 of this volume, prevention is certainly not always going to be more cost-effective than treatment in producing health benefits. For these reasons the question of what an optimal balance of prevention and treatment would look like remains unclear. To begin to dissipate some of this empirical fog, two basic considerations are addressed in the first section of the volume.

Miller, Roehrig, Hughes-Cromwick, and Turner (Chapter 2 of this volume) refine the empirical picture of what we are actually currently spending on preventive services as compared to treatment. Recently this team (Miller et al. 2008) determined that excluding public health research, our actual expenditures as a percent of the health care dollar varied from 7.4% (1996) to 8.5% (2002). Because their estimate of the percentage of health care expenditures devoted to prevention is notably higher than the 1–3% commonly alleged, their analysis raises the prospect that we are not as far from a maximally effective balance between prevention and treatment as most critics contend. If an ounce is one-sixteenth (6.35%) of a pound, then we are already spending above the "ounce of prevention" referred to in Benjamin Franklin's iconic off-the-cuff statement quoted earlier. However, even if we spend 8% on prevention, increased coverage for, and resource investment in, prevention may still be called for. We may need to spend more on prevention to effect optimal health—including optimal health in the most cost-effective way. Some, such as Dee Edington,[18] advocate spending 20% of the health care dollar on prevention, including worksite wellness programs and occupational safety and health services, which are not included in the estimates of Miller et al.

Beyond the observations of Miller et al. on what is left out of their economic analysis, Russell (Chapter 3 of this volume) and Wallace (Chapter 4 of this volume) remind us that much of prevention occurs in nonclinical settings: highway, occupational, food, and water safety, safety engineering of cars and other accident-potential instruments, postmarket drug monitoring, construction codes, health education in schools, etc. Furthermore, Russell makes a clear distinction between what may be cost-*saving* vs. cost-*effective* in prevention. She tackles some of the challenges of cost-effectiveness analyses and explains how some of the things we think save money in prevention indeed are not more cost-effective (and often less cost-effective) than many treatments for the same diseases.

Wallace divides prevention into four spheres: environmental control, personal behaviors, policy and practice decisions, and clinical interventions. The 8% captured by Miller et al include only the last of these in their study.

18. Stated at an oral presentation at a plenary session of the American College of Preventive Medicine annual meeting, February 23, 2009, and reasserted at a meeting at the Altarum Institute, Ann Arbor, MI, June 3, 2009. For further discussion of Edington's approach to this question, see Edington (2009).

By "policy and practice decisions" Wallace means how local, state, and federal agencies develop and implement policies from evidence-based prevention information. The actual impact of community-wide programs, Wallace notes, once implemented, is often very difficult to determine.

But an even bigger problem, according to Wallace, is that many of our clinical recommendations for prevention arise from observational studies, not from randomized trials, and are subject to confounding variables that may not yet be understood. This means that some of our interventions, either on the clinical or community level, may not be having the effect(s) we want. He notes that even so, clearly we have reduced the incidence of our number one killer, heart disease, as well as several cancers. We know, of course, that we do not always need to understand the mechanisms of diseases in order to prevent them (or of their interventions) (Gerstman 2003, 290). Nevertheless, having randomized controlled trials of community interventions would give us better evidence of the effectiveness of prevention interventions in the field, particularly now that we know that various socioeconomic/cultural groups may respond differently to different intervention methods. Wallace also highlights the fact that we often do not know how various prevention interventions may interact with each other, how preventive services effect (or are affected by) existing illness or disease interventions in individuals, and how best to communicate preventive interventions to individuals and the public.

Diana B. Petitti was co-chair of the U.S. Preventive Services Task Force in the fall of 2009 at the time of significant conflict over its mammography screening recommendations. In her provocative and compelling Chapter 5 of this volume she offers a perspective that recommends an equivalence strategy—not necessarily with dollars, but with evidence. Treatment has often been held to looser and less carefully crafted evidence-based standards than prevention. In attacking this "double standard" she defends the use of evidence for rational decision making, urging that the requisite evidence should not be diminished for prevention, rather it should be enhanced for treatment. In the process she provides a political lens on the uses and abuses of scientific evidence to make policy.

These contributions by Miller et al., Russell, Wallace, and Petitti are only beginning steps in gaining a more refined empirical picture of the clinical effectiveness, cost, and relative efficiency of prevention. To end the first section, Faust (Chapter 6) rounds out the picture by articulating some of the historical reasons as to why prevention has often been left out of insurance coverage, and why it was so often ignored by mainstream medicine. He notes, however, that many of these barriers were removed by the passage of the health care reform act of 2010, also known as PPACA.

THE PATIENT PROTECTION AND AFFORDABLE CARE ACT OF 2010 (PL 111-148)

The Patient Protection and Affordable Care Act of 2010 (PPACA) is the result of the first year of the Obama administration's efforts to reform health insurance in the United States. The act eliminates pre-existing condition exclusions, removes limits on annual and lifetime insurance coverage (caps), permits greater portability of insurance, prohibits premium rates discrimination because of health status or gender,[19] prohibits plans from rescinding coverage, guarantees coverage acceptance and renewal, prohibits participant and provider discrimination, and permits states to develop their own health insurance exchanges that enable individuals without employer-based affordable health insurance coverage to purchase insurance, with subsidies if they qualify. Furthermore, PL 111-148 requires all U.S. residents to purchase and maintain insurance policies; not doing so causes the individual to have to pay a fine.

From the viewpoint of Treatment Priority or Equivalence, PL 111-148 has redressed many of the preventive care services exclusions that previously marked Medicare, Medicaid, and private health insurance. Prevention provisions enacted in the law include the following:

- Preventive services that qualify to meet the mandate for insurance coverage must include all clinical services determined to carry an A or B grade by the Task Force for Clinical Preventive Services, and all vaccines recommended by the Centers for Disease Control and Prevention (CDC) for Medicare and Medicaid.[20]
- In 2011, cost sharing for mandated preventive services in Medicare and Medicaid is eliminated, and incentives to encourage Medicare and Medicaid beneficiaries to complete behavior modification programs are added.
- In the private sector "qualified health benefits plans" are required to provide the same preventive services coverage as Medicare without

19. Discrimination may occur based only on individual/family status, geographic area, age, and tobacco use. It may not occur because of a physical or mental illness, prior claims experience, prior receipt of treatment or diagnostic tests, genetic information, or disability (United States Congress 2010, Section 2705).

20. An "A" grade recommends the service with a high certainty that "the net benefit is substantial." A "B" grade recommends the service with a "high certainty that the net benefit is moderate or there is moderate certainty that the net benefit is moderate to substantial." (The "Task Force for Clinical Preventive Services" is a renaming of the U.S. Preventive Services Task Force.)

cost sharing (no co-pays or deductibles), including maternity, well baby care, and well child care. The elimination of cost sharing for preventive measures, when cost sharing for treatment is still allowed, constitutes priority for prevention.

- Medicaid is required to cover tobacco cessation services for pregnant women.
- Premium discounts and rebates "or other reward[s]" under a wellness program are permitted as long as the program does not discriminate on health status. At the same time it limits the incentive to a maximum of 30% of premium cost.
- A "Prevention and Wellness Trust" for carrying out prevention research, evaluation, and program delivery is established with funds from the Federal treasury, increasing from $2.4 billion to $4.3 billion from 2010 through 2018.
- By 2012 nutritional labeling of standard menu items at chain restaurants (20 or more locations) and vending machines is required, regulated by the Food and Drug Administration (FDA) and superseding state or local labeling regulations.
- A $5 billion federal Prevention and Public Health Fund is established for community infrastructure, such as bike paths, playgrounds, and hiking trails, to increase physical activity and build healthier communities (Kamerow 2010).
- Every 2 years the Department of Health and Human Services must develop a "National Prevention and Wellness Strategy" using evidence-based clinical and community prevention and wellness activities. This is done through a National Prevention, Health Promotion, and Public Health Council specifically charged with providing recommendations on "the most pressing health issues confronting the United States," including "the reduction of tobacco use, sedentary behavior, and poor nutrition." The Council's role is designed to increase the efficiency and effectiveness of existing regulatory bodies.

Additionally the act rectifies the deficit in funding for preventive medicine residencies by authorizing such funding for schools of public health, medicine, or through accredited hospitals or state/local/tribal health departments. The funding is still authorized, however, through the Health Services and Resources Administration, the procurement of whose funds involves an annual struggle to separate residency funding from authorized funding for other public health workforce specialties—nurses, health administrators, veterinarians, etc.

These changes in prevention coverage are revolutionary for health plans and our nation. Although we could conclude that a major rebalancing of prevention in relation to treatment finally has occurred, we must remember that PPACA also strengthened insurance for treatment in several important ways:

- The elimination of underwriting criteria (pre-existing condition exclusions) and lifetime caps on coverage predominantly benefits treatment.
- Mental health and substance abuse benefits now have to be provided at parity with medical/surgical benefits (Sections 1311 and 1312).
- Provider nondiscrimination eliminates exclusion of types of providers by health plans if the state licenses those providers and the benefits provided are within the scope of practice of the state.
- Cost sharing is more limited under plan coverage.
- The Secretary of Health and Human Services is permitted to define the "essential" health benefits packages that all health plans must provide. Given special interest groups' past successes in getting their (often) single issues covered we can expect the list of essential health benefits to broaden over the coming years; most special interest groups advocate for enhanced treatments.[21]
- Although many dispute his numbers, the U.S. federal actuary for Medicare and Medicaid estimated that PPACA's expanded health insurance coverage would increase expenditures in Medicare and Medicaid by approximately $930 billion from 2010 to 2019 (Foster 2009).[22] The amounts of these expenditures that can be allocated to the strengthened prevention or treatment benefits are not easily teased out, but the majority of the effect will likely result in increases in treatment, though in a different ratio than currently occurs between prevention and treatment.
- Furthermore, as noted previously, when financing for physician payments for treatment through Medicare is at risk, some members of Congress first look to the Prevention and Public Health Fund to make up the difference—arguably, another indication of Treatment Priority.

21. Some special interest groups do advocate for more prevention. The most successful prevention-related lobbying campaigns have been for breast and cervical cancer screening and tobacco control in public places.

22. This amount does not include offsetting potential savings by PPACA either through initiatives to encourage more efficient provision of care or revenue enhancements through taxes or other income. However, it also does not include the additional costs of insurance plans through employers and other nongovernmental agencies.

A THOUGHT EXPERIMENT: TO PREVENT OR
TO ALLEVIATE HARM?

Before reviewing the second part of the volume on normative analysis, a thought experiment can perhaps help focus the central moral question about priorities. Although there are limitations to thought experiments as intuitive approaches to philosophy and policy (see Faust's Chapter 7 of this volume), they can engage people to explore their own preferences, intuitions, and justifications.[23]

Bill, John, or the Public's Health

You are a versatile and accomplished solo primary care physician working in a backwater rural area. You have two long-established male patients—full brothers, John and Bill—sitting in your waiting room. Your secretary has made an error and scheduled both to be seen at the exact same time as your last appointment of the day. Furthermore, you have a firm scheduled departure from the office after this last appointment to meet another extremely important and longstanding commitment, and your schedule is booked so far in advance that you would not be able to see John again for at least 3 months for a prevention visit. Assume that if John has to wait 3 months to get started on his prevention program he will have passed the threshold at which his risk factor changes would have made a substantive difference in his risk for future heart disease. Additionally, the chairman of the local board of health has called for a teleconference for the purposes described below (option 3). You have time to see either Bill *or* John, but not both, *or* to participate in the board of health teleconference. There are no other possibilities. The details on these three options are presented:

Option 1—See Bill, age 62, who is having epigastric discomfort that (he doesn't know yet, but you do from test results just in) is really ischemic heart disease. He smoked until age 44 and has had hypertension since age 51. If you evaluate and treat him now, giving him the proper, effective, and efficient treatment for his ailment, you will attenuate his progressing heart disease and assist him on the road to rehabilitation. Instead of dying at age 63 from an acute heart attack and its sequelae, Bill will likely live reasonably happily to age 75, with minimal discomfort from his heart disease until the last 2 years of his life, when he will experience gradually reduced capacity and become disabled

---

23. This thought experiment has been presented at several other venues since the initial 2004 presentation at ACPM referred to at the beginning of the Introduction. Faust (2005) previously published this thought experiment in an abbreviated form.

before dying. His treatment over his remaining lifetime, all things considered, will cost (in 2010 dollars) $250,000.

Option 2—See John, age 50. John is concerned and worried about his family history of heart disease. His father died at age 58 from ischemic heart disease and he suspects his brother, Bill, already has it. During this appointment he is expecting to have his risk factors for heart disease assessed, and then start on a program to reduce these risk factors. He has a good record of being a compliant patient. If you evaluate and help him now, providing him with the proper assistance to reduce his risk factors for future heart disease, you will as likely help him avoid lethal heart disease as you are likely to save Bill from dying relatively soon by treating him: instead of dying at age 63 from a heart attack John would have had at age 62, he will live reasonably happily to age 75, with minimal discomfort from his heart disease until the last 2 years of his life, when he will experience gradually reduced capacity and become disabled before dying. His treatment over his remaining lifetime, all things considered, will cost (in 2010 dollars) $250,000.

Option 3—Take the local health department board teleconference call. The board has been seeking, and has now been tentatively approved for, a grant of $250,000 that can be used only for the purposes for which it was sought—to provide a community-wide heart attack prevention program that has the statistical likelihood of saving 12 years of life in one unknown individual in the community. You know from prior community prevention studies that if you take the call and then vote to accept this grant, one unknown person will successfully gain 12 years. If you don't sit in on the teleconference the board of health will not have a quorum and will not be able to accept the grant. If the board does not accept the grant today at this teleconference time (a time that conflicts with seeing John or Bill) the grant will be lost forever, and one unknown person who will not have changed his or her risk factors will die prematurely.

For the purposes of this thought experiment there is nothing else to know about Bill, John, or the health department's grant program. The following are the rules of the experiment:

1. You must choose *only one* of the three options.
2. Neither Bill nor John can return to see you in your office in the foreseeable future; this is your (and anybody else's) only chance to influence their care.
3. The net amount of suffering and pleasure that all recipients of services (either through your direct care or through the health department) would have in life by the ends of their lifetimes is equal in the three scenarios.

4. There is no appeal to the grantor to the health department for a delay in taking the vote. If you do not participate in this call, the department will lose the $250,000 grant.
5. If you do not see Bill or John, no one else is available to evaluate or treat them for their current concerns, nor is anyone else available for the required quorum to approve the health department grant.
6. You will earn the same income and gain the same quantitative satisfaction from participating in any of the three options.

What Will You Do? See Bill? See John? Take the Health Department's Call?

As we made clear earlier, utilitarian calculations are certainly not the only reasons we give priority to treatment over prevention in resource utilization, and may not even be the main reasons. This thought experiment attempts to remove utilitarian factors by stipulating that all three options involve equal additional years of life and equivalent costs, and thus to provoke respondents to consider other factors that are important in the decision to treat, prevent, or fulfill their obligations to the public's health. Such considerations *beyond* effectiveness or efficiency are likely to be the basis for any priority that people believe treatment has.

MORAL ANALYSIS AND ARGUMENT

A thought experiment such as Bill, John, or the Public's Health only sets the stage. As interesting and germane as it may be, the preferences it elicits do not constitute normative argument or analysis. Moral inquiry goes further: How *should* the respondents feel? What choice *should* they make?

How do we approach a question such as whether society or providers are as morally obligated to assist people with preventing illness and disease as they are with helping them with treatment for existing illness? Moral philosophers have long seen a basic division that, although it may oversimplify the world of ethical theory, is useful in pursuing this volume's topic. *Utilitarian* theories of right action ask us to reason on the basis of how much good (in this case, human well-being) can reasonably be expected to be achieved by the behavior in question.[24] *Deontological* theories ask us to reason on the basis of a few

---

24. There are several different dimensions of a utilitarian theory: what constitutes the goodness or badness of a resulting state of affairs, whether it is the reasonably expected or actual

fundamental principles of right and wrong that focus on some aspect of the inherent nature of an action, not the good or bad results it is likely to achieve.

Although we will note an exception to the following assertion later, a utilitarian, focusing on the value of results, typically defends the position previously defined as Equivalence. Without settling the larger argument at the level of basic moral theory as to whether utilitarianism or some sort of deontological view is fundamentally the correct form of moral reasoning, the ethicists contributing to this volume attempt something more manageable. They fill in the moral landscape by asking somewhat less ultimate ethical questions, such as what deontological arguments for treatment's priority survive criticism from within the relatively friendly domain of *non*utilitarian reasoning?

The Chapters by Faust, Daniels, and Menzel in the second section of this volume explore different issues around this moral landscape. Faust (Chapter 7) concludes that two factors drive plausible arguments for Treatment Priority: compassion and its large contributing factor, vividness, which in turn is composed of spatial and temporal proximity. These proximity variables exert a disproportionate influence on our moral imagination of envisioning future harm, and therefore on our desire to take action now to minimize future harm, particularly where current harm is so pervasive and needs alleviation. Faust notes that any policy of resource allocation is dependent on more than simply cost–benefit or cost–effectiveness analyses. It also includes (as argued by Robert Solomon, Martha Nussbaum, and others) judgments from our emotions—we are moved by the little girl whose undeserved circumstance has her in the well needing rescuing at the cost of millions of dollars in equipment, manpower, and effort. These, in turn, have an effect on both our intuitions and our behaviors. Using short cases Faust tests out some of our moral intuitions about the relevance of proximity and its associated vividness to see how stubborn and fundamental these intuitions may be.

Daniels (Chapter 8) explores whether the respects in which candidates for treatment are worse off than people who are candidates for prevention allows them to be appropriately protected by principles of justice that emphasize fair equality of opportunity. After concluding that much prevention is indeed included in what people owe each other by way of accessible basic care, he argues that one aspect that characterizes the treatment situation compared to the prevention situation is morally relevant and tilts toward priority for treatment: the higher concentration of risk in a particular individual, in contrast to a wider dispersion of risk over more people. Both how high the risk for

consequences that should count, the scope of the beings whose "well-being" needs to be counted, etc. Substantive differences in these dimensions create a huge number of variations. Some do not even typically go by the label "utilitarian." We gloss over these differences.

an individual has to be before this factor becomes relevant, however, and the weight that any resulting priority for treatment should have remain open to considerable, legitimate moral disagreement. Daniels argues that such inevitable disagreements about the allocation of resources between treatment and prevention can be resolved only through a fair deliberative social process that abides by conditions of publicity and standards of reasonableness.

Menzel (Chapter 9) explores several arguments for Treatment Priority that he concludes are weak, but then focuses his primary attention on two that seem more worthy. One claims it would be unfair to people who are already ill if we shifted to a policy of Equivalence: they would be disadvantaged, not only because competition for treatment would then be greater, but because they can no longer benefit as much from increased emphasis on prevention. Ultimately this argument fails, Menzel claims, but it does capture one of the important moral barriers to adopting a policy of Equivalence.

A second worthy argument, in Menzel's view, is rooted in an empirical fact about how people value life and health; this argument is familiar to many in psychology and economics. If we look at people's actual preferences, whether elicited or implicit, we find that people place greater value on a good state of affairs achieved from a situation of relatively high risk than they do on the same good state of affairs achieved from a situation of lower risk. A situation calling for treatment is usually one in which an individual is at greater risk than people are when they are candidates for prevention. Thus, if we pay careful attention to the degree of value in the well-being that good health constitutes when it results from treatment, as opposed to the amount of value present in the same good health achieved by prevention, we see that the former *value* is typically greater, though the *health* achieved is objectively the same. This argument in favor of Treatment Priority, in contrast to the initial argument about unfairness to the already ill, is utilitarian. It makes a claim about the comparative value of results—here, the subjective preference-based value of results. Menzel concludes that this argument also runs into difficulties that render it less than conclusive and only selectively applicable.

In his separate Chapter 11 of this volume, Menzel pursues a further consideration about the value of life and health that complicates views on the relationship between prevention and treatment. In health economics and comparative cost-effectiveness studies, a standard practice is to discount future health benefits back to present value. There is ample justification for such a practice within the theoretical structure of economics, but does it have a moral justification? Although a dollar spent or saved now is worth more than a dollar spent or received years into the future, why should we think that an additional *year of life* or *health improvement* gained by someone 10 years from now has any less human and moral value than an additional year of life preserved for someone now? From an ethical perspective, the alleged parallels between discounting health benefits and discounting money are either mysterious or overdrawn. The matter is important: discounting health benefits that appear only years into the future will systematically disadvantage prevention, as its benefits usually come to fruition later than the benefits of treatment. Menzel provides a comprehensive ethical appraisal of this controversy.

Major normative issues in the relationship between treatment and prevention are manifest in U.S. law. Pope (Chapter 10 of this volume) reviews some of the most important laws (often slow in their historical development) that feature prevention of health problems, examines normative problems raised by these laws and others that can be predicted to follow, and explores whether the common law has a built-in bias toward treatment as opposed to prevention. His discussion touches on a large variety of health issues with which the law intersects: smoking, obesity, alcohol abuse, diabetes, sexually transmitted disease, tanning beds, distractive texting, etc.

For most of U.S. history, Pope observes, public health laws were aimed at preventing discrete harm to others—for example, mandatory vaccinations, isolation, and quarantine to prevent the spread of contagious diseases. The individual whose freedom was overridden posed a direct threat to society. Today, in contrast, the greatest threats to public health come from self-regarding behaviors. For example, within the constraints of existing laws, individuals who become obese rarely pose any direct health threat to others. Therefore, he argues, interfering with the liberty of such individuals demands a fundamentally different moral justification: either a theory of justified paternalism or a theory of the power of overall societal welfare to justify coercion of the individual. Pope examines both justifications of contemporary developments in public health law.

Because of space limitations, many other issues in normative ethics that affect the prevention/treatment discussion are not addressed in this volume. One is the extent to which, in ethical reasoning, values should be aggregated across a group of individuals. Smaller individual gains for a larger number of people, when added together, can surpass in value larger individual gains for a smaller number of people. Whether such aggregation is ethically appropriate becomes a major bone of contention between utilitarians and most deontologists. The case for prevention—at least the case for Equivalence—often aggregates prevention's benefits among a large number of people. The demand for treatment tends to come from particular individuals in need. Doubts about aggregation are deeply embedded in some deontological objections to Equivalence. Another question that frequently surfaces in applied ethics, only considered peripherally by Faust (Chapter 7) in this volume, concerns "role morality." Are physicians, for example, because of their unique role or the valuable cultural traditions of their profession, under greater obligation to alleviate harm than they are to prevent harm?

RELIGIOUS AND CULTURAL TRADITIONS

Effective ethical arguments and policy making are not made in sealed chambers of rationality—in the real world they reach people imbued with traditions and cultures. Traditions inform our ethical premises and reasoning, and certainly impact on health policy decision making. Thus, we would be remiss in not understanding what traditions have to say about the treatment–prevention distinction. The third section of this volume is not a merely interesting aside but represents an important dimension of the relationship between prevention and treatment in our society.

The five contributions focus on the perspectives of four different Western religious traditions—Jewish, Catholic, Protestant, and Seventh-Day Adventist—and of selective Asian traditions. They help us better understand the relative values that different cultures and religious worldviews place on the prioritization of prevention and treatment.

The authors were asked to address a number of questions:

- Does their tradition explicitly address the question of whether treatment or prevention takes priority? If so, how does it do so, and if not, can it be argued on the basis of more complex interpretation that it does so implicitly?
- Do any of the proverbs, aphorisms, standard texts, or other sources used in the tradition explicitly address the treatment–prevention relationship or relate to it implicitly?
- How might the tradition's non-text-based teachings address the priority question?
- Do contemporary reflections—including the author's own—conducted within the general framework of the tradition provide any insight on priority?

Jotkowitz and Glick (Chapter 12 of this volume) open this section by discussing the methods Judaism uses to come to consensus on ethical issues. *Halachah*, literally "the way," is Jewish law based upon the written law, the *Torah* (the first five books of the Old Testament), and the oral law, the *Mishnah* and the *Talmud*. From *halachic* principles and casuistry have evolved interpretations of issues such as resource allocation between prevention and treatment. Jotkowitz and Glick show us where prevention and treatment are discussed separately in biblical and contemporary texts and responsa, the recorded decisions by various authoritative groups of rabbis. They note, however, that the *balance* between prevention and treatment is not specifically addressed in these *halachic* sources. Their reading between the lines of *halacha* and responsa leads them to side with Freedman (1977): saving a life takes precedence over prevention *for individuals*. They also note, though, that resource allocation through community-wide deliberation needs to take all of society's needs into account. Thus, there is precedent for a utilitarian calculation in this case, using evidence-based medicine and cost-effectiveness analyses to encourage the health of the society as a whole. They proceed to analyze the Bill/John/Public Health thought experiment from different precedents in Jewish sources and responsa, again finding that there is a difference in interpretation depending on whether an individual in reasonable proximity to the physician is at immediate risk, or whether a total community is at risk.

Catholicism's answers on ethical questions come from a different set of sources than Judaism's: Biblical scripture beyond the *Torah*, teachings of bishops and the Pope, Natural Law theory as developed in various traditional writings such as those of Aquinas, and "experience and reason" more generally. The Catholic Christian tradition related by Kenny (Chapter 13 of this volume) has a longstanding commitment to alleviating harm for people currently suffering and marginalized, which overwhelms considerations of prevention. Christ's healing ministry is a much stronger emphasis in Catholicism than is health promotion or prevention. Another factor diminishing attention to health promotion is a certain emphasis on asceticism toward the body in the history of Catholicism. More recently, though, the Church has validated the need for human beings to consider the body as important in honoring God, and therefore keeping it in good form. Moreover, in its search for social justice, including the amelioration of poverty, strong concerns of the Church for reducing risk for disease have emerged.

Kenny notes that the hospital as an institution was an offspring from Christ's ministry to the sick as well as tending to and comforting the disadvantaged. In contemporary Catholicism the tradition is summarized in the Ethical and Religious Directives for Catholic Health Services (U.S.) or the Health Ethics Guide (Canada); neither has any discussion of prevention or health promotion. At the same time the revised 2009 Catechism affirms a balance for prevention and the needs of the community; it counsels avoiding excesses of food, alcohol, and nonprescription drugs, and the elimination of tobacco entirely, while urging that indulgence and addiction should not be a reason for discrimination in access to medical services.

Kenny notes that the emphasis in Catholicism on certain virtues such as temperance and prudence should bode well for an emphasis on prevention, but finds less evidence of actual Church advocacy and activism because of differences between public health activities and moral theology, particularly around the use of contraceptives, immunizations for human papillomavirus (HPV), and vaccines developed from aborted fetuses. However, in some significant exceptions the Church has strongly advocated prevention because of Catholic liberation theology: harm reduction through needle exchange in England and Australia, for example. She calls for improved imagination in Catholic theology in resetting priorities about prevention.

Given the dissident origin and continuing pluralistic character of Protestantism, its traditions on the subject are more difficult to capture and summarize than Jewish and Catholic ones, as noted in this volume by Lutheran social ethicist Aana Marie Vigen (Chapter 14). Emblematic of the independence of individual thought in Protestantism, she articulates her own direct engagement with the topic from within a theological framework rather than from claims about historical tradition. Three themes, she argues, will shape a Protestant approach to prevention, treatment, and their relationship: the radical encounter of human finitude with divine grace; understanding health, healing, and illness holistically as a part of all of life; and the demanding call to love neighbor and stranger, along with God, above all else. Living out such themes on a question such as priorities between prevention and treatment requires a detailed analysis of social context; in turn, those contexts are so varied that no general claim about relative priorities can be made. Christian considerations of *social* justice will give prominence to the social determinants of health and thus raise the importance of "primordial" prevention. *Global* justice will also affect the priorities discussion: even if prevention (especially primordial prevention) should have greater priority than it typically does, injustice can occur when *basic treatments* that are urgent for a developing nation's population, and relatively inexpensive from a global perspective, get overlooked amid an emphasis on prevention.

At least one religious group has a tradition that speaks very distinctly to the prevention–treatment relationship: the Protest denomination of Seventh-day Adventists. Branson (Chapter 15 of this volume) describes the distinctive history of the central place of prevention in the communal life of Seventh-day Adventists. Although Adventists began by celebrating miraculous healings, they soon adopted distinct practices of health reform. The denomination's founders sent selected members to be trained at the most reputable medical institutions such as Bellevue Medical Center in New York and the University of Michigan School of Medicine. One result was John Harvey Kellogg's founding of the Battle Creek Sanitarium in Michigan, soon to become the nation's largest health care facility. There the treatments of "regular medicine," including surgery, were performed, while simultaneously health-promoting lifestyle

measures were stressed, including the lighter breakfast products of the associated Kellogg Cereal Company and the nutritional value of soybeans. Eventually
the prestige of Adventists' hospitals threatened to outrun a waning emphasis on
prevention, but the church continued to require its own members to abide by
certain health promoting practices. As Branson notes, research on the lifestyle
and health practices of Adventists and their longevity has resulted in major studies that have significantly influenced U.S. public policies on smoking and diet.

To help explain this fascinating history Branson explores the theological
sources of Seventh-day Adventist teachings about healthful living. Readers gain
an understanding of how health promotion became a central part of a living
religion, both as a concern in its own right and in comparison with the advanced
developments in curative medicine that were not disparaged.

One non-Euro-American tradition is represented in this section. Chan
(Chapter 16) describes the relative emphases on prevention and treatment in
modern Hong Kong, influenced not only by Western acute care medicine but
the traditional emphasis on prevention in Chinese medicine. Although this
emphasis gave way to Western acute care medicine in the twentieth century,
recently prevention has regained ground in Hong Kong. Chan attributes this
trend to recovery of the utilitarian considerations that all along had been prominent in Confucian and Chinese tradition. Among the evidence Chan cites to
justify his claim are interesting comparative data from identical survey questions addressed to Hong Kong as compared to U.S. populations.

VOLUME LIMITS

There are, of course, many interesting and important matters related to the prioritization of prevention and treatment that this volume does not address.

We generally limit our discussion to born human beings. We do not enter
into debates about fetal personhood or whether suffering and deprivation can
be attributed to the unborn. Prevention and treatment are certainly not completely removed from that debate. Work done on the *in utero* embryo, such as
through minimally invasive fetoscopic surgery, cystoscopic laser treatments,
and open fetal surgery for rare and life-threatening conditions, could be classified as prevention of suffering for the future born, or these procedures can be
considered treatment interventions of anatomically abnormal fetuses. Similarly,
prevention could include the use of preimplantation genetic diagnosis to select
only healthy embryos, preventing genetically diseased or abnormal embryos
from being incubated and born. Thus, arguments over prevention may venture
into the ontological debate about whether disease can be prevented before there
is a numerical or psychological entity with personhood. We note that some

prenatal interventions, however, still remain clearly preventive (for example, maternal folic acid nutritional supplementation to minimize neural tube defects) and some remain clearly curative (such as fetal surgery).

Furthermore, we do not deal with cross-generational issues. We are not asking if the preservation, prevention, or treatment of a 20-year-old person is worth more than the preservation, prevention, or treatment of an 80-year-old person. Although our thought experiment does compare a 50 year old and a 62 year old, we consider these brothers to be essentially within the same generation. In either case, the malady prevented or treated occurs at age 62–63. We are also not asking contentious age-related questions such as whether the 50-year-old person has more to contribute to society, or whether that should matter morally. Moreover, we have not asked our authors to worry about future generations, but only the current body politic.

These are some of the volume's limits. Beyond the substance of the volume's particular sections and chapters we have two overarching hopes for readers: first, that readers are provoked into many further reflections about the relationship between prevention and treatment, far beyond what we can envision, and especially in the many intersections between empirical data, moral analysis, and religious/cultural tradition. Second, especially for readers within the worlds of health policy and clinical prevention, that the relative importance of prevention and treatment will begin to be seen as a moral issue, not only a discussion and debate about economic and health-related consequences.

REFERENCES

Braveman, P.A., Egerter, S.A., and Mockenhaupt, R.E. 2011. Broadening the Focus: The Need to Address the Social Determinants of Health. *American Journal of Preventive Medicine* 40 (1S1):S4–S18.

Brock, D., and Wikler, D. 2009. Ethical Challenges in Long-Term Funding for HIV/ AIDS: the Moral Imperative for Shifting Priorities from Treatment to Prevention. *Health Affairs* 28 (6): 1666–76.

Cjeka Search and the American College of Physician Executives. 2009. *Physician Executive Compensation Survey*. Tampa FL: American College of Physician Executives.

CMS Legislative Summary of H.R. 1, *Medicare Prescription Drug, Improvement, and Modernization Act of 2003*, Public Law 108–173. 2004. Available at http://www.cms. hhs.gov/MMAUpdate/downloads/PL108-173summary.pdf, accessed June 1, 2011.

Committee on Training Physicians for Public Health Careers, Board on Population Health and Public Health Practice. 2007. In L.M. Hernandez and A. WeziMunthali, Eds., *Training Physicians for Public Health Careers*. Washington DC: National Academy of Sciences Press.

Cutter, M.A.G. 2003. *Reframing Disease Contextually*. Boston: Kluwer Academic Publishers, No. 81 in Philosophy and Medicine series.

Daniels, N. 1985. *Just Health Care*. New York: Cambridge University Press.

———. 2008. *Just Health: Meeting Health Needs Fairly*. New York: Cambridge University Press.

Dhruva, S.S., Phurrough, S.E., Salive, M.E., and Redberg, R.F. 2009. CMS's Landmark Decision on CT Colonography—Examining the Relevant Data. *New England Journal of Medicine* 360 (26):2699–2701.

Edington, D. 2009. *Zero Trends: Health as a Serious Economic Strategy*. Ann Arbor: University of Michigan Health Management Resource Center.

Evans, H.M. 1988. The Limits of Preventive Medicine. *International Journal of Moral and Social Studies* 3 (3):255–66.

Faust, H.S. 2005. Prevention vs. Cure: Which Takes Precedence? *Medscape Public Health & Prevention* 3 (1-May). Available at http://www.medscape.com/viewarticle/504743, accessed June 1, 2011.

Foster, R.S. 2009. Estimated Financial Effects of the "Patient Protection and Affordable Care Act of 2009," as Proposed by the Senate Majority Leader on Nov. 18. In Office of the Actuary ed., Health and Human Services, Centers for Medicare and Medicaid Services. Baltimore, MD.

Freedman, B. 1977. The Case for Medical Care, Inefficient or Not. *Hastings Center Report* 7 (2):31–39.

Fries, J.F. 1980. Aging, Natural Death, and the Compression of Morbidity. *New England Journal of Medicine* 303 (3):130–35.

Gerstman, B.B. 2003. *Epidemiology Kept Simple*. Hoboken, NJ: Wiley-Liss.

Godlee, F. 2005. Preventive Medicine Makes Us Miserable. *British Medical Journal* 330 (Apr.):7497.

Greenberg Quinlan Rosner [company]. 2009. Americans Overwhelmingly Support Investment in Prevention, May 18. Available at http://healthyamericans.org/assets/files/health-reform-poll-memo.pdf, accessed June 1, 2011.

Jonsen, A. 1986. Bentham in a Box: Technology Assessment and Health Care Allocation. *Law, Medicine and Health Care* 14 (3-4): 172–4.

Kaiser Family Foundation/Harvard School of Public Health. 2009. The Public's Health Care Agenda for the New President and Congress. Available at http://www.kff.org/kaiserpolls/7853.cfm, accessed June 1, 2011.

Kamerow, D. 2010. Prevention and the New U.S. Health Reform Act. *British Medical Journal* 340:c2116.

Kliff, S. 2010. Doc Fix New Weapon vs. Health Reform. Politico.com, Dec. 5. Available at http://dyn.politico.com/printstory.cfm?uuid=B7C7A0C9–025C-BB83–3165CCC3DCA2F19F, accessed January 5, 2010.

Lasagna, L. 1964. The Hippocratic Oath: Modern Version. Boston, MA: Tufts University. Available at http://www.pbs.org/wgbh/nova/doctors/oath_modern.html, accessed June 1, 2011.

Last, J.M. 2001. *A Dictionary of Epidemiology*, 4th ed. New York: Oxford University Press.

Liebowitz, A.A., Parker, K.B., Rotheram-Borus, M.J. 2011. A US Policy Perspective on Oral Preexposure Prophylaxis for HIV. *American Journal of Public Health* 101(6):982–985.

Lockridge, R.S. 2004. *Seminars in Dialysis* 17 (2):125–30.

Malm, H. 2002. "Do This, It Could Save your Life!" and Other Problematic Claims in Preventive Medicine. *APA Newsletter* 1 (2):3–9.

Menzel, P.T. 1983. *Medical Costs, Moral Choices: A Philosophy of Health Care Economics in America.* New Haven, CT: Yale University Press.

———. 2011. The Value of Life at the End of Life: A Critical Assessment of Hope and Other Factors. *Journal of Law, Medicine and Ethics* 39 (2):215–223.

Miller, G., Roehrig, C., Hughes-Cromwick, P., and Lake, C. 2008. Quantifying National Spending on Wellness and Prevention. *Beyond Health Insurance: Public Policy to Improve Health. Advances in Health Economic and Health Services Research* 19:1–24.

National Academy of Sciences, Committee on Training Physicians for Public Health Careers, Board on Population Health and Public Health Practice. 2007. In. L.M. Hernandez and A. WeziMunthali, Eds., *Training Physicians for Public Health Careers.* Washington, DC: National Academy of Sciences Press. Available at http://books.nap.edu/openbook.php?record_id=11915&page=R1, accessed June 1 2011.

Nattinger, A.B., and Goodwin, J.S. 1992. Screening Mammography for Older Women, A Case of Mixed Messages. *Archives of Internal Medicine* 152:922–25.

Nussbaum, M. 2000. *Women and Human Development: The Capabilities Approach.* New York: Cambridge University Press.

Olsen, J.A. 1993. Time Preferences for Health Gains: An Empirical Investigation. *Health Economics* 2:257–65.

Osborne, M., and Evans, T.W. 1994. Allocation of Resources in Intensive Care: A Transatlantic Perspective. *The Lancet* 343:778–80.

Pareto, V. 1906. *Manuele di Economia Politica.* English translation: *Manual of Political Economy,* A. Schwier and A. Page, Eds. New York: August M. Kelly, 1971.

Porter M.E. 2009. A Strategy for Health Care Reform—Toward a Value-Based System. *New England Journal of Medicine* 361 (2):109–12.

Rawls, J. 1971. *A Theory of Justice.* Cambridge, MA: Harvard University Press.

Rose, G. 1992. *The Strategy of Preventive Medicine.* Oxford: Oxford University Press.

Rubin, R. 2009. Health Suffers in Recession: It's Preventive Care That Often Gets Cut First. *USA Today,* June 25. Available at http://today.uchc.edu/headlines/2009/jun09/recession.html, accessed June 1, 2011.

Salive, M.E. 2009. Personal Email Communication to Halley S. Faust, July 23, 2009. [At the time of his communication and the publication of this book Dr. Salive is Director of the Division of Medical and Surgical Services, Centers for Medicare and Medicaid Services. Baltimore, MD.]

Schreiner, G.E. 2000. How End-Stage Renal Disease (ESRD) Medicare Developed. *American Journal of Kidney Diseases* 35 (4):S37–S44.

Tappenden, P., Jones, R., Paisley, S., and Carroll, C. 2007. Systematic Review and Economic Evaluation of Bevacizumab and Cetuximab for the Treatment of Metastatic Colorectal Cancer. *Health Technology Assessment* 11 (12):1–128.

United States Congress. 2010. *The Patient Protection and Affordable Care Act, H.R. 3590.* Washington, DC: Government Printing Office.

Woolf, S.H. 2008. The Power of Prevention and What It Requires. *Journal of the American Medical Association* 299 (20):2437–39.

PART ONE

Evidence, Policy, and History

2

What Is Currently Spent on Prevention as Compared to Treatment?

GEORGE MILLER, PhD, CHARLES ROEHRIG, PhD,
PAUL HUGHES-CROMWICK, MA, AND ANI TURNER, BA ∎

BACKGROUND

There is a widely held perception that the U.S. health care system needs to transition from a culture of reactive treatment of disease to one of proactive disease prevention and wellness promotion. Addressing this perceived need requires metrics and methods to measure spending on prevention as a basis for understanding the current distribution of funds between prevention and treatment, and to promote discussion regarding both the amount that should be spent on prevention and how that amount would best be distributed among prevention activities.

To provide a basis for these metrics and methods, we developed a taxonomy of prevention activities, designed methods to measure expenditures associated with each of these activities, and produced an estimate of the portion of the National Health Expenditure Accounts (NHEA)—the U.S. government's official source of national health care expenditures—that is devoted to prevention. Our original work (Miller et al. 2008) produced a time series of expenditure estimates for each year from 1996 through 2004. In this chapter, we revise and extend these results through 2008 and describe preliminary work to investigate prevention spending outside the NHEA and to explore the trade-offs between spending on prevention and on treatment.

Estimates of expenditures on prevention cited in the literature (Faust 2005; Lambrew and Podesta 2006; Lubetkin et al. 2003; McGinnis, Williams-Russo, and Knickman 2002; OECD 2009; Satcher 2006; Shodell 2006; Woolf 2006, 2009) range between 1 and 5% of U.S. health care spending. Most of these estimates can be traced to a study conducted in 1991 (Brown et al. 1991) whose content is not readily available except in a short summary (Brown et al. 1992). Without access to the detailed report, it is difficult to understand the definitions, assumptions, and methods that led to these estimates. Our work provides updated estimates that use precise definitions, a transparent methodology, and a subdivision of the estimates into components to aid researchers in applying their own concepts of prevention activities.

METHODS

One of the challenges in estimating prevention expenditures is defining what is meant by prevention. We characterize prevention activities using the standard three categories of primary, secondary, and tertiary prevention. Although many researchers use these terms, they are not used consistently and are not always defined precisely. Our definitions are consistent with those introduced in Chapter 1 of this volume, which are similar to those employed by a number of other researchers. Our estimates exclude tertiary prevention, most of whose activities involve treatment of medical conditions.

Categories of primary and secondary prevention activities whose expenditures we have quantified are depicted within the NHEA framework in Figure 2.1. Three of the five principal components of the NHEA include prevention elements: Personal Health Care, Public Health Activity, and Research. (We ignore a small portion of the Administration and Net Cost of Private Health Insurance component that is devoted to prevention.[1]) These three components contain four categories of preventive activities: medical, dental, public health, and research. Within these categories, we estimate prevention expenditures separately for each of the eight elements shown at the bottom of the figure.

---

1. PricewaterhouseCoopers (2006) estimates that of the roughly 14% of health insurance premiums devoted to the net cost of private insurance, 5 percentage points are allocated to health promotion, wellness, and prevention programs plus all of the following activities: marketing and sales, communications with consumers regarding benefits, disease management programs, care coordination, and investments in health information technology. This implies that our omission is a small amount, though it may be growing in importance with recent employer actions.

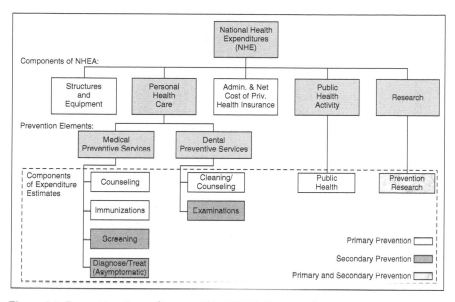

Figure 2.1 Prevention Expenditures within NHEA Framework.

Our approach for the elements within each of the four categories is summarized below. Details of our estimation methods can be found in Miller et al. (2008).

- Medical preventive services include patient counseling, immunization, screening for disease, and diagnosis and treatment of asymptomatic patients to arrest potential problems identified during routine screening. These are partitioned into primary and secondary prevention as a function of the stage of the medical condition that is being prevented. Counseling and immunization of patients with no known disease constitute primary prevention, screening for disease in an asymptomatic patient is secondary prevention, and diagnosis and treatment of risk factors or early-onset disease in asymptomatic patients is secondary prevention. We estimated expenditures for these services via a "bottom-up" analysis in which we identified specific clinical preventive services and derived associated expenditure estimates from a variety of sources. Major sources included publically available national datasets such as the Medical Expenditure Panel Survey (MEPS) and the National Ambulatory Medical Care Survey and the National Hospital Ambulatory Medical Care Survey (NAMCS/ NHAMCS). We recognize that our definition of secondary prevention results in some uncertainties as to whether some activities (particularly those that follow a positive screening result) constitute prevention or treatment. In practice, it is difficult to determine whether many of the activities that would otherwise follow a positive screen were instead initiated by the patient presenting with symptoms (which would cause us to classify the activities as treatment rather than prevention). We have therefore omitted some of these follow-up costs from our calculations. However, our data sources allow us to discern whether treatment for asymptomatic disease or risk factors (such as hypertension) is associated with patients with symptomatic disease (such as coronary heart disease)—which we do not count as prevention, or with no such disease—which we include as secondary prevention.

- Dental preventive services include cleaning and counseling, characterized as primary prevention, and dental examinations and x-rays, which represent screening and are counted within secondary prevention. We used MEPS data and dental billing data to estimate the portions of NHEA dental services expenditures devoted to each of these types of services.

- Public health activities are generally designed to prevent disease and injuries by promoting healthy lifestyles, supporting healthy environments, and preparing for public health crises such as disease epidemics and other natural and man-made disasters. These activities are generally population based, and are not aimed directly at individuals. Because most of these activities can be considered primary prevention, we assigned all public health expenditures captured within the NHEA to primary prevention. Although this probably results in a slight overstatement of primary prevention expenditures, the lack of data on state and local government expenditures for public health activities (Sensenig 2007) precluded our exclusion of the limited public health expenditures that constitute treatment rather than prevention, and prevented us from allocating some of the total to secondary prevention.

- Research activities are included if they are related to preventive services. We used estimates from the National Institutes of Health (NIH) to identify the fraction of NHEA research expenditures devoted to prevention. Due to data limitations, we did not attempt to distinguish between primary and secondary prevention research activities.

RESULTS

Our expenditure estimates for each year from 1996 through 2008 are shown in Table 2.1. They are expressed as a percent of total NHEA expenditures in

Table 2.2. These numbers differ somewhat in the earlier years from those reported in Miller et al. (2008) because of recent revisions to some of the underlying data. This is especially true for research spending, for which NIH has revised its method for estimating the percent of its research portfolio devoted to prevention. Our results suggest that NHEA expenditures devoted to prevention grew from $81.3 billion in 1996 to $204.8 billion in 2008, in current dollars. As a share of the NHEA, this represents an increase from 7.5% in 1996 to 8.6% in 2008. This share previously peaked at 8.6% in 2002 and then declined between 2003 and 2005 due to reductions in public health spending as a percent of NHEA. Primary prevention represents slightly more than half the expenditures, consisting largely of public health spending—the largest prevention element.

Our estimate that 8.6% of 2008 NHEA expenditures goes to prevention is nearly three times as large as the commonly cited figure of 3% (Brown et al. 1992), but depends on the definitions used. For example, our estimate falls to 8.3% when research is excluded, 5.3% when consideration is limited to primary prevention plus screening, 4.4% for primary prevention alone, and 3.1% if we count only public health expenditures.[2]

Figure 2.2 depicts historical levels of spending on prevention interventions (including all classes of prevention described above except research), prevention research, treatment interventions, and treatment research within the NHEA.[3] Spending on treatment interventions is plotted using the vertical scale to the right of the graphs; the other three classes of expenditures are plotted using the scale to the left. The figure illustrates the extent to which historical expenditures have been dominated by treatment, and the small fraction of total expenditures that has historically been devoted to research, particularly research into prevention. It is interesting to note that spending is greatest where the results are most immediate (treatment interventions) and lowest where the results are most delayed (prevention research).

2. There is evidence that public health spending has been influenced by changes in crisis preparedness funding following the attacks on September 11, 2001. It is difficult, however, to precisely track this spending since it is allocated across multiple governmental entities. One group estimates that federal spending for public health preparedness has fallen 27% (in real terms) since fiscal year 2005 (Trust for America's Health 2010).

3. The figure omits two of the five principal components of the NHEA shown in Figure 2.1 that we do not allocate either to prevention or to treatment—Structures and Equipment, and Administration and Net Cost of Private Insurance—because of the difficulty in identifying the extent to which these expenditures support prevention versus treatment activities. These two components accounted for 11.6% of national health expenditures in 2008.

Table 2.1. Estimates of Annual Expenditures by Prevention Element (Billions of Dollars)

Prevention Activities	Expenditures by Year (Billions of Dollars)													Annual Growth
	1996	1997	1998	1999	2000	2001	2002	2003	2004	2005	2006	2007	2008	
Medical preventive services														
Counseling	3.3	3.6	4.0	3.9	4.4	4.7	5.5	5.6	6.0	6.4	6.8	7.2	7.5	7.1%
Immunizations	3.4	3.6	3.8	4.1	4.3	4.9	5.7	6.1	6.6	7.1	7.5	7.9	8.3	7.8%
Screening	8.4	9.2	10.0	9.9	10.9	11.9	14.1	14.7	15.8	16.9	17.9	19.0	19.9	7.4%
Diagnosis/treatment (asymptomatic)	17.3	20.2	21.8	24.4	27.5	30.9	35.5	39.8	44.4	48.5	51.7	55.8	57.4	10.5%
Dental preventive services														
Dental cleaning/ counseling	7.5	8.2	8.7	9.4	9.9	11.0	12.3	12.9	13.9	14.7	15.5	16.5	17.4	7.3%
Dental examinations	6.2	6.8	7.3	7.8	8.3	9.2	10.3	10.8	11.6	12.3	13.0	13.8	14.5	7.3%
Public health	32.4	34.8	37.5	40.7	43.0	47.5	51.9	53.7	54.0	56.2	62.6	68.8	72.9	7.0%
Research	2.8	3.1	3.4	3.7	4.0	4.5	5.1	5.5	6.1	6.4	6.5	6.6	6.8	7.7%
Total*	81.3	89.5	96.5	103.9	112.4	124.5	140.3	149.3	158.3	168.4	181.5	195.7	204.8	8.0%

*Discrepancies in totals are due to rounding.

Table 2.2. ESTIMATES OF ANNUAL EXPENDITURES BY PREVENTION ELEMENT (PERCENT OF NHEA)

Prevention Activities	Expenditures by Year (Percent of NHEA)												
	1996	1997	1998	1999	2000	2001	2002	2003	2004	2005	2006	2007	2008
Medical Preventive Services													
Counseling	0.3%	0.3%	0.3%	0.3%	0.3%	0.3%	0.3%	0.3%	0.3%	0.3%	0.3%	0.3%	0.3%
Immunizations	0.3%	0.3%	0.3%	0.3%	0.3%	0.3%	0.3%	0.3%	0.3%	0.3%	0.3%	0.3%	0.3%
Screening	0.8%	0.8%	0.8%	0.8%	0.8%	0.8%	0.9%	0.8%	0.8%	0.8%	0.8%	0.8%	0.8%
Diagnosis/ treatment (asymptomatic)	1.6%	1.8%	1.8%	1.9%	2.0%	2.1%	2.2%	2.2%	2.3%	2.4%	2.4%	2.4%	2.4%
Dental Preventive Services													
Dental cleaning/ counseling	0.7%	0.7%	0.7%	0.7%	0.7%	0.7%	0.7%	0.7%	0.7%	0.7%	0.7%	0.7%	0.7%
Dental examinations	0.6%	0.6%	0.6%	0.6%	0.6%	0.6%	0.6%	0.6%	0.6%	0.6%	0.6%	0.6%	0.6%
Public health	3.0%	3.0%	3.1%	3.2%	3.1%	3.2%	3.2%	3.0%	2.8%	2.8%	2.9%	3.0%	3.1%
Research	0.3%	0.3%	0.3%	0.3%	0.3%	0.3%	0.3%	0.3%	0.3%	0.3%	0.3%	0.3%	0.3%
Total*	7.5%	7.8%	8.0%	8.1%	8.2%	8.3%	8.6%	8.4%	8.4%	8.3%	8.4%	8.6%	8.6%

*Discrepancies in totals are due to rounding.

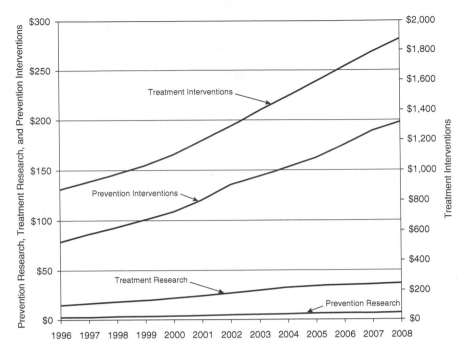

Figure 2.2 Historical Trends in Spending on Treatment Interventions, Prevention Interventions, Treatment Research, and Prevention Research (Billions of Dollars).

EXTENSIONS

Prevention Expenditures Outside the NHEA

Although our estimates of spending on prevention within the NHEA are nearly triple the previous estimates commonly cited, there are other types of expenditures that could be considered prevention, but that fall outside the health accounts. In a recent study of prevention spending in the Netherlands, researchers found that only 20% of their estimate was included in that nation's health accounts (deBekker-Grob et al. 2007). Prevention spending outside the health accounts funded activities such as environmental safety, traffic safety, domestic waste disposal, and enforcement of rules regulating the use of drugs, alcohol, and tobacco. A previous U.S. study found 56% of prevention expenditures included in the NHEA (Brown et al. 1991). Principal non-NHEA expenditures captured in this study funded nutrition programs and water and sewage treatment.

The NHEA represent a long-standing benchmark of U.S. health spending, so it will remain useful to examine the proportion of NHEA expenditures directed toward prevention. This answers the question of "how much of our health dollars is going to prevention versus treatment?" The NHEA also provide a convenient definitional limit to the scope of activities included in the estimates. However, given that prevention activities aim to avoid or minimize the use of the health care delivery system, and given our understanding of the importance of determinants of health that lie outside the delivery system, it makes sense to expand our perspective beyond the official estimates of spending on health care goods and services. This expanded estimate would address the broader question of "how much are we, as a society, investing in protecting and promoting our health?"

As we expand our view outside the NHEA, defining the boundaries of prevention spending becomes more difficult. Distinctions between healthy behavior and recreation, between creating opportunities for better health and more general social welfare programs, and between creating healthier environments and community infrastructure investments quickly become blurred. Data availability may also be a challenge. We can identify the data sources used to estimate the NHEA, although it can be difficult to separate the component we have defined as prevention. Once we move outside the NHEA, however, we may find that adequate data are not available to estimate some categories of spending.

Thus, there are two major difficulties in moving beyond the NHEA: (1) developing a rationale for defining what is included as spending on prevention, and (2) obtaining data to estimate non-NHEA spending. Our focus here is on the first challenge: conceptually defining the boundaries of spending on prevention outside the NHEA. Investigation of data sources and the organization of funding programs may lead to later refinement of our category definitions.

As an initial attempt to categorize spending outside the NHEA, we have defined three tiers of spending that are progressively broad in definition. These tiers would be mutually exclusive and cumulative. Initial estimation work would focus on the first tier, but the other two are presented to extend the rationale to the broadest boundaries.

A reasonable "first tier" expansion of our prevention spending estimates outside the NHEA could apply the following criterion:

Tier 1 Criterion: Expenditures Outside the NHEA with a Primary Purpose of Health Protection, Health Promotion, or Preventive Health Services

We recognize that many goods and activities serve multiple purposes, but under this criterion we are asking ourselves if the primary purpose is maintaining or improving health. For example, government activities directed toward transportation safety may fall outside the usual definition of health spending but can be argued to be primarily directed toward preventing injury or death and so would be included here. Similarly, many activities under the heading of "safety"—worksite safety inspections, food safety guidelines and inspections, and air and water quality monitoring—can be argued to be primarily directed toward preventing illness, injury, or death and thus would be considered part of our national investment in wellness and prevention under this definition. Programs that provide food, an essential requirement for basic health, to those that cannot afford it would also be included. (A more precise understanding of the expenditures already included in the public health component of the NHEA, particularly from the Food and Drug Administration, may be required.)

Individual purchases that promote physical fitness, such as health club memberships, health coaching, or exercise equipment, can be made for social reasons or to improve appearance, but one could argue that the primary purpose is to maintain or improve health, either by increasing muscle strength, improving cardiovascular health, or promoting weight loss.

TIER 2 CRITERION: EXPENDITURES OUTSIDE THE NHEA WITH A PRIMARY PURPOSE OTHER THAN HEALTH, BUT WITH A DIRECT PREVENTION-RELATED HEALTH BENEFIT

Tier 2 would add spending for goods or activities for which health promotion or protection is not the primary purpose, but that directly benefit health. For example, investments in bicycle paths may be intended primarily to serve either transportation or recreational purposes, but they also reduce barriers to incorporating regular exercise into the lives of both adults and children and so would fall into this category. Training and participation in a particular sport would be considered primarily recreation, but would be included in this tier as having a direct health benefit. Law enforcement activities would also be included here since they serve other purposes (justice, protection of property) but also directly prevent physical injury or death. In general, since spending within this tier, by definition, also serves another primary purpose, ideally we would estimate and include only the proportion of spending in each category that is associated with prevention.

TIER 3 CRITERION: EXPENDITURES OUTSIDE THE NHEA WITH A PRIMARY PURPOSE OTHER THAN HEALTH AND NO DIRECT HEALTH BENEFIT, BUT A BENEFIT TO AN ESTABLISHED DETERMINANT OF HEALTH

The third tier would include spending that is not aimed directly toward health but is directed toward another type of determinant of health. So, we might include spending on programs that support education, improve the availability of affordable housing, and so on, as very early preventive health investments, even though their primary purpose is not health promotion or disease prevention. This category may be too broad for a baseline definition of prevention spending, but it may be useful in highlighting the importance of investment in nonhealth factors that may have a large impact on health status.

This tier is the most difficult to define, since even the identification of the determinants of health and their relative importance may be debated. In some sense, almost all aspects of our behavior and environment have some bearing on our mental or physical well-being. Although correlations between health status and characteristics such as level of education and socioeconomic status have been established, the nature of the causal relationships is not yet clearly understood. A detailed and critical review of the literature on determinants of health (Evans and Stoddart 1990, 2003; Kindig 2006) could narrow the focus in this tier to those determinants with the most significant and well-established impact on health.

To illustrate our tiered approach to defining categories of prevention expenditures outside the NHEA, Table 2.3 presents examples that fall under each of the three criteria. As research moves from conceptual, taxonomic considerations to empirical estimation, attention would need to be paid to ensure that expenditures were neither missed nor double counted, including differentiating intermediate goods accounting from final demand accounting (inputs versus outputs). We also recognize that goods and services that fall within these

Table 2.3. Examples of Spending Outside NHEA under Expanding Criteria

Funding	TIER 1: Primary Purpose Health Protection, Health Promotion, or Preventive Health Services	TIER 2: Primary Purpose Other Than Health, But Strong Health Benefit	TIER 3: Primary Purpose Other Than Health, No Strong Health Benefit, But Benefit to a Determinant of Health
Personal spending	Consumer cost of safety features (e.g., auto air bags) Health coaching Home exercise equipment Health club membership Helmets—bike, ski, motorcycle Weight loss programs Smoking cessation programs	Training and participation in particular sports	Postsecondary education

(Continues)

Table 2.3. EXAMPLES OF SPENDING OUTSIDE NHEA UNDER EXPANDING
CRITERIA (CONTINUED)

Funding	TIER 1: Primary Purpose Health Protection, Health Promotion, or Preventive Health Services	TIER 2: Primary Purpose Other Than Health, But Strong Health Benefit	TIER 3: Primary Purpose Other Than Health, No Strong Health Benefit, But Benefit to a Determinant of Health
Federal government	Food safety monitoring Environmental Protection Agency Women, Infants, and Children (WIC) Supplemental Nutrition Program Consumer Products Safety Commission Supplemental Nutrition Assistance Program (SNAP), formerly Food Stamps Occupational safety and worksite inspections National Highway Traffic Safety Administration	Law enforcement Drug control and prevention Public housing	Financial aid for higher education Employment assistance/job retraining Department of Housing and Urban Development— programs to promote affordable housing Early childhood programs
State and local government	Environmental quality monitoring and improvement—air and water Water and sewer authorities Education (K–12)—health curriculum Education (K–12)—physical education	Bike paths Sports parks Law enforcement Education—sports programs	Education (K-12) Early childhood programs Employment assistance/job retraining Financial aid for higher education
Industry/ nonprofit/ foundations	Employee wellness programs Soup kitchens Ergonomic design in workplace Worksite safety	Homeless shelters	Programs to increase literacy Programs to increase high school graduation rates Habitat for Humanity

additional categories of spending, particularly those with a dual purpose, could expand to the point at which they become absurd and infeasible to estimate, and so will require further scrutiny to assess their real contribution to disease prevention and health promotion.

We characterized our estimates of prevention spending within the NHEA in terms of the percent of health care spending devoted to prevention. When the estimate is expanded to include spending outside the NHEA, identifying the denominator to use in characterizing prevention expenditures as a percent of a larger class of spending becomes problematic. It is perhaps more meaningful under these circumstances to characterize the relation between prevention and treatment spending as the ratio of one to the other. Thus, for example, the data plotted in Figure 2.2 for the year 2008 would suggest that spending on prevention (including prevention research) equals 10.7% of spending on treatment (including treatment research), leading to an observation that for every 10 dollars devoted to treatment, we spend slightly more than 1 dollar on prevention. Given that spending outside the NHEA that is devoted to treatment is small, the inclusion of non-NHEA spending in our estimate would cause the numerator of this ratio to increase while the denominator remains roughly constant.

Cost-Effectiveness Trade-offs between Prevention and Treatment

Although a principal objective of this chapter is to update and clarify estimates of spending on prevention, our quantification of expenditures does not address whether the money has been well spent. The cost-effectiveness of an investment in health care, measured as the investment's discounted incremental cost divided by its discounted incremental effectiveness (typically expressed in terms of quality-adjusted life years saved by the investment), is generally used to describe the investment's efficiency. It is clear that some prevention interventions are highly cost-effective, whereas the benefits of other interventions do not seem to be justified by their costs. In fact, Cohen, Neumann, and Weinstein (2008) observe that the variation in cost-effectiveness across different preventive interventions is similar to that found for different treatment interventions, suggesting that opportunities for improving the overall cost-effectiveness of health expenditures through the reallocation of resources exist both within and between the broad categories of prevention and treatment.

However, there is some evidence that prevention activities are currently underfunded: our analysis suggests that many recommended preventive services are not being performed. If all services recommended by the U.S. Preventive Services Task Force (USPSTF) (U.S. Preventive Services Task Force

2009) were fully delivered to their target populations, we estimate that total expenditures listed in Table 2.1 for counseling, immunizations, and screening would more than triple, that total expenditures on all prevention activities would increase by roughly 40%, and that the percent of the NHEA devoted to prevention would increase from 8.6% to nearly 12%. Yarnall et al. (2003) draw a similar conclusion, suggesting that full satisfaction of USPSTF recommendations would require 7.4 hours per working day of the average primary care physician. They conclude that "time constraints limit the ability of physicians to comply with preventive services recommendations."

Furthermore, even if the current emphasis on funding treatment rather than prevention is appropriate, preventive measures that save health care expenditures-which include fewer than 20% of the interventions reviewed by Cohen et al. (2008)-have the effect of reducing the cost-control pressures on treatment and therefore deserve emphasis. Examples of such cost-saving preventive measures include childhood immunizations, aspirin chemoprophylaxis for the prevention of heart disease, tobacco-use screening and counseling, pneumococcal immunization for older adults, and vision screening for older adults (Maciosek et al. 2006).

A final note on this topic concerns an emerging perspective that technical cost-effectiveness studies do not give full credit to the benefit side of preventive activities by insufficiently capturing worker productivity across the full continuum of labor force participation, absenteeism, "presenteeism," etc., and across the life-course, e.g., preventive activities that enable workers to delay retirement. This is not to say that researchers do not attempt to capture these benefits of preventive activities in their cost-effectiveness studies, but rather that they are impeded from complete benefit evaluation due to data limitations. These issues are further explored by Cohen and Neumann (2009), Center for Studying Health System Change (2009), Loeppke (2008), and Manton et al. (2009).

Although much research is needed before we have a comprehensive understanding of the optimal allocation of expenditures to prevention, a useful extension of our work would be to develop and apply methods to improve our understanding of the trade-offs associated with alternative allocation of expenditures between prevention and treatment activities. For example, as illustrated by Russell (2000), the adoption of new, more effective, and more costly treatment therapies for a condition can either increase or decrease the cost-effectiveness of measures designed to prevent the condition. Russell notes that this observation has important implications for the allocation of research funds to developing new preventive measures.

A dynamic model of the impact of alternative investments in treatment and prevention (including investments in research to develop new treatment and prevention interventions) would be a useful tool in increasing our understanding of these interactions and trade-offs. Such a model would represent the time path of clinical effectiveness (measured in terms of quality-adjusted life years realized) associated with a given population that benefits from a corresponding time path of spending on health care interventions (broken into prevention and treatment) and health research (also categorized by prevention and treatment). The health research spending involves creating more effective interventions in the areas of prevention and treatment. The model would explicitly treat the time lags in effectiveness realized with a given pattern of spending, the diminishing returns associated with increased spending of each type, and the effects of discounting of future costs and effectiveness on the cost-effectiveness of a given allocation of funds among the four types of activities.

Previous research has led to some simple models that address the trade-offs between treatment and prevention. As noted above, Russell (2000) develops a simple relationship to show how the cost-effectiveness of prevention changes with the introduction of a new treatment therapy. Homer and Hirsch (2006) develop a simple systems dynamics model of chronic disease prevention that they use to illustrate the effects of different levels of investment in "onset prevention" (by which they presumably mean primary prevention) versus "complications prevention" (secondary and tertiary prevention). Heffley (1982) uses a simple Markov model and optimization theory to identify the optimal allocation of resources between treatment and prevention. All of these models were developed for illustrative purposes rather than detailed research, none of them explicitly addresses the allocation of resources to research into new treatment and prevention alternatives, and none of them examines the impact of discounting of future costs and effectiveness (an important issue in health services research, as noted below). It appears that there remains a need for new modeling that represents in greater detail the impact of alternative investments in treatment and prevention. We are currently extending the work reported here to develop and apply such a model. The model describes the flow of members of a population among alternative states of health as a function of specific patterns of spending.

Rates used to discount future expenditures and effectiveness in cost-effectiveness analysis can affect the relative cost-effectiveness of an investment in treatment compared to an investment in prevention. Although there are economic arguments for the standard practice of discounting costs and effectiveness at the same rate, typically 3% per year (Gold et al. 1996), the practice remains controversial (Brouwer et al. 2005, Menzel in this volume, Chapter 11). This issue is significant when comparing the cost-effectiveness of treatment measures with those for prevention, because the time lags between expenditures and the realization of their impact tend to be greater for preventive measures than for treatment. This becomes especially true when comparing research (particularly research into prevention) with existing treatments, because the time lags between investments in research and the realization of their results in medical practice in the form of improved health outcomes are especially long. Such long time lags tend to make investments appear less efficient because the effectiveness denominator is discounted more heavily than the cost numerator in the cost-effectiveness ratio.

DISCUSSION

Limitations of our methods and data, which could contribute to either overstatement or understatement of actual prevention spending, have been described elsewhere (Miller et al. 2008). In summary, our assumption that all public health expenditures in the NHEA represent primary prevention might lead to an overstatement of expenditures. However, our omission of some (low volume) types of screening and of treatment of some diseases that might be viewed as secondary prevention (such as osteoporosis treatment for individuals who have not yet suffered a fracture) will tend to lead to understatement. Similarly, our inability to determine whether some diagnostic and treatment activities that might result from positive screening results (and which would therefore constitute secondary prevention) were instead initiated by a patient presenting with symptoms (which would constitute treatment) has caused us to omit them from our estimates, also tending to understate prevention expenditures. Furthermore, as noted earlier, our partitioning of NHEA expenditures into the two categories of treatment and prevention has omitted two components of the NHEA that we allocate to neither. Because small portions of these relatively small components might reasonably be assumed to contribute to prevention, our methods tend to understate prevention expenditures slightly. (For similar reasons, they also tend to understate our estimates of treatment expenditures shown in Figure 2.2.) Finally, our treatment of research expenditures is consistent with that of the NHEA, in which industrial research to develop new interventions (such as pharmaceuticals) or new equipment used for diagnosis and treatment are included in the costs of existing interventions (because this is how industry recovers these costs) rather than as research per se. Capturing these expenditures as research would increase our estimates of research and decrease those associated with prevention and treatment interventions.

In spite of these limitations, we have attempted to update and clarify estimates of spending on prevention using precise definitions, transparent methods, and detailed presentations that allow other researchers to include or exclude components of spending that are consistent with their needs.

Although the magnitude of our estimates depends on the components that are included, the estimates tend to exceed the values commonly quoted in the literature.

We also provide preliminary thoughts on methods to expand the estimates beyond the NHEA and to address whether health care dollars are appropriately allocated between treatment and prevention. Although much remains to be done before we obtain a thorough understanding of these issues, we hope the findings of our research to date contribute to a more informed discussion of our nation's allocation of health care resources.

REFERENCES

Brouwer, W.B.F., Niessen, L.W., Maarten, J.P., and Rutten, F.F.H. 2005. Need for Differential Discounting of Costs and Health Effects in Cost Effectiveness Analyses. *BMJ* 331:446–48.

Brown, R., Corea, J., Luce, B., Elixhauser, A., and Sheingold, S. 1992. Effectiveness in Disease and Injury Prevention. Estimated National Spending on Prevention—United States, 1988. *Morbidity and Mortality Weekly Report* 41 (29):529–31.

Brown, R.E., Elixhauser, A., Corea, J., Luce, B.R., and Sheingold, S. 1991. *National Expenditures for Health Promotion and Disease Prevention Activities in the United States.* Battelle: The Medical Technology Assessment and Policy Research Center.

Center for Studying Health System Change. 2009. The Dollars and Sense of Prevention: A Primer for Health Policy Makers. Washington, DC, June 9. Available at http://www.hschange.com/CONTENT/1066/?conf=26, accessed June 13, 2011.

Cohen, J., and Neumann, P. 2009. The Cost Savings and Cost-Effectiveness of Clinical Preventive Care. *Research Synthesis Report No. 18.* Princeton, NJ: Robert Wood Johnson Foundation.

Cohen, J., Neumann, P., and Weinstein, M. 2008. Does Preventive Care Save Money? Health Economics and the Presidential Candidates. *The New England Journal of Medicine* 358 (7):661–63.

deBekker-Grob, E., Polder, J., Mackenback, J., and Meerding, W. 2007. Towards a Comprehensive Estimate of National Health Spending on Prevention (the Netherlands). *BioMed Central Public Health* 7:252.

Evans, R.G., and Stoddart, G.L. 1990. Producing Health, Consuming Health Care. *Social Science Medicine* 31 (12):1347–63.

———. 2003. Consuming Research, Producing Policy? *American Journal of Public Health* 93 (3):371–79.

Faust, H.S. 2005. Prevention vs. Cure—Which Takes Precedence? *Medscape Public Health & Prevention*, May 27. Available at www.medscape.com/viewarticle/504743, accessed June 13, 2011.

Gold, M., Russell, L., Siegel, J., and Weinstein, M. 1996. *Cost-Effectiveness in Health and Medicine.* New York: Oxford University Press.

Heffley, D.R. 1982. Allocating Health Expenditures to Treatment and Prevention. *Journal of Health Economics* 1:265–90.

Homer, J.B., and Hirsch, G.B. 2006. System Dynamics Modeling for Public Health: Background and Opportunities. *American Journal of Public Health* 96 (3):452–58.

Kindig, D.A. 2006. A Pay-for-Population Health Performance System. *JAMA* 296 (21):2611–13.

Lambrew, J.M., and Podesta, J.D. 2006. Promoting Prevention and Preempting Costs. A New Wellness Trust for the United States, October 5. Center for American Progress.

Loeppke, R. 2008. The Value of Health and the Power of Prevention. *International Journal of Workplace Health Management* 1 (2):95–108.

Lubetkin, E.I., Sofaer, S., Gold, M.R., Berger, M.L., Murray, J.F., and Teutsch, S.M. 2003. Aligning Quality for Populations and Patients: Do We Know Which Way to Go? *American Journal of Public Health* 93 (3):406–11.

Maciosek, M.V., Coffield, A.B., Edwards, N.M., Flottemesch, T.J., Goodman, M.J., and Solberg, L.I. 2006. Priorities Among Effective Clinical Preventive Services, Results of a Systematic Review and Analysis. *American Journal of Preventive Medicine* 31 (1):52–61.

Manton, K.G., Gu, X., Ullian, A., Tolley, H.D., Headen, A.E., and Lowrimore, G. 2009. Long Term Economic Growth Stimulus of Human Capital Preservation in the Elderly. *Proceedings of the National Academy of Sciences* 106 (50):21080–85.

McGinnis, J.M., Williams-Russo, P., and Knickman, J.R. 2002. The Case for More Active Policy Attention to Health Promotion. *Health Affairs* 21 (2):78–93.

Miller, G., Roehrig, C., Hughes-Cromwick, P., and Lake, C. 2008. Quantifying National Spending on Wellness and Prevention. *Beyond Health Insurance: Public Policy to Improve Health. Advances in Health Economics and Health Services Research* 19: 1–24.

OECD. 2009. *Health at a Glance—OECD Indicators, 2009.* Available at www.oecd.org/ health/healthataglance, accessed June 13, 2011.

PricewaterhouseCoopers. 2006. *The Factors Fueling Rising Healthcare Costs 2006.* Prepared for America's Health Insurance Plans. Available at http://www.affordableaccessto-healthcare.org/LinkClick.aspx?fileticket=yayr/xrWY4Q=&tabid=105&mid=538, accessed June 13, 2011

Russell, L.B. 2000. How Treatment Advances Affect Prevention's Cost-Effectiveness: Implications for the Funding of Medical Research. *Medical Decision Making* 20: 352–54.

Satcher, D. 2006. The Prevention Challenge and Opportunity. *Health Affairs* 25 (4): 1009–11.

Sensenig, A.L. 2007. Refining Estimates of Public Health Spending as Measured in National Health Expenditures Accounts: The United States Experience. *Journal of Public Health Management Practice* 13 (2):103–14.

Shodell, D. 2006. Paying for Prevention. *Medscape Public Health & Prevention.* Available at www.medscape.com/viewarticle/544651, accessed June 13, 2011.

Trust for America's Health. 2010. *Ready or Not? Protecting the Public's Health from Diseases, Disasters, and Bioterrorism, 2010.* Available at http://healthyamericans.org/ assets/files/TFAH2010ReadyorNot%20FINAL.pdf, accessed June 13, 2011.

U.S. Preventive Services Task Force. 2009. *The Guide to Clinical Preventive Services, 2009.* Rockville, MD: Agency for Healthcare Research and Quality.

Woolf, S.H. 2006. The Big Answer: Rediscovering Prevention at a Time of Crisis in Health Care. *Harvard Health Policy Review* 7 (2):5–20.

———. 2009. A Closer Look at the Economic Argument for Disease Prevention. *JAMA* 301 (5):536–38.

Yarnall, K.S.H., Pollak, K.I., Ostbye, T., Krause, K.M., and Michener, J.L. 2003. Primary Care: Is There Enough Time for Prevention? *American Journal of Public Health* 93 (4):635–41.

3

Prevention vs. Cure

An Economist's Perspective on the Right Balance

LOUISE B. RUSSELL ■

Whenever the subject of health care costs comes up in the national debate, the idea that the United States spends too little on prevention is sure to come up as well. For decades, there have been those who have urged the nation to spend more on prevention, arguing that we are missing major opportunities not only to improve people's health, but also to save money on a grand scale. The theme returned in 2008, as the presidential candidates put forth proposals for health reform, and again in 2009 and 2010, as Congress got down to the business of passing reform legislation.

By this argument, the allocation of medical spending between prevention and cure is out of balance and has been for a long time. Too little is spent on prevention and too much on cure. Many speakers and writers have cited the statistic that the United States devotes only 3% of its medical expenditures to prevention. Such a small number automatically confers credibility on the idea that important opportunities are being missed.

When I first became aware of this theme in the late 1970s, I was puzzled and intrigued. Here was an investment that looked like a sure thing. According to the advocates, the health benefits of prevention were large and came at no cost, since the costs were offset by savings in treatment. Prevention was usually characterized as being riskless as well. Yet then, and now, people were apparently not investing in it to anything like the extent that seemed reasonable to the advocates. As an economist, I was skeptical of this argument. If prevention was such a good deal, and the information to support its claims was solid and widely available, how could it be that so many were missing out? I wrote a book,

Is Prevention Better than Cure?, published by Brookings in 1986, that addressed the issue. And in that book I reported that, with rare exceptions, studies did not show that prevention reduced medical costs.

In 2007 I wrote a report for the National Coalition on Health Care in which I reviewed recent studies published in the top medical journals to see whether the situation had changed (Russell 2007). It had not. It remains the case that the majority of preventive interventions do not reduce medical costs, but instead add to them—usually at the same time that they improve health. Good health is gained, but at a cost. In February 2008, *The New England Journal of Medicine* published a review of hundreds of recent cost-effectiveness studies that came to the same conclusion (Cohen, Neumann, and Weinstein 2008).

In this chapter I present evidence to help answer three questions: Does prevention reduce medical costs? Does the United States spend only 3% of its health dollars on prevention? Should it spend more? (And if so, on what?) Much of the evidence comes from cost-effectiveness studies, so I also explain how cost-effectiveness analysis is used to evaluate medical interventions, whether preventive or therapeutic.

The evidence comes, almost exclusively, from interventions that public health experts would term primary or secondary prevention (e.g., U.S. Preventive Services Task Force 1989; Chapter 1 of this volume). I will not discuss tertiary prevention as it is too often difficult to draw a clear line between tertiary prevention and treatment.

HOW COST EFFECTIVENESS ANALYSIS EVALUATES PREVENTION (AND TREATMENT)

Cost-effectiveness studies compare the costs and health effects of medical interventions. Thus an early and crucial decision in any analysis is what should be compared with what. For a preventive intervention, the comparator may be waiting and treating the disease after it occurs. For example, vaccination is typically compared with no vaccination, in which case the disease is treated after it happens. Or a study can compare alternative approaches to prevention, such as different types of drugs for reducing blood pressure (Edelson et al. 1990), or different frequencies of screening (Eddy 1990; Frazier et al. 2000).

As part of the analysis, cost-effectiveness studies estimate and compare the costs of each alternative. Costs are assessed from the perspective of the medical sector in most studies. An evaluation of drugs for hypertension, for example, would typically count the costs of medications, laboratory tests, physician and staff time, hospital stays, and other goods and services supplied by the medical sector. The medical sector perspective falls short of providing all the information needed for making good decisions in the public interest. Drawing on economic welfare theory, the Panel on Cost-Effectiveness in Health and Medicine recommended the societal perspective for national and community decisions (Gold et al. 1996; Russell et al. 1996; Weinstein et al. 1996; Siegel et al. 1996). Medical sector costs are, however, exactly what is needed to address the claim so often made for prevention—that it reduces medical costs.

Table 3.1 shows a cost-effectiveness analysis that evaluated the costs (and effects) of two interventions designed to improve the health of asthma patients (Lahdensuo et al. 1998). Because the patients already had asthma, the two interventions qualify as tertiary prevention, or even treatment, but I like this example because it shows the essentials of a cost-effectiveness analysis very simply and clearly. The costs of the self-management intervention appear in the first column and the costs of traditional care in the second column. The third column shows the differences—costs of self-management minus those of traditional care—thus identifying where there are net savings and where there are net increases in cost. In this case, although self-management saves on some items (drugs, physician visits, hospital care), it costs more for others (counseling and peak flow meters).

Table 3.1 also shows that patients on the self-management intervention benefited by an extra 14.9 incident-free days over the year, per patient, compared

Table 3.1. ANNUAL COSTS AND INCIDENT-FREE DAYS PER PATIENT: GUIDED SELF-MANAGEMENT AND TRADITIONAL CARE FOR ASTHMA, 1997 DOLLARS*

Cost Items/Incident-Free Days	Self-Management	Traditional	Difference
Counseling	348	179	169
Peak flow meter	32	0	32
Drugs	613	623	−10
Physician visits	47	80	−33
Hospital stays	33	52	−20
Total Costs	1074	935	138
Incident-Free Days	359.2	344.3	14.9

Cost-effectiveness ratio: $3,380 per incident-free year**

*Costs were converted from 1994 Finnish marks, the monetary unit of the original article, to 1997 U.S. dollars with the 1994 mark–dollar exchange rate and the medical Consumer Price Index. I have left them in 1997 dollars because I have used the table in other papers and want readers to know that this is exactly the same table.

**The cost-effectiveness ratio was calculated by dividing 365, the number of days in a year, by 14.9, the extra incident-free days per patient from self-management, to get the number (24.4966) that converts 14.9 days to one incident-free year. Per patient costs, $138, were then multiplied by the same number, 24.4966, to get the cost per incident-free year, $3380.

with patients who received traditional care. Incident-free days are the days during the study year in which the patient experienced no incident related to asthma: no admissions to the hospital; no unscheduled visits to a doctor, outpatient clinic, or emergency department; no days lost from work; not even any courses of oral antibiotics or prednisolone. This is a very different measure from the quality-adjusted life-year that is commonly used in cost-effectiveness analysis and that I describe later. Among other differences, the measure used in the asthma study makes no attempt to put the different incidents on a common scale, although clearly a day in the hospital is much more serious than a day on prednisolone or a day with an unscheduled visit to the doctor. Thus the study's results are not fully comparable with those in Tables 3.2 and 3.3 and Figure 3.1.

Accepting this unique measure of health, self-management cost $138 more per patient than traditional care, but also gave each patient 14.9 more incident-free days during the year, or two more incident-free weeks. The result is that the self-management intervention added to total medical spending, at a rate of $3380, in 1997 dollars, for each year free of asthma-related incidents. In 2007 dollars, the base used for the rest of the cost-effectiveness ratios in this chapter, the cost would be $5035 per incident-free year. As the later examples will make clear, the self-management intervention is a bargain. Even so, it adds to medical costs—it does not reduce them. The treatment savings are more than offset by the costs of the intervention.

Each cost-effectiveness ratio compares two alternatives that could be applied to the same health problem. Often, the comparison is between a new approach, preventive or therapeutic, and the standard approach to the same problem, which again may be preventive or therapeutic. In the example, self-management was compared with traditional management for asthma, which can be viewed as two treatments or two types of tertiary prevention. Cost-effectiveness ratios have been calculated to compare bypass surgery with medication for heart disease, both treatments (Pliskin et al. 1981); different schedules of cervical cancer screening, both preventive (Eddy 1990); and medication for blood pressure with waiting to treat heart disease and stroke when it appears, a preventive approach compared with treatment (Edelson et al. 1990). The structure of the analysis is always the same: measure the costs and the health effects of the two approaches and then calculate the difference in costs and the difference in health effects, as illustrated in Table 3.1.

In cost-effectiveness analysis, health effects are always measured in some way that is natural to health, such as incident-free days, as in the asthma study, or cases of disease. The more specific the measure to the intervention, however, the more difficult it is to compare that intervention with others that have different effects on health. The quality-adjusted life year (QALY) was developed to bridge the gap. QALYs estimate the health associated with each intervention by weighting each year of life on a scale from 0 to 1, depending on how healthy the person is during that time; 0 represents death and 1 represents perfect health. The weighted years of life are then summed to get the total QALYs for an intervention. Any state of health can be placed on the 0–1 continuum and the result, total QALYs, combines changes in lifespan, and changes in the quality of life, in a single measure that summarizes all the changes in terms of an equivalent number of years of perfect health.

Thus the health effects of any intervention can be measured in QALYs—the equivalent number of healthy years—and compared with the health effects of any other intervention, whether the interventions are for the same or different conditions. When QALYs are used to measure health, the cost-effectiveness ratio is sometimes called the cost-utility ratio. The studies I cite in the rest of this chapter typically use QALYs to measure health, or, occasionally, just years of life unadjusted for quality. I will use the term "healthy year" rather than QALYs or quality-adjusted life-years. I will describe the cost-effectiveness ratio as the additional cost required to achieve an additional healthy year or, more simply, as the cost of a healthy year.

Better health—more QALYs—can be used for many purposes: paid work, volunteer work, schooling, childcare, household upkeep, or simply enjoying life. Cost-effectiveness analyses typically do not attempt to predict or value those uses, but simply measure health as health. The cost-effectiveness ratio compares interventions in terms of the cost required to produce a healthy year, treating all healthy years as equal. If users want to treat health gains that might be used in paid work as more valuable than those used for other purposes, or health gains to young adults as more valuable than gains for older adults, they are free to do so, but cost-effectiveness analyses do not take that step. Cost-effectiveness analyses do not identify individuals, so they do not include the value that might be assigned to individuals by those who do, or do not, care about them. Nor do cost-effectiveness analyses distinguish between health gains brought by prevention and those brought by treatment. What matters in cost-effectiveness analysis is how much health an intervention produces, not how the health is produced, who gets it, or how it is used.

Most cost-effectiveness analyses also differ from the asthma example in that they estimate the costs and health effects of an intervention over the remaining lifetime of the patients, not just for a single year. Depending on the intervention, costs and benefits can stretch many years into the future—80 or 90 years in the case of interventions that take place in childhood. The full value of the intervention, and its full cost, may not be adequately represented in an analysis that covers a shorter time period.

The timing of costs and benefits over a lifetime can be very different for different interventions. Childhood vaccinations involve upfront costs for the vaccination, but the health gains from preventing disease also begin soon after the vaccination and stretch far into the future. By contrast, medication for high blood pressure involves repeated small costs for many years, with gains in health and life not evident until some years after the medication is first prescribed. Bypass surgery involves major upfront costs, follow-up costs over subsequent years, a short-term loss of quality of life (and possibly of life itself) due to the surgery, followed by an improvement in quality of life after patients recover and a gain in length of life that may not be experienced for some years.

To adjust for these differences in timing, costs and benefits are discounted. The process of discounting reflects the logic that people prefer to pay costs later rather than now, so that future costs count less than present costs, and they prefer to receive benefits now rather than later, so that future benefits count less than present benefits. In other words, they have a preference for the timing of costs and benefits, called, reasonably enough, "time preference." The logic of discounting also draws on the productivity of resources: resources can be spent now or invested to produce more resources in the future. If they are spent now, that future return is lost, which thus is a cost of spending them now. By discounting costs and benefits, analysts summarize them in terms of their "present values," that is the dollars and QALYs that, if received immediately, would be equivalent to the costs and QALYs that are, in reality, spread over many years.

Cost-effectiveness analyses typically discount costs and health effects at the same rate. Based on the recommendation of the Panel on Cost-Effectiveness in Health and Medicine, published in 1996, the discount rate used in most published studies is a real rate of 3% per year (Gold et al. 1996, 309; Lipscomb, Weinstein, and Torrance 1996). "Real" means that the discount rate does not include an allowance for inflation, which is consistent with the practice of conducting cost-effectiveness analyses in real dollars (all costs in a study are measured in the price level of a single year). The Panel based its choice of 3% on the widely accepted shadow price of capital approach, which is based on the idea that consumption, now or in the future, is the purpose of all economic activity, and that the discount rate should reflect the rate at which people are willing to trade present for future consumption (Lipscomb et al. 1996). The panel recommended that cost-effectiveness analyses take the public-interest perspective, called the societal perspective by economists, and this approach to choosing the discount rate is consistent with the public-interest perspective.

Discounting costs and health at the same rate has been the practice for decades. But over those same decades there have been debates about various aspects of the practice, such as whether the discount rate should vary, instead of being constant, or whether health should be left undiscounted. The discounting of health seems particularly objectionable to some people, who believe that it somehow represents a failure to take health seriously enough, although they are comfortable with the idea of discounting costs. Interested readers might want to consult the Panel's chapter on time preference (Lipscomb et al. 1996), and Chapter 11 by Menzel in this volume, which consider these arguments and others in detail. But they might start by asking themselves the following: Do I truly have no preference between two interventions, one of which costs $100,000 now and produces 10 years of healthy life this year, and the other of which also costs $100,000 now and produces 10 years of healthy life 15 years from now? (I have simplified the example by putting costs now, so that they do not need to be discounted, and attention can focus on discounting, or not discounting, health.) If the healthy years are not discounted, the two interventions are equivalent in value, both yielding a year of healthy life for $10,000. At a discount rate of 3%, the first intervention produces 10 years of healthy life, still a cost of $10,000 per healthy year, whereas the second produces 6.42 healthy years at a cost of $15,576 per healthy year. They are no longer equivalent. Discounting costs, but not health benefits, implies that we do not prefer benefits sooner rather than later, but are willing to wait, even indefinitely.

The final product of a cost-effectiveness analysis is a cost-effectiveness ratio. That ratio shows the *additional* cost of producing an *additional* year of healthy life by using one intervention rather than another. *It does not show the value of a year of healthy life—either to an individual or to a policy maker.* It does provide a lower bound for that value: if the intervention is chosen, it is reasonable to infer that the decision maker valued the health gained at least as highly, probably more highly, and possibly much more highly, than the cost of achieving it. If an individual with asthma chooses, for example, to spend the money to self-manage his or her asthma following the program in Table 3.1, we can infer that he or she values an incident-free year at more than $3380 in 1997 dollars, or $5035 in 2007 dollars. We cannot infer the full value the person places on an incident-free year—only that it is more than the cost required to gain an incident-free year with the self-management intervention.

Economics prescribes that a rational decision maker—someone who is trying to get the most benefit from the resources at his or her disposal—will invest in goods and services until the benefit from the last dollar spent on each good or service is the same. Economists refer to this benefit as "utility," but it can also be thought of as satisfaction, or even happiness. The utility of expenditure is something that only the decision maker knows. It is the value the decision maker places on what is purchased—a healthy year in cost-effectiveness analysis. The cost-effectiveness ratio shows the cost required to purchase that healthy year with the specified intervention. The decision maker brings a value for that healthy year to the decision.

Available resources set the overall level of spending, of course. An individual's resources are determined by his or her income, which limits his or her ability to pursue utility. If the individual has spent all of his or her income and has chosen a health service that costs $50,000 for a year of healthy life, but has no money left for services that bring a year of healthy life at only $20,000 and $30,000, respectively, he or she could gain greater satisfaction by choosing differently. He or she would, in fact, gain 2 years of healthy life rather than 1 year for the same expenditure. If he or she is well aware of this, and nonetheless chooses the $50,000 option, that suggests that the value of that intervention to him or her involves more than just another healthy year. Perhaps the option is more attractive in other ways, as might be the case if the $50,000 option addresses a particularly dreaded disease.

Cost-effectiveness analysts readily grant that health is not everything people care about, and that not all aspects of health are captured by a cost-effectiveness analysis. For this reason, the Panel on Cost-Effectiveness in Health and Medicine advised that cost-effectiveness analysis "is an aid to decision making, not a complete procedure for making resource allocation decisions in health and medicine, because it cannot incorporate all the values relevant to such decisions" (Gold et al. 1996, 305; Russell et al. 1996). Nonetheless, decisions that appear to be very much at odds with the principle of equal benefit per dollar deserve careful examination. At the national level, as at the level of the individual, if an intervention that is very expensive per year of healthy life is chosen, and one that is very inexpensive is not, someone should ask why.

DOES PREVENTION REDUCE MEDICAL COSTS?

The first question I promised to address is whether prevention reduces medical costs, as is so often claimed. Why does this claim seem so intuitively right?

One reason is that when we think of prevention, we tend to think of the individual who benefits and the moment at which he or she benefits—or would benefit. Exactly this situation was presented in a radio advertisement I heard a few years ago. The ad's narrator described a man about to undergo bypass surgery, mentioned the cost of the surgery, and asked, "Wouldn't this man be better off if he had embraced prevention earlier in life? And wouldn't the medical sector be better off because the expense of the surgery would have been avoided?"

But the ad overlooked the many years the man would have had to take those medications and the costs that would have been incurred during those years.

It also overlooked the many other people who would have had to take medications for many years, but who would not have needed bypass surgery even without the medications. Prevention addresses risks. It must be given to everyone at risk even though not everyone will develop the disease without intervention. Among all those at risk, medical science does not yet know how to distinguish those who will benefit from those who will not. Some people ultimately benefit and others do not. But costs are incurred for all of them.

Another reason is that people look at the initial costs, such as the cost of screening, without counting the subsequent costs necessary to produce better health outcomes. They consider, for example, how inexpensive it is to check blood pressure. Or the low cost of advertisements that urge people to get their blood pressure checked. But neither the ads nor the blood pressure checks produce better health by themselves. That requires additional expenditures to do something about elevated blood pressure levels—visits to the doctor, prescription medications, laboratory tests to monitor the effects of the medications, and so on. Screening produces information. Ads disseminate information. But unless that information leads to action, which requires additional resources, there is no improvement in health.

Consider the example of cholesterol screening followed by statins, when needed, to reduce elevated levels. A classic example of secondary prevention, statins treat a risk factor for heart disease in order to reduce the risk of heart disease itself. To calculate the total costs of this intervention, the analyst must track the costs of screening, medications, physician visits, laboratory tests, and, in addition, the hospitalizations and other treatment that occur because statins are not 100% effective. These costs must be tracked over the lifetimes of all people with a particular risk profile, defined in terms of gender, age, initial cholesterol level, blood pressure, smoking, and so on. The total costs of prevention for these people, and the associated years of healthy life, are then compared with the costs and healthy years of the alternative—treating heart disease after it occurs—to determine the cost-effectiveness of reducing cholesterol with statins.

Table 3.2 shows the results of an analysis of statins for people aged 55–64 (Prosser et al. 2000). The authors analyzed statins' cost-effectiveness for patients with different risk profiles. Aside from gender and age, the low-risk group had elevated low-density lipoprotein (LDL) cholesterol as their only risk factor. The high-risk group also smoked and had low high-density lipoprotein (HDL) cholesterol and hypertension. Note that the study begins at the point at which individuals have been identified as having elevated LDL levels and thus excludes the costs of the initial screening required to identify them.

Each cost-effectiveness ratio in Table 3.2 compares (1) the costs and health effects of prevention (statins) for patients with the specified risk profile and (2) the costs and health effects of waiting until heart disease occurs in the same patients and treating it then. To calculate the ratio, the costs of treatment are

Table 3.2. Cost-Effectiveness of Statins in People Aged 55–64, 2007 Dollars*

No Heart Disease at Baseline, High LDL Cholesterol	Cost per Healthy Year
Men, LDL 160–189	
Diastolic BP <95, nonsmoker, HDL >49	344,000
Diastolic BP ≥95, nonsmoker, HDL >49	239,000
Diastolic BP ≥95, smoker, HDL <35	165,000
Women, LDL 160–189	
Diastolic BP <95, nonsmoker, HDL >49	539,000
Diastolic BP ≥95, nonsmoker, HDL >49	299,000
Diastolic BP ≥95, smoker, HDL <35	224,000
No Heart Disease at Baseline, Very High LDL Cholesterol	**Cost per Healthy Year**
Men, LDL ≥190	
Diastolic BP <95, nonsmoker, HDL >49	210,000
Diastolic BP ≥95, nonsmoker, HDL >49	141,000
Diastolic BP ≥95, smoker, HDL <35	88,000
Women, LDL ≥190	
Diastolic BP <95, nonsmoker, HDL >49	389,000
Diastolic BP ≥95, nonsmoker, HDL >49	239,000
Diastolic BP ≥95, smoker, HDL <35	180,000
Heart Disease at Baseline	**Cost per Healthy Year**
Men	5,800
Women	12,600

*Numbers updated to 2007 dollars using the medical CPI. BP, blood pressure; LDL, low-density lipoprotein; HDL, high-density lipoprotein.

subtracted from the costs of statins (put another way, the treatment savings are subtracted from the costs of prevention) and the healthy years produced by treatment are subtracted from the healthy years produced by statins. The result, since statins cost more than treatment, but also produce more healthy years, is the *additional* cost for each *additional* healthy year produced by statins.

Two points are revealed by the table. First, statins do not, in general, reduce medical costs—they add to them, in many cases substantially. For example, the first number in the table, $344,000 (2007 dollars), shows that for men aged 55–64 without heart disease at baseline, whose LDL cholesterol is between 160 and 189 but who have no other risk factors–their blood pressure is normal, they do not smoke, and their HDL cholesterol is in the good range—statins cost an additional $344,000 for each healthy year gained compared to the alternative of treating heart disease when it occurs. Second, the additional cost, per year of healthy life gained, varies enormously with the individual's risk profile. Statins are very cost-effective for people who have already been diagnosed with heart disease, only $5800 for each additional healthy year in men, and $12,600 in women. In fact, the article states that statins are cost-saving for some high-risk subgroups of men with heart disease, although it does not identify the subgroups. Statins are much less cost-effective for people who do not have heart disease, ranging as high as $539,000 per healthy year for women aged 55–64 whose only risk factor is LDL cholesterol in the 160–189 range and $344,000 for men with the same risk profile. In general, statins are more cost-effective for men than women and for people with several risk factors for heart disease than for those with only elevated LDL levels. The article shows that they also tend to be more cost-effective for older people than for younger people.

Table 3.3 presents a range of common preventive interventions, and in a somewhat different way: it shows the number of healthy years of life that could be purchased for $1 million spent on that intervention. The numbers come from studies published in the major medical journals and are also included in my National Coalition on Health Care report (Russell 2007). Presenting cost-effectiveness results this way helps to focus on the primary goal of health spending: longer life and better health. It answers the question, if an additional $1 million were available, how much good health could be purchased by spending it on this intervention?

The table makes the same two points as the study of statins: (1) prevention rarely reduces medical costs and can add substantially to them; and (2) how prevention is targeted makes a big difference to its cost-effectiveness. For example, screening white men for colorectal cancer just once, at age 55, would bring 577 healthy years for $1 million compared with not screening. By contrast, spending an additional $1 million to screen women for cervical cancer every year would bring 0.3 of a healthy year compared with screening every 2 years instead. The more cost-effective the intervention, or the way of using the intervention, the more healthy years can be gained by spending $1 million on it. The gain depends on factors such as the effectiveness of the intervention and the incidence and severity of the disease. A given intervention is generally more cost-effective when targeted to high-risk groups than to low-risk groups because high-risk groups are more likely to experience the disease and thus are more likely to benefit from attempts to prevent it.

Finally, Figure 3.1, created from data supplied by the authors of the *New England Journal of Medicine* article mentioned earlier (Cohen et al. 2008), shows the distribution of cost-effectiveness ratios for 279 comparisons involving preventive interventions. (It also shows ratios for more than 1000 treatment comparisons—I will return to those later.) These ratios were taken from articles that were published between 2000 and 2005 and included in the Tufts-New England Medical Center registry of cost-effectiveness analyses; studies must meet certain quality standards to be included in the registry. In the figure interventions are grouped according to how much the intervention added to medical costs compared to the alternative: from those that improved health and cost less than

Table 3.3. Years of Healthy Life for an Expenditure of $1 million, 2007 Dollars

	Years/$1 Million
Varicella (chickenpox) vaccine, preschool children*	186
BP medication, age 35–64, no heart disease*	23
Hydrochlorothiazide (diuretic)	
Prazosin hydrochloride (alpha blocker)	6
Cholesterol-lowering medications	
Low-risk men 45–54	2
High-risk men 45–54	12
Aspirin to prevent heart disease	
Men 45, 10-year risk 2.5%	87
Men 45, 10-year risk 5.0% or higher	Cost-saving
Cervical cancer screening"	
Every 3 years vs. no screening	24
Every 2 years vs. every 3 years	0.8
Annually vs. every 2 years	0.3
Colorectal cancer screening*	
White men, sigmoidoscopy once at 55	577
White men, sigmoidoscopy every 10 years vs. at 55	47
Mammography	
All women aged 50–79, every 2 years	33
Magnetic resonance imaging (MRI) for women with BRCA1	
Mammography alone	49
Mammography plus MRI	2
Proteinuria screening from age 50	
Normal blood pressure (BP), no diabetes	3
High blood pressure and diabetes	44
Diabetes screening	
Age 55 with high BP vs. no screening	20
All adults 55 vs. those with high BP	2
HIV screening	
Prevalence 1.0%	29
Prevalence 0.1%	15
Abdominal aortic aneurysm screening, men 60–74	46
Diet/exercise to prevent diabetes in high-risk adults	5
Smoking cessation, average of 15 programs	192

*Studies used years of life unadjusted for quality; all others used QALYs.

the alternative at the bottom ("cost-saving"), to those that added less than $10,000 for each additional healthy year compared to the alternative (<$10K), up to interventions that added more than $1 million per healthy year compared to the alternative (>$1 million), and, at the top, those that not only added to medical costs but made people's health worse.

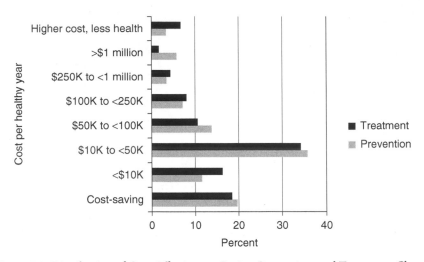

Figure 3.1 Distribution of Cost-Effectiveness Ratios, Prevention, and Treatment. Chart created from the original data, supplied by the authors.

For now, focus just on the cost-effectiveness ratios for prevention, the lighter bars. The lowest bar ("cost-saving") shows that just under 20% of preventive interventions were cost-saving, that is, they improved health and their medical costs were less than the alternative. (Depending on the issues addressed by the analysis, the alternative could be treatment or another type of prevention for the same condition.) More than 80% of the preventive interventions fall higher on the chart—they increased medical costs compared to the alternative.

Again, the answer to the question raised in this section is clear: the majority of preventive interventions do not reduce medical spending and some are very expensive. As a rule then, with prevention as with so much else, it costs more to get more. The evidence of hundreds of studies over the past four decades has consistently shown that most preventive interventions add more to medical spending than they save, although at the same time they do improve health (Russell 2009).

DOES THE UNITED STATES SPEND ONLY 3% ON PREVENTION?

For many years, it has been widely agreed that the United States allocates only 3% of its total health spending to prevention. Some speakers and writers put the number a little higher, some a little lower (Miller et al. 2008). This is another element of the prevention/health debate that has puzzled me. Considering all the well-child and prenatal visits, all the screening tests, and all the preventive checks—blood pressure measurement, weight and height, questions and advice from doctors—that go on during doctors visits, whatever the reason for the visit, and all the people who are on blood pressure medications and statins, how is this number even plausible? The number is about equal to the percentage spent by state health departments and reported in the National Health Expenditure Accounts, so, in occasional discussions with others, I wondered if that might be its source.

Researchers at the Altarum Institute in Ann Arbor, Michigan, have identified the most commonly cited source for this number as a study that was published in 1992, but only in the form of an executive summary (Miller et al. 2008; Brown et al. 1992). The number is based on data for the year 1988 and thus predates the growth in preventive measures such as the use of statins over the 1990s. More importantly, it apparently excludes most of what goes on in private doctors' offices, hospitals, and clinics. Although the published summary gives few details of how the estimate was developed, it does explain that two-thirds of the amount was direct spending by federal, state, and local governments.

The Altarum researchers have put together more accurate estimates of prevention's share of national health spending for the late 1990s through 2007 (Miller et al. 2008; Miller et al., Chapter 2 of this volume). They carefully and conservatively estimated expenditures for primary prevention (including public health spending), screening and other secondary prevention, dental prevention, and prevention-related research. Their final estimates, when all those categories are combined, show that prevention accounted for 8–9% of national health spending during this period, depending on the year. Prevention-related research accounted for about half a percentage point of this amount and dental prevention for about 1.5 percentage points.

Although they are considerably higher than the much-quoted 3%, these estimates are still conservative. For example, the authors could not measure the bits and pieces of prevention that go on during physician visits for other purposes, such as the routine measurement of blood pressure, so did not include them.

But step back for a moment, away from the medical sector, and look at the larger view. Highway and car design have improved enormously over the years—from two-lane roads that crowned in the middle to highways that are graded to keep cars on the road around turns and that separate traffic with median strips; from Tin Lizzies to cars with reinforced roofs, seat belts, and air bags. This is prevention too, and it is designed to keep people out of the medical sector altogether. The same is true of water treatment, pollution control, standards for food handling, workplace safety measures, building construction codes, health education in schools, parental time spent teaching children to brush their teeth and fasten their seatbelts, and many, many other activities. All are prevention and are designed to keep people out of the medical sector.

In the interest of intelligent resource allocation, it is essential to look beyond the medical sector to these other activities. The medical sector's main job is to treat injury and illness. No other sector shares that job. But many other sectors share the job of prevention. Most of the activities that prevent injury and illness, and most of the resources spent on them, are in these other sectors. Thus the important question is whether the United States is spending enough on prevention more broadly, wherever it takes place, not whether it is spending enough on the relatively narrow range of preventive activities that falls within the purview of the medical sector. It may be, for example, that health would be better served by repairing our crumbling infrastructure (Herbert 2010)—water systems, bridges, and train tracks—than by screening more people for cancer or prescribing more statins.

This wider view includes an important resource that is used for both prevention and treatment, but that is rarely considered as a cost: people's unpaid time. All those parents teaching, and reminding their children to brush their teeth and use their seatbelts; taking their children and themselves and their elderly parents to medical visits; caring for sick children kept home from school; enforcing bedtimes; going to the gym to take care of their own health; and so on. Although medical and public health recommendations proceed almost as though people's time were unlimited, it is a scarce resource. Lack of time prevents people from following some recommendations. A preference for spending their limited time elsewhere dissuades them from others.

The American Time Use Survey identifies a large part of the time that people spend on medical care, preventive and therapeutic, outside of institutions (Russell 2007). Conducted by the U.S. Bureau of Labor Statistics, the survey asks a nationally representative sample of Americans 15 years old and older how they spent their time during one day, a 24-hour period. Days are sampled continuously throughout the year. The first 2 years of the survey, 2003–2004, showed that, on any given day, 11.3% of adults spent time on health-related activities, including self-care, care related to the health of children or other adults, and outpatient medical services. These adults spent an average of 1 hour and 48 minutes on various health-related activities. Over the course of a year, that daily average adds up to 74 hours for every person 15 years old or older, almost two 40-hour workweeks per person. And that's not all: for example, time spent teaching kids about tooth brushing and seatbelts falls under other general categories, such as time spent with children for educational and recreational purposes, and cannot be separately identified.

SHOULD THE UNITED STATES SPEND MORE ON PREVENTION?

The 3% figure is used to argue that the United States spends too little on prevention. But the percentage of total health spending, no matter what it is, is no basis for concluding that prevention deserves more resources, or, by extension, that treatment deserves fewer. Neither prevention nor treatment is a single, homogeneous commodity. Each candidate intervention must be judged on its own merits.

The point bears repeating: each intervention, whether preventive or therapeutic, should be judged on its own merits. Those merits are relative. They depend on the alternatives, on what would be done if the intervention in question were not used. As Table 3.1 shows, the cost-effectiveness of self-management for asthma depends not only on how effective self-management is, but also on how effective traditional care is, not only on the costs of self-management, but also on those of traditional care. Traditional care already produced 344 incident-free days per patient per year; self-management produced 15 more. It also cost $138 more per patient than traditional care. The result was a very cost-effective intervention at only $3380 in additional costs for each additional incident-free year (1997 dollars). If self-management had been less effective, or more expensive, its cost per incident-free year would have been higher. But it is equally true that if traditional care had been more effective, or less expensive, the cost per incident-free year of choosing self-management would also have been higher.

Cost-effectiveness compares alternative approaches to a problem and the cost-effectiveness ratio changes when important features of either alternative change. The merits of statins are relative to those of the treatment available for heart disease and stroke after they occur. If treatment for heart disease and stroke becomes more effective, statins have less to contribute and their cost-effectiveness declines. If the cost of statins increases, while the cost of treatment stays the same, the cost-effectiveness of statins again declines. At current prices, statins cost more than treatment, much more in some groups, for each healthy year gained (Table 3.2). At a cost of 10 cents per pill they could be cost-saving compared to treatment (Pletcher et al. 2009).

The cost-effectiveness of any intervention, preventive or therapeutic, depends on what it is compared to, so the comparator should represent a realistic choice. The current standard of care is often the comparator. The cost-effectiveness ratio is then defined and described in terms of the intervention of interest— self-management or statins, for example—compared to the current standard. Or the comparator can be defined by a progression of reasonable alternatives, such as the cost-effectiveness of screening for cervical cancer at different frequencies (Table 3.3); no one in high-income countries would consider not screening a reasonable alternative. In that case, the cost-effectiveness of each screening interval depends on the costs and effects of the next interval. If, as is typically the case, cervical cancer is slow growing, annual Pap smears cost a lot for each additional healthy year. If the disease were to become more aggressive annual Pap smears would be more cost-effective compared with screening less often because more new cases of disease would appear in the space of a year.

Evaluating interventions one by one then, is there evidence that more resources should be devoted to prevention? The argument that more should be spent on prevention implies that preventive interventions that produce additional healthy years at low cost are being ignored in favor of treatments that produce additional healthy years at high cost. Is this the case? Here I will return to the perspective of the medical sector, only reminding readers that the answer should eventually consider the wider scope of preventive activities as well and the many activities that are, or could be, carried on outside the medical sector.

Figure 3.1 again provides a useful overview. It is based on a large sample: 279 cost-effectiveness ratios in which a preventive intervention was the focus of interest, and 1221 ratios in which a treatment was, from 599 cost-effectiveness studies published between 2000 and 2005. Because the articles are recent, they are likely to represent relatively new interventions, rather than well-established ones. The chart makes it easy to consider the cost-effectiveness of prevention and cure by putting them side by side, grouping those options that may be cost-saving at the bottom, then those that cost less than $10,000 per healthy year, and so on, all the way to those that increase costs and worsen health at the top.

If the United States invests too little in prevention, cost-effectiveness analyses would show many more cost-saving and low-cost options for prevention than for cure—options that are not being used. But the two distributions look remarkably similar. Between 18% and 20% of the preventive interventions have the potential to be cost-saving. A similar percentage of treatment interventions is also potentially cost-saving. As the cost per healthy year gained increases, the share of preventive interventions is sometimes a little lower, sometimes a little higher, than the share of treatments. Both prevention and treatment offer some interventions that are exceptionally expensive—more than $1 million per healthy year—or downright worthless, adding to costs and making people worse off. In fact, Figure 3.1 and Tables 3.1–3.3 show that although people may think that prevention reduces medical spending, they clearly do not make that a requirement for spending on it. The interventions shown in Tables 3.2 and 3.3 are all widely used, yet most of them add to medical spending and some are quite expensive. The evidence suggests that, rhetoric aside, we are as ready to invest in prevention—at least in the medical sector—as in treatment.

Although the shapes of the two distributions are probably right, they may be optimistic. Both prevention and treatment are probably less effective and more expensive than the chart shows. Why? First, cost-effectiveness analyses tend to be optimistic in their estimates of the health effects of an intervention. They base their estimates on the best possible evidence, such as randomized controlled trials. Trials employ a standard of care that is not always realized in the community. As a simple example, *JAMA* recently reported that most doctors and their staffs do not take blood pressure measurements correctly (Mitka 2008). Incorrect measurements can lead to treatment for people who do not need it. In addition, due in part to a lack of studies to support such estimates, cost-effectiveness analyses tend to neglect the adverse effects of interventions. When those adverse effects take the form of a shorter lifespan, they are captured in the overall mortality associated with an intervention. But when they take the form of less serious side effects or injuries, they are not automatically captured—sometimes not even recognized as related to the intervention. To what extent these adverse effects detract from the health gains of a preventive or therapeutic intervention is not a matter that can be addressed in general, but is specific to each intervention and the way it is used.

Second, by focusing solely on medical sector costs, cost-effectiveness analyses underestimate an intervention's costs. Patients' time, the time of unpaid caregivers, and costs billed outside the medical sector are rarely counted in analyses of either prevention or treatment. Of course, because cost-effectiveness ratios are based on the differences between two alternatives, including these other costs could reduce the net for some interventions, depending on which alternative incurs more. But, until they are counted, it is not possible to know for sure. My expectation is that because prevention so often involves a screening process that requires time from many people to select the smaller number likely to benefit, counting these costs will usually increase the costs of prevention more than those of treatment, and thus the net cost of prevention. This expectation has been borne out by a few studies that measure patients' time (Jonas et al. 2008; Russell and Safford 2008). But here again, the lack of data for the majority of interventions means we cannot know for sure.

Why do these costs matter if our concern is to reduce medical spending? They matter because efficient resource allocation needs to count the full costs of interventions, not just those that pertain to a particular part of the economy. Reducing costs in the medical sector while raising them elsewhere is cost shifting and may be less, not more, efficient when overall resource allocation is considered. Furthermore, patients and caregivers are influenced by these costs. Decisions about preventive interventions will not be optimal, and interventions will not realize their full potential, if these crucial stakeholders are deterred by the magnitude of costs that are ignored by medical decision makers.

Third, by tradition, studies of vaccines often value healthy years of life gained at the future wages that could be earned with those years (Russell 2007). When they report that a vaccine is cost-saving they include these future wages among the cost offsets. Referring back to my earlier discussion of cost-effectiveness methods, these studies project the portion of the health gain that is likely to be used for paid work and value that portion at the potential earnings, in addition to reporting it as part of the total health gain, thus counting it twice. Whatever the merit of this approach, it does not show whether the vaccine reduces medical costs because it is not limited to medical costs.

Given what is known, are there guidelines that might suggest how to invest most effectively in prevention? Where might prevention be most likely to save money—accepting that those instances will be relatively restricted and will not lead to a general reduction in medical spending? See Russell (2009) for more discussion of the factors that affect the cost-effectiveness of prevention, but two particularly important points follow.

Cost-effectiveness analyses show that both prevention and cure are most efficient when targeted to those who benefit most. The cholesterol example presented earlier showed that statins are more cost-effective for high-risk people than for low-risk people. The same is true for many other interventions, including many forms of screening. The tendency in the medical sector, however, has been the other way—to lower cut points for risk factors and to extend screening to lower-risk groups. Note that there is nothing inherently wrong with this approach as long as no more cost-effective ways to improve health are available.

There is also some evidence for targeting the underserved. Because they have not received services regularly in the past, the prevalence of silent disease and undiagnosed risk factors is higher among them than in the general population (Russell 1993a, 1993b). For example, a study published in the *Journal of the American Medical Association* in 1988 showed that because of the long accumulation of treatable conditions, cervical cancer screening was cost-saving among poor elderly women who had not had a Pap smear in recent memory (Mandelblatt and Fahs 1988). By contrast, annual Pap smears are very expensive compared to screening less frequently (Table 3.3; Eddy 1990). Not many new cases of disease develop in a year's time.

Prevention is not a solution to the health care cost problem. Some preventive interventions reduce medical spending, in some circumstances, but the majority, in most circumstances, do not. The same is true of cure. Each intervention needs to be evaluated individually. Sometimes the next best investment is prevention and sometimes treatment. The goal should be to find the most effective mix, the one that makes the best use of our resources to improve health and extend life, whether through prevention or treatment. The evidence from cost-effectiveness studies suggests that the balance between prevention and cure, at least in the medical sector, may not be so far wrong after all.

REFERENCES

Brown, R., Corea, J., Luce, B., Elixhauser, A., and Sheingold, S. 1992. Effectiveness in Disease and Injury Prevention: Estimated National Spending on Prevention— United States, 1988. *Morbidity and Mortality Weekly Report* 41 (29):529–31.

Cohen, J.T., Neumann, P.J., and Weinstein, M.C. 2008. Does Preventive Care Save Money? Health Economics and the Presidential Candidates. *The New England Journal of Medicine* 358 (7):661–63.

Eddy, D.M. 1990. Screening for Cervical Cancer. *Annals of Internal Medicine* 113 (3):214–26.

Edelson, J.T., Weinstein, M.C., Tosteson, A.N.A., et al. 1990. Long-Term Cost-Effectiveness of Various Initial Monotherapies for Mild To Moderate Hypertension *Journal of the American Medical Association* 263 (3):407–13.

Frazier, A.L., Colditz, G.A., Fuchs, C.S., and Kuntz, K.M. 2000. Cost-Effectiveness of Screening for Colorectal Cancer in the General Population. *Journal of the American Medical Association* 284 (15):1954–61.

Gold, M.R., Siegel, J.E., Russell, L.B., and Weinstein, M.C., Eds. 1996. *Cost-Effectiveness in Health and Medicine.* New York: Oxford University Press.

Herbert, B. 2010. What's Wrong with Us? *The New York Times,* February 16.

Jonas, D.E., Russell, L.B., Sandler, R.S., Chou, J., and Pignone, M. 2008. Value of Patient Time Invested in the Colonoscopy Screening Process: Time Requirements for Colonoscopy Study. *Medical Decision Making* 28 (1):56–65.

Lahdensuo, A., Haahtela, T., Herrala, J., Kava, T., Kiviranta, K., Kuusisto, P., et al. 1998. Randomised Comparison of Cost Effectiveness of Guided Self Management and Traditional Treatment of Asthma in Finland. *British Medical Journal* 316 (7138):1138–39.

Lipscomb, J., Weinstein, M.C., and Torrance, G.W. 1996. Time Preference. In M.R. Gold et al., Eds., *Cost-Effectiveness in Health and Medicine* (pp. 214–46). New York: Oxford University Press.

Mandelblatt, J.S., and Fahs, M.C. 1988. The Cost-Effectiveness of Cervical Cancer Screening for Low-Income Elderly Women. *Journal of the American Medical Association* 259 (16):2409–13.

Miller, G., Roehrig, C., Hughes-Cromwick, P., and Lake, C. 2008. Quantifying National Spending on Wellness and Prevention. *Beyond Health Insurance: Public Policy to Improve Health.* Advances in Health Economics and Health Services Research: Emerald Group Publishing Limited, 1–24.

Mitka, M. 2008. Many Physician Practices Fall Short on Accurate Blood Pressure Measurement. *Journal of the American Medical Association* 299 (24):2842–43.

Pletcher, M.J., Lazar, L., Bibbins-Domingo, K., et al. 2009. Comparing Impact and Cost-Effectiveness of Primary Prevention Strategies for Lipid-Lowering. *Annals of Internal Medicine* 150 (4):243–54.

Pliskin, J.S., Stason, W.B., Weinstein, M.C., et al. 1981. Coronary Artery Bypass Graft Surgery: Clinical Decision Making and Cost-Effectiveness Analysis. *Medical Decision Making* 1 (1):10–28.

Prosser, L.A., Stinnett, A.A., Goldman, P.A., et al. 2000. Cost-Effectiveness of Cholesterol-Lowering Therapies According to Selected Patient Characteristics. *Annals of Internal Medicine* 132 (10):769–79.

Russell, L.B. 1986. *Is Prevention Better than Cure?* Washington, DC: The Brookings Institution.

———. 1993a. The Role of Prevention in Health Reform. *The New England Journal of Medicine* 329 (5):352–54.

———. 1993b. Too Much for Too Few: What Cost-Effectiveness Tells Us about Prevention. In W.D. Skelton and M. Osterweis, Eds., *Promoting Community Health: The Role of the Academic Health Center* (pp. 70-79). Washington, DC: Association of Academic Health Centers.

———. 2007. *Prevention's Potential for Slowing the Growth of Medical Spending.* Washington, DC: National Coalition on Health Care. Available at http://www.ihhc-par.rutgers.edu/downloads/RussellNCHC2007.pdf accessed February 8, 2011.

———. 2009. Preventing Chronic Disease: An Important Investment, But Don't Count on Cost Savings. *Health Affairs* 28 (1):42–45.

Russell, L.B., Gold, M.R., Siegel, J.E., Daniels, N., and Weinstein, M.C. 1996. The Role of Cost-Effectiveness Analysis in Health and Medicine. *Journal of the American Medical Association* 276 (14):1172–77.

Russell, L.B., Yoko Ibuka, and Katharine G.A., Health-Related Activities in the American Time Use Survey, *Medical Care,* 2007;45(7), July:680–685.

Russell, L.B., and Safford, M.M. 2008. The Importance of Recognizing Patient's Time as a Cost of Self-Management. *The American Journal of Managed Care* 14 (6):395–96.

Siegel, J.E., Weinstein, M.C., Russell, L.B., and Gold, M.R. 1996. Recommendations for Reporting Cost-Effectiveness Analyses. *Journal of the American Medical Association* 276 (16):1339–41.

U.S. Preventive Services Task Force. 1989. *Guide to Clinical Preventive Services: An Assessment of the Effectiveness of 169 Interventions.* Baltimore, MD: Williams & Wilkins.

Weinstein, M.C., Siegel, J.E., Gold, M.R., Kamlet, M.S., and Russell, L.B. 1996. Recommendations of the Panel on Cost-Effectiveness in Health and Medicine. *Journal of the American Medical Association* 276 (15):1253–58.

4

The Evidence Base for Clinical Prevention

An Incomplete Story

ROBERT B. WALLACE, MD, MSC ■

THE NATURE AND SCOPE OF PREVENTION

In the first chapter of this volume, Faust and Menzel explain the basic definitions of primary, secondary, and tertiary prevention. These approaches to clinical prevention are well defined. However, to understand the full scope of prevention, other dimensions deserve to be noted, largely to emphasize that much of prevention does not take place in the clinical setting. One additional construct, for example, is *primordial prevention* (Farquhar 1999), in which the biological or environmental underpinnings and risk factors for potential disease occurrence have been eliminated, such as would be the case if there were no tobacco available in the environment. Primordial prevention could have an important role in disease prevention, and does not take place in the clinic. This chapter summarizes the nature and extent of scientific evidence underpinning clinical prevention, reviews how proven interventions are actually delivered in the United States, catalogs the limitations of this evidence, and discusses the implications of these limitations for the place of prevention services in clinical practice.

Preventive interventions can be thought of in several ways. *Clinical prevention* is very much tied to access to medical care with all its incumbent factors, as well as to the general judgments and actions of health professionals.

Although access to clinical prevention, the theme of this volume, is by definition the result of an interaction with health professionals, even many clinical
preventive interventions may not be delivered in the conventional way. Some
interventions, such as influenza vaccines, may be acquired in community centers, grocery stores, senior centers, and pharmacies. Dieticians, high school
teachers, orthotists, physical therapists, and psychologists may give high-qual-
ity prevention advice. In addition, a very important prevention dimension is
self-directed preventive behaviors, such as promoting personal exercise and a
healthy diet and seeking self-administered smoking cessation programs. Such
behaviors have diverse origins that may not lie within formal health services.

Another important dimension of prevention, perhaps the most important, is
the set of interventions that does not require either individual or clinical behaviors, but that has been "engineered" into our social, physical, and economic
environments. Examples include installing airbags in autos and guard rails
along dangerous highway segments, inspecting buildings during construction,
screening canned foods during processing for *botulinus* toxin, recalling dangerous toys, wearing protective gear during hazardous occupations, installing residential fire alarms, ensuring multiple operating exits in public buildings, and
providing adequate police protection to minimize crime against individuals.
These policies and practices are very important to health maintenance and protection, but are often not considered part of preventive practice; many of these
are fully beyond the reach of both the health care system and even the public
health system. Although beyond the scope of this discussion, the ability to
account for the cost and health outcomes of these environmental interventions
is extremely difficult (Weatherly et al. 2009).

Thus, preventive interventions could be thought of as having three general
domains: (1) environmental modification and control, (2) personal behavior
alterations, and (3) services obtained in the clinical setting. However, one final,
global preventive dimension worth considering relates to prevention-relevant
policy and practice decisions. Policy decisions by states and the federal government as well as by other medical organizations may have critical downstream
implications for applying prevention, especially those related to the provision
of health insurance and the structure of health services. An example is the
recent "pay-for-performance" movement, in which small bonuses are offered to
health systems and practitioners if certain clinical or preventive utilization
goals are met (Frieden and Mostashari 2008). Also, community knowledge and
culture may alter the acceptance of various interventions, or the propensity of
individual health practitioners to offer them to patients. For example, parental
resistance to many widely used childhood vaccines continues to be an important public health problem. Clinical practice technology may also determine
the application of clinical preventive interventions. The use of computerized

decision support has been shown in several instances to increase the utilization of preventive services (Garg et al. 2005).

Potent industrial forces can intentionally subvert some prevention programs. Historically, the resistance of the auto industry to installing seat belts (Nader 1965) and the activities of the tobacco industry to resist the passage of legislation to limit second-hand smoke exposure is now well documented (Landman and Glantz 2009), and the activities of many industries to influence environmental risk assessments are available in the public record. Most assuredly, prevention takes place in a political and policy context, and all the forces should be recognized. Thus, not surprisingly, policy decisions on the appropriate application of prevention in the clinic and community are not solely related to the availability and interpretability of scientific evidence.

THE EVIDENCE BASE FOR PRIMARY AND SECONDARY PREVENTION

The scientific basis for primary and secondary prevention is derived from the same fundamental sources that help direct clinical treatments. Good prevention starts with the important advances that come from basic science, which are then translated to individuals and populations. The scientific evidence for prevention is fundamentally derived in two ways: (1) observational epidemiological studies, in which the people are studied in their "normal habitat," and outcomes related to various exposures and behaviors are monitored over time, and (2) randomized trials, in which preventive interventions are applied to populations, and outcomes are monitored according to the assigned intervention. The second source of evidence for prevention is deemed a more definitive level of scientific evidence, but both types have problems in interpretation and translation into clinical or population prevention policy (Flather, Delahunty, and Collinson 2006), as well as for therapeutic matters (Williams 2010). Randomized trials are perhaps more applicable to clinical preventive interventions because the interventions themselves take place in individual persons in the clinical setting. It is much more difficult to randomize populations or communities and assign interventions to large groups. The process of identifying effective primary and secondary preventive interventions has been an important part of the scientific and political trend in medical practice called "Evidence-Based Medicine" (EBM) (Sackett et al. 2000; Petitti in Chapter 5 of this volume). EBM has had a critical role in encouraging clinical policies to be based on available scientific studies, and preventive medicine has been an important force in defining the EBM process. Prevention's role in this methodology will likely raise its profile in the coming decade.

Much of the detail of how EBM is applied to prevention is well explained in the works of the U.S. Preventive Services Task Force (USPSTF 2009a) and the Canadian Task Force on Preventive Health Care (CTFPHC 2009) (see also Chapter 5 in this volume by Petitti). The EBM process begins with identifying important potential preventive interventions that have not yet been well evaluated. In the USPSTF, the interventions are generally considered in three classes: (1) counseling interventions, (2) disease screening, and (3) chemopreventive and vaccine applications. Then, a structured and comprehensive literature search is made to access relevant scientific reports. These reports are then screened for their relevance and scientific quality; those "surviving" reports are then submitted to structured evidence summaries and sometimes meta-analyzed (subjected to pooled statistical analysis where feasible). The quality of the evidence is graded in two important ways: (1) the primary study methods are graded, with well-conducted randomized trials receiving the highest value, with decreasing regard for epidemiological (observational) studies, and the least regard for expert opinion, and (2) the evidence itself is graded to assess how well it lends itself to clinical policy recommendations. Finally, a summary recommendation is promulgated as a "clinical guideline." Such guidelines are intended to be advisory to primary care physicians and the recommendations may range from strong endorsement for an intervention to a strong proscription. In between are more modest recommendations, positive or negative, and the all-too-often situation in which the evidence garnered is deemed inadequate or contradictory.

Many individual, potential clinical preventive interventions have been rigorously evaluated, with detailed summarization of the evidence through structured algorithms, systematic reviews, and other methods of evidence summary, to very good end. In fact, those clinical preventive interventions that are recommended for primary care practice have been used as indicators of the overall quality of care of those practices.

However, it is with some irony that most of the evidence for long-term disease prevention associated with "healthier" personal behaviors and lifestyles promulgated in clinical practice, such as optimal diet, regular exercise, avoidance of smoking, and protective sexual practices, comes from observational epidemiological studies, with their decreased strength of evidence (USPSTF 2009a), and not from randomized trials. Studies of lifestyle and behaviors tend to have consistent findings, and they form the basis for many of the hygienic practices we recommend in public health and clinical practice venues. However, these studies are largely observational, subsuming a set of methodological limitations that generate concerns about the level of scientific proof. One general problem with such studies is confounding, where, for example, a particular healthy behavior may be an indicator of some other health-giving factor.

For example, exercising may be a sign of wealth sufficient to purchase exercise club memberships and trainers. Thus, consuming diets rich in fruits and vegetables may also be indicative of affluence, safer residential environments, and social and employment opportunities that may lead to healthier outcomes. Another problem with observational studies is the difficulty in measuring the "exposures" of interest. Diet is notoriously difficult to assess in detail, particularly when so much is from manufactured foods or restaurants, in which the constituents are often impossible to identify. Measurement issues also arise in surveying or otherwise assessing sensitive personal issues such as sexual behaviors or illicit substance abuse practices. An overriding methodological issue in prevention studies is that putatively positive or adverse exposures that may lead to altered disease occurrence may have taken place many decades prior to the clinical event. Validating the nature and extent of those exposures is extremely problematic.

With respect to environmental interventions, the evidence is probably the weakest because of the difficulty of experimentally modifying environmental situations, likely more challenging than even lifestyle modifications. Some environmental interventions are based on uncommon but dramatic and tragic events or outbreaks, such as the collapse of an inadequately constructed building, botulism from inadequate food canning processes, or a water-borne outbreak from a municipal water supply. Such events lead to policies that are welcomed as intuitively correct even in the absence of scientific studies in the usual sense. The evidence that higher levels of air particulates (soot) cause cardiovascular disease and stroke is based largely on toxicological and ecological data (Brook 2007; Polichetti et al. 2009), but the growing evidence base mandates a particulate-related air pollution risk analysis and management policy even in the absence of critical studies. It is likely that the community and public environmental controls and policies currently in place have a collectively important preventive role, but quantifying the community health impact can be extremely difficult.

As noted, an extremely important element of prevention takes place in the community, and the evidence for community or public health-based preventive interventions is mostly based on observational methods because of the difficulties of experimental, randomized research in the community setting. The efficacy of community-based interventions, such as public health education programs, condom distribution, low-fat dietary recommendations, or air pollution control, is often much more difficult to prove or refute, and the logistical barriers to conducting rigorous, outcomes-based research or randomized trials in community settings are legion. To deal with the dilemma of marshalling firm evidence, the Guide to Community Preventive Services (GCPS 2009), sponsored by the U.S. Centers for Disease Control and Prevention, has attempted to evaluate these interventions in a manner analogous to clinical preventive interventions. However, because the level of scientific evidence is often of lesser quality and credibility than is available for clinical EBM, policies are often promulgated based on more indirect or less rigorous scientific evidence. It is likely that the promulgation of community or public prevention policies errs on the side of health and safety likelihood, even in the absence of fully developed evidence, the so-called "precautionary principle" (Chaudry 2008; Petrenko and McArthur 2009).

There are substantive struggles to obtain evidence on prevention. For example, that the prevalence of cigarette smoking in the United States has more than halved since the mid-1960s is unquestioned, but reasons for that drop are complex and difficult to discern; proof of individual public policies on tobacco control may be incomplete. There are no randomized trials determining the effect of increasing the cigarette tax on chronic disease outcomes. Another example involves the U.S. Consumer Products Safety Commission or other government agencies, which may order a product withdrawn from the market based on a relatively small number of adverse events, such as aspirating improperly attached parts of dolls or deaths from three-wheel all-terrain vehicular crashes. Despite the compelling logic and likely utility of such actions, there may be little quantitative evidence of community outcomes for such interventions. These may be appropriate and important public policy decisions based more on community values than on methodologically rigorous studies. Sometimes these policies may flounder because these values vary among communities.

Despite the limitations of observational evidence, and other issues in translating science to effective prevention policy, it should not be lost that many important scientific accomplishments have resulted in triumphs in evidence-based primary and secondary prevention. Dramatic control of risk factors for cardiovascular disease, both in the clinic and the community, has resulted in great strides in preventing heart attack and stroke (Fang et al. 2007; Tu et al. 2009). Exercise interventions have been shown to deter the onset of glucose intolerance and adult-onset (Type II) diabetes (Manson et al. 1992; Hawley 2004; Orozco et al. 2008). Clinical hypertension treatment has clearly decreased the occurrence of several vascular diseases (Hajjar, Kotchen, and Kotchen 2006). Effective screening and treatment programs have decreased deaths from some important cancers. Appropriate nutrition supplements have improved child development. Many effective vaccines have controlled otherwise fatal or extremely harmful infectious diseases of both children and adults, and have also been useful in controlling some important cancers that are caused by infectious agents. Although not yet successful, vaccine technology has been applied to the control of Alzheimer's disease (Foster et al. 2009).

Having acknowledged important victories in preventing diseases, it is still apparent that economic forces may drive some of the scientific priorities that translate to clinical treatments in preference to clinical or community preventive interventions. For example, some community environmental interventions require alterations in business and industrial practices. Here, evidence for the interventions may be modest and indirect, leading to substantial political resistance. Conversely, there may be greater economic incentives to fully fund research that leads to clinical treatments, because if these are successful, the investment can be recouped from the health care system. Many potentially effective clinical and community preventive interventions, such as lifestyle or other behavioral interventions, have little likelihood of bringing a direct "return on investment," and their development must often come from limited government research programs. Even preventive interventions with salable products may not receive adequate investments unless there is government intervention in the private sector, such as for the production of many vaccines.

HOW SUCCESSFUL IS THE UNITED STATES IN APPLYING PRIMARY AND SECONDARY PREVENTION?

Given that there is ample evidence for the efficacy of many clinical preventive interventions and that the United States spends more per capita on health services than any other nation on earth, we might ask how well clinical prevention is delivered in the United States in contrast to other countries in the developed world. There are several ways to address this question, but most cross-national analyses depend heavily on only vital statistics. More refined national data systems that document the occurrence of diseases, conditions and preventive practices do not universally exist or are not comparably constructed to allow easy comparison—for example, for determining the rates of vaccine delivery to geographically defined populations or the receipt of cancer screening tests. For many effective interventions, there are also likely to be national differences in clinical guidelines directing the utilization of those applications.

International comparisons of mortality usually focus on selected causes of death that as a group go under various names, such as preventable, amenable, avoidable, or premature mortality. The calculation may be as simple as contrasting adjusted mortality rates. *Preventable, avoidable,* and *amenable* mortality generally involves those primary causes of death that would not exist or would be much less frequent if complete preventive services were universally available in the health care system (Nolte and McKee 2008). *Premature mortality* is a calculation used by the World Health Organization and many national governments, and is often expressed as the cumulative excess years of potential life lost due to all-cause mortality or specific diseases, which may differ somewhat in different analyses, and are beyond the scope of this discussion. No one really believes that "preventable" mortality, such as infant deaths or deaths from heart attack, can really be totally prevented, but for some important conditions, such as coronary disease, substantial mortality salvage is possible. But it is also true that many preventable conditions occur commonly, even among populations with complete access to and receipt of effective preventive care. In other situations, the causes of "preventable" deaths may in large measure be beyond any health system, such as deaths from firearms, which are related to various cultural practices, laws, and political policies.

However, despite the arguments that could be made at the margin of these prevention indicators, the stark reality is that the United States often does not fare well among industrialized nations for a wide range of preventive service indicators, and health and social policy makers have much to do in providing access to effective interventions. One commonly cited indicator of health is the international comparison of infant mortality rates, in which in recent years the United States has ranked worse than at least two dozen other countries, most less affluent. Another indicator of health is rates of preventable deaths; of selected industrialized countries, the United States was ranked 14th (Nolte and McKee 2008).

THE LIMITS OF PREVENTION

When arguments are made concerning fiscal priorities for primary and secondary prevention, it is important to understand the limitations of prevention applications, both in the clinical setting and in the larger community. Although some preventive interventions such as immunizations have had an enormous impact on population morbidity and mortality, much more progress and research are needed to address these limitations. This section highlights some of the gaps in our understanding and in the delivery of various interventions, making the promulgation of clinical guidelines and effective prevention policy a great challenge. Whether these gaps can explain some of the international differences noted above is uncertain.

Gaps in Knowledge of the Causes of Many Important Diseases and Conditions

The scientific basis for prevention depends on the diseases and conditions in question. As noted above, many important conditions can be prevented or deferred by risk factor management or screening for the condition at an early stage, or by changing behaviors that lead to disease occurrence. These include chronic conditions such as diabetes, heart attack and stroke and some some important cancers, and the transmission or early detection and treatment of certain communicable diseases such as tuberculosis, human immunodeficiency virus (through condom use), measles, or influenza; the evidence for these interventions is relatively robust. However, there are many other important conditions within the United States and other nations for which few disease-causation mechanisms or risk factors or causes have ever been defined, such as most mental illnesses, drug addiction and alcohol abuse, many cancers, disabling arthritic conditions, allergic and atopic diseases (e.g., asthma), most birth defects, collagen-vascular diseases (e.g., lupus, scleroderma), and neurodegenerative diseases such as multiple sclerosis, Parkinson's disease, and Alzheimer's disease. Thus, the ability to suggest even hypothetical preventive interventions, biologically, behaviorally, or clinically, is extremely limited for the great, cumulative morbidity and mortality burden with these conditions. Without such knowledge, broadly effective prevention is impossible. Thus, one critical pathway to better disease prevention is to increase support for basic research that defines the causes of important clinical conditions.

A significant issue is the relation of disease occurrence and mortality to individual and population socioeconomic status (SES). SES is typically measured by educational attainment, employment type, and general affluence, and the relation of SES to health status is widely demonstrated with little disagreement. For most important diseases and conditions, incidence rates vary closely and inversely with SES. One reason is related to access to more frequent and higher quality medical care, including primary and secondary preventive services. Other factors that are likely to be important are the relation of SES to more healthful behaviors, general environments, and safer workplace environments. However likely these explanations appear, the extent of the relation of SES to health status as being mediated by individual preventive service access and related practices is far from proven, and should be the subject of further incisive research. Thus, it is possible that there are many important but yet undiscovered health-giving forces that correlate with SES. It may follow from this discussion that, although unproven, one way to improve levels of health status and decrease disparities of health status and outcomes among individuals and populations is to improve the general economic status, even if the mechanisms are not fully understood. We should note that general population-level improvements in economic status may not affect all individuals to the same degree or in the same manner, and the effects of such an intervention on health behaviors may be expected to be similarly heterogeneous (Berkman 2009).

Gaps in the Ability to Administer Effective Interventions

Even when we have sufficient knowledge that various interventions can potentially decrease the occurrence of disease and adverse outcomes, there is substantial difficulty delivering these interventions in the clinical or community setting. For example, the adverse effects of overweight and obesity have been clearly documented (Brown et al. 2009), but both community and clinical approaches to the primary prevention of obesity or the control of existing cases have been modest at best (Galani and Schneider 2007; Lemmens et al. 2008). For example, Figure 4.1 shows low levels of adherence to dietary and exercise behaviors to reduce risks for cardiovascular disease.

Another example is cigarette smoking. Clinical smoking cessation program success among active smokers is modest, particularly in avoiding recidivism; long-term cessation rates are even more modest (Cahill and Perera 2008; Eisenberg et al. 2008). The same may be said for exercise and dietary interventions as well. There have also been great difficulties in delivering important vaccines intended for the general population, where the adverse event rates are very low and the efficacy is very high. Some of this is likely due to the

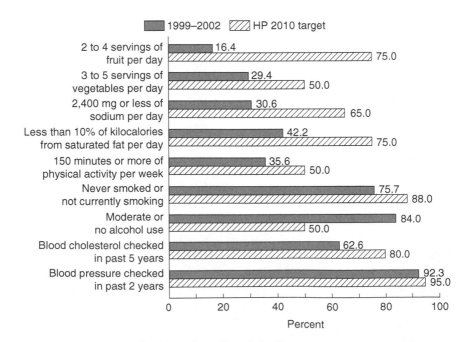

Figure 4.1 Percentage of Adults Who Followed Cardiovascular Disease Prevention Recommendations: United States, 1999–2002 (Wright, Hirsch, and Wang 2009).

lack of access to effective preventive care, but cultural resistance to vaccines in the American population has been well documented (Dias and Marcuse 2000).

Evidence-based clinical prevention guidelines have delineated what "works" in terms of specific interventions. However, to say that certain interventions are "effective" is to belie what is contained in the guideline scientific summaries— that even under the best of clinical trial circumstances many interventions have limited efficacy. Effective reduction of blood lipids does not prevent all heart attacks and strokes, nor does effective blood pressure control. Even highly effective vaccines used to prevent important childhood illnesses sometimes have less than full efficacy. This is also true of condoms for prevention of sexually transmitted diseases and prenatal care for prematurity. In the case of cancer screening in clinical practice, the value of screening for breast cancer has been repeatedly questioned. It has been estimated that on balance screening mammography leads to only a 20% reduction in breast cancer-related mortality among those who partake of screening (Esserman, Shieh, and Thompson 2009). Furthermore, there is still debate as to whether mammography improves outcomes among women 40–50 years and above 75 years of age (USPSTF 2009b). The efficacy of mammography has never been fully evaluated in women over age 70 years with carefully conducted randomized trials. Yet by some bodies, the American Cancer Society and the American College of Radiology, mammography is still recommended to all women 40 years of age and above. Of note, different medical organizations have promulgated different preventive guidelines, despite using the same evidence base. Similarly, questions about screening for prostate cancer have been raised (Amling 2006), although this has always been controversial and not ever recommended in an unqualified manner by most expert groups and associations. A central issue here is that even when a preventive intervention has been "proven" in principle, such "proof" is not the same as level of effectiveness, and patients should be educated as to how much "prevention" they are really receiving from any given intervention.

The Unknown Effectiveness of Combined Preventive Interventions

It is widely believed in health care delivery that creating efficient systems to deliver multiple preventive interventions systematically will lead to an improvement in overall acceptance and utilization rates. There is likely to be some fiscal efficiency obtained from developing a system in which clinical preventive interventions are "packaged" or "bundled" into programs that are targeted to specific age, sex, and other risk-factor-appropriate groups. However, despite the intuitive appeal both from economic and health outcome perspectives, it is not known whether the systematic application of multiple proven interventions across the lifespan leads to the net benefits that would be expected from the individual interventions. This is not an argument against the practice of systematic preventive service delivery, but a plea for empirical demonstration of its effectiveness. It is possible that the net outcomes may be less than expected because of individual variation in response to the interventions or the issue of competing risk (Wolbers et al. 2009); or it may be greater than expected because of rigorous attention to all effective interventions. Knowing how well the systematic approach works can lead to better prioritization of intervention packages.

The "Problem" of Prevention in the Face of Existing Illness

By definition primary prevention and secondary prevention are targeted at individuals who are generally healthy and without any clinical evidence of the disease for which the intervention is targeted. The reality of medical practice is that primary and secondary preventive maneuvers are often performed among patients with existing clinical conditions. In fact, with the increasing technical ability to detect earlier forms of disease, more and more individuals sustain disease diagnoses with less functional consequences. Such patients also receive many preventive interventions irrespective of concurrent "comorbid" diagnoses. Whether such standard and proven interventions actually have the same efficacy among those with existing conditions is uncertain, because such persons are often excluded from efficacy trials of many of these interventions. However, using synthetic estimates of preventive efficacy, recent frameworks for evaluating this efficacy in the face of existing illness have appeared as a guide to what might be expected in this clinical situation (Braithwaite, Fiellin, and Justice 2009).

That technological advancements have allowed identification of earlier disease manifestations and even "predisease" has led to a cogent argument that the lines between disease risk and occurrence have been blurred for many conditions, such as diabetes or breast cancer (Aronowitz 2009). One consequence of this is the change in the natural history and clinical behavior of various conditions and pathophysiological processes. Though this may be good for preventing overt, harmful illnesses, the ability to detect earlier biological states of some conditions may necessitate reevaluation and restudy of the efficacy of current primary and secondary preventive interventions, since they may be intervening in a different stage of a disease's natural history.

The Adverse Effects of Preventive Interventions and Related Medical Services

It is widely demonstrated that preventive interventions may have adverse effects on individual health. Such effects may range from uncommon adverse reactions to vaccines (Zhou et al. 2003) to the hazards of prophylactic aspirin consumption or mechanical bowel perforation due to colonoscopy (PHSRG 1989; Hart et al. 2000; Panteris, Haringsma, and Kuipers 2009). Most of the adverse effects of preventive interventions are rare or at least uncommon, because the nature of prevention generally dictates that the net health effect must be very positive. However, adverse effects are still important health effects and must be addressed in economic calculations of preventive efficacy. Less easy to measure are the potential adverse psychological effects of prevention. For example, the practice of "blaming the victim" for his or her own unhealthy behaviors when disease occurs has received comment (Crawford 1977). Family strife has been reported when children, who are taught in school of the hazards of smoking, become emotionally upset because one or both of their parents are smokers. Another type of psychological adverse effect is the false belief that a negative screening test means that the individual is not at risk and need not practice preventive behaviors, such as improving healthy exercise or dietary habits. Such effects are difficult to quantify and require further study.

The ethos that preventive interventions should be safer than clinical treatments, a view to which this author subscribes, suggests that clinicians practicing prevention should be less tolerant of adverse effects ("First, do no harm") than they are for therapies. Holding prevention to a higher standard of efficacy is also in keeping with the concept of "cost-benefit." There is a very important reason for this approach to preventive: most patients who receive these interventions will never really need them. An additional reason to treat prevention modalities differently than therapies is that for the most part prevention modalities trade immediate harms (adverse effects) for potential future benefits that are often hard to quantify. Some attempts at quantifying this issue have, however, been made. For example, the "Number Needed to Prevent (NNP)," or somewhat more incorrectly, the "Number Needed to Treat (NNT)," has been used to assess the value of some prevention measures. If a patient has a bacterial pneumonia treated with an antibiotic, many if not most patients might be expected to respond and benefit from that medication, while the NNP a case of cervical cancer by vaccinating girls aged 12 years against human papillomavirus (HPV) has been estimated to be about 324 if the vaccine maintains lifelong efficacy, and substantially higher if it does not (Brisson et al. 2007). In the end, valuing the costs and benefits of such prevention modalities as this vaccine is quite complex, and it begs for highly accurate information, on both the short-term and long-term, favorable and adverse outcomes of the intervention at hand.

IMPLICATIONS AND A PERSPECTIVE ON THE VALUE OF PREVENTION VERSUS TREATMENT

There are several implications of the above discussion that direct a perspective on the extent and role of primary and secondary prevention in clinical practice. An important initial point is that a substantial portion of prevention does not take place in clinical practice. Rather, much of it takes place in the community, including schools, the workplace, and recreational areas, and is driven by managing the general, physical, and social environment. This is not to demean the role of clinical prevention, but to emphasize that most individuals want to live and thrive by preventing as many of the causes of morbidity and mortality that are possible, not merely those that may be prevented in the clinical setting. This is also the goal of population health, to diminish the *overall* rates of death and disease.

It also follows from this overall health goal that economic assessments of the amount or proportion of funds dedicated to primary and secondary prevention in practice must deal with the more general economic and societal investment in prevention and how much we get back for it. Similar to the situation in clinical prevention, cost accounting the total societal investment in prevention is challenging and requires much arbitrary estimation of the costs and net health impact—the "return on investment." For example, how much do we get back from constructing a guardrail on a roadside curve to prevent careening down a steep embankment? How many lives are saved by having a U.S. Department of Agriculture officer visually inspect an animal carcass in a slaughterhouse, or by reducing the level of sulfur dioxide in the ambient air by 10%? How much do we invest and get back from constructing and utilizing health clubs and gymnasia? Ironically, many community social and environmental interventions have never been fully evaluated for the cost–benefit of their execution, in part because there is a less evidentiary rationale for them than would be applied to clinical interventions. Yet we invest an enormous amount of resources in environmental and other community prevention programs.

If the evidence for many environmental interventions is meager, there are great challenges in making economic decisions on utilizing clinical preventive interventions. An important issue is whether the strength of evidence for these interventions should have the same standard as for therapies applied in clinical practice. It is difficult to provide a precise quantification of the level of evidence quality for comparative purposes, mostly because these summary measures, although derived from objective studies, are in the end largely subjective. How do we make a clinical decision when the level of evidence in favor of an intervention is an "A" (good) versus a "B" (fair)? Similarly, the methodology to rank various interventions in terms of net health effect is incomplete, making the selection of the best or most effective preventive interventions from a large menu challenging, and even harder if comparing a preventive intervention with a clinical treatment. So it may be difficult to determine if, for example, the quality of evidence that leads to screening and prevention for a particular metabolic birth defect has the same health yield as a heart transplant.

An additional problem with evaluating primary and secondary preventive interventions, where evidence is incomplete, is changing or inadequate public information and communication. The general media provide a continuing barrage of new study reports with actual or implied changes in prevention guidelines and recommendations. Recently, there was a furious, politically tinged debate in the public media over the newly proffered recommendation by the USPSTF to abandon routine mammographic screening in women 40–49 years of age (Sack 2009; Petitti in Chapter 5 of this volume). Similarly, there is a periodic debate on the hazards of dietary cholesterol and fat consumption, the health value of various dietary supplements, and whether walking is a health-giving exercise. All of this serves to induce confusion and cynicism about prevention, and possibly reduce the motivation to engage in interventions for which there is clear evidence of efficacy.

Another consideration as to the decision on allocating preventive versus treatment resources in clinical practice is to consider the fundamental imperatives of healing, partly explored by Faust in Chapter 7 of this volume. Associated with this imperative is the seeming ubiquity of healers in nearly all historical and contemporary societies. Healing systems and healers, although often not unified, are basically part of every culture and likely emerged because of the universal experience of having to deal with suffering, disease, and death. It seems possible, though admittedly speculative, that there are evolutionary dimensions to societies' designation of healers and healing systems, whether related to ritual, religion, or other evolved, more technologically sophisticated social systems. Whatever the biological and philosophical underpinnings, it is possible that healing is in our DNA. Although treatment methods by healers in early primitive healing societies have been described, there is less literature on the role prevention may have had. Such an inquiry would be welcome, though likely difficult at best.

One perhaps superficial way to begin to address the nature of this proposed healing imperative is to study the clinical care utilization behaviors of prevention and public health professionals relative to their therapeutically oriented colleagues. A study that this author has always wanted to do is to compare the consumption of therapeutic resources by preventive medicine physicians and their families with those of primarily treatment-oriented physicians and their families, particularly when health misfortunes strike. The answer might provide some insight into the primacy of healing relative to preventive services.

Despite the great virtues and successes of primary and secondary prevention, one characteristic of healing that is basically not true of prevention is that it attempts to address current, deeply experienced personal health problems. Healing does not require anywhere near as much consideration of "investing" in the uncertainties of future health status as does prevention, and the application of resources for some potentially unseen future gain, particularly when most or all the of the prevention resources have to be spent "now." Many individuals understand the prevention credo and are future oriented, but many others do not have the full understanding, or have chosen not to accept this future orientation (see Faust, this volume, Chapter 7, and Menzel, this volume, Chapter 9). Some of these concepts have dimensions that are addressed in economic theories, and may have similar psychological and behavioral commonalities. Comprehending and evaluating this future orientation are critical to where prevention sciences will take us.

CONCLUSIONS

Clinical prevention has had an important effect on preventing disease, disability, and death. The prevention sciences have also been in the forefront of bringing new research methods into clinical practice, such as summarizing study evidence and promulgating clinical guidelines. A large amount of prevention also takes place in the community and in the environment; any overall assessment of preventive versus curative medicine must take this into account. Despite the successes of clinical prevention, the evidence base for prevention is far from complete, and much more research is needed to conduct the necessary studies and to evaluate both the individual as well as the aggregate interventions applied in the clinical setting. One of the most challenging aspects of this evaluation is to document better the long-term positive and adverse effects of these interventions in order to enhance prevention and to establish better clinical policy.

REFERENCES

Amling, C.L. 2006. Prostate-Specific Antigen and Detection of Prostate Cancer: What Have We Learned and What Should We Recommend for Screening? *Current Treatment Options in Oncology* 7 (5):337–45.

Aronowitz, R.A. 2009. The Converged Experience of Risk and Disease. *The Milbank Quarterly* 87 (2):417–42.

Berkman, L.F. 2009. Social Epidemiology: Social Determinants of Health in the United States: Are We Losing Ground? *Annual Review of Public Health* 30:27–41.

Braithwaite, S.R., Fiellin, D., and Justice, A.C. 2009. The Payoff Time: A Flexible Framework to Help Clinicians Decide When Patients with a Comorbid Disease Are Not Likely to Benefit from Practice Guidelines. *Medical Care* 47 (6):610–17.

Brisson, M., Van de Velde, N., de Wals, P., and Boily, M.C. 2007. Estimating the Number Needed to Vaccinate to Prevent Diseases and Death Related to Human Papillomavirus Infection. *CMAJ* 177 (5):464–68.

Brook, R.D. 2007. Is Air Pollution a Cause of Cardiovascular Disease? Updated Review and Controversies. *Reviews on Environmental Health* 22 (2):115–37.

Brown, W.V., Fujioka, K., Wilson, P.W.F., and Woodworth, K.A. 2009. Obesity: Why Be Concerned? *The American Journal of Medicine* 122 (S1):S4–S11.

Cahill, K., and Perera, R. 2008. Competitions and Incentives for Smoking Cessation. *Cochrane Database of Systematic Reviews* 3: Document number CD004307.

Chaudry, R.V. 2008. The Precautionary Principle, Public Health, and Public Health Nursing. *Public Health Nursing* 25 (3):261–68.

Crawford, R. 1977. You are Dangerous to Your Health: The Ideology and Politics of Victim Blaming. *International Journal of Health Services* 7 (4):663–80.

CTFPHC (Canadian Task Force on Preventative Health Care). 2009. Available at http://www.phac-aspc.gc.ca/cd-mc/ctfphc-gecssp-eng.php, accessed June 13, 2011.

Dias, M., and Marcuse, E.K. 2000. When Parents Resist Immunizations. *Contemporary Pediatrics* 7 (Jul):1–4.

Eisenberg, M.J., Filion, K.B., Yavin, D., Bélisle, P., Mottillo, S., Joseph, L., Gervais, A., O'Loughlin, J., Paradis, G., Rinfret, S., and Pilote, L. 2008. Pharmacotherapies for Smoking Cessation: A Meta-Analysis of Randomized Controlled Trials. *CMAJ* 179 (2).135–44.

Esserman, L., Shieh, Y., and Thompson, I. 2009. Rethinking Screening for Breast Cancer and Prostate Cancer. *JAMA* 302 (15):1685–92.

Fang, J., Alderman, M.H., Keenan, N.L., and Croft, J.B. 2007. Declining U.S. Stroke Hospitalization since 1997: National Hospital Discharge Survey, 1988–2004. *Neuroepidemiology* 29 (3–4):243–49.

Farquhar, J.W. 1999. Primordial Prevention: The Path from Victoria to Catalonia. *Preventive Medicine* 29 (6):S3–S8.

Flather, M., Delahunty, N., and Collinson, J. 2006. Generalizing Results of Randomized Trials to Clinical Practice: Reliability and Cautions. *Clinical Trials* 3 (6):508–12.

Foster, J.K., Verdile, G., Bates, K.A., and Martins, R.N. 2009. Immunization in Alzheimer's Disease: Naïve Hope or Realistic Clinical Potential? *Molecular Psychiatry* 14 (3):239–51.

Frieden, T.R., and Mostashari, F. 2008. Health Care as if Health Mattered. *JAMA* 299 (8):950–52.

Galani, C., and Schneider, H. 2007. Prevention and Treatment of Obesity with Lifestyle Interventions: Review and Meta-Analysis. *International Journal of Public Health* 52 (6):348–59.

Garg, A.X., Adnican, N.K., McDonald, H., Rosas-Arellano, N.P., Devereaux, P.J., Beyene, J., Sam, J., and Haynes, R.B. 2005. Effects of Computerized Clinical Decision Support Systems on Practitioners Performance and Patient Outcomes. *JAMA* 293 (10):1223–38.

GCPS (Guide to Community Preventive Services). 2009. *The Community Guide*. Last reviewed June 22, 2009. Available at http://www.thecommunityguide.org/index.html, accessed June 13, 2011.

Hajjar, I., Kotchen, J.M., and Kotchen, T.A. 2006. Hypertension: Trends in Prevalence, Incidence, and Control. *Annual Review of Public Health* 27:465–90.

Hart, R.G., Halperin, J.L., McBride, R., Benavente, O., Man-Son-Hing, M., and Kronmal, R.A. 2000. Aspirin for the Primary Prevention of Stroke and Other Major Vascular Events: Meta-Analysis and Hypotheses. *Archives of Neurology* 57 (3):326–32.

Hawley, J.A. 2004. Exercise as a Therapeutic Intervention for the Prevention and Treatment of Insulin Resistance. *Diabetes/Metabolism Research and Reviews* 20 (5):383–93.

Landman, A., and Glantz, S.A. 2009. Tobacco Industry Efforts to Undermine Policy-Relevant Research. *American Journal of Public Health* 99 (1):45–58.

Lemmens, V.E.P.P., Oenema, A., Klepp, K.I., Henriksen, H.B., and Brug, J. 2008. A Systematic Review of the Evidence Regarding Efficacy of Obesity Prevention Interventions Among Adults. *Obesity Reviews* 9 (5):446–55.

Manson, J.E., Nathan, D.M., Krolewski, A.S., Stampfer, M.J., Willett, W.C., and Hennekens, C.H. 1992. A Prospective Study of Exercise and Incidence of Diabetes Among US Male Physicians. *JAMA* 268 (1):63–67.

Nader, R. 1965. *Unsafe at Any Speed: The Designed-In Dangers of the American Automobile*. New York: Grossman.

Nolte, E., and McKee, C.M. 2008. Measuring the Health of Nations: Updating an Earlier Analysis. *Health Affairs* 27 (1):58–71.

Orozco, L.J., Buchleitner, A.M., Gimenez-Perez, G., Roqué i Figuls, M., Richter, B., and Mauricio, D. 2008. Exercise or Exercise and Diet for Preventing Type 2 Diabetes Mellitus. *Cochrane Database of Systematic Reviews* 3: Document number CD003054.

Panteris, V., Haringsma, J., and Kuipers, E.J. 2009. Colonoscopy Perforation Rate, Mechanisms and Outcome: From Diagnostic to Therapeutic Colonoscopy. *Endoscopy* 41 (11):941–51.

Petrenko, A., and McArthur, D. 2009. Between Same-Sex Marriages and the Large Hadron Collider: Making Sense of the Precautionary Principle. *Science and Engineering Ethics* 16 (3):591–610.

PHSRG (Physician's Health Study Research Group). 1989. Final Report on the Aspirin Component of the Ongoing Physicians' Health Study. Steering Committee of the Physicians' Health Study Research Group. *New England Journal of Medicine* 321 (3):129–35.

Polichetti, G., Cocco, S., Spinali, A., Trimarco, V., and Nunziata, A. 2009. Effects of Particulate Matter (PM_{10}, $PM_{2.5}$ and PM_1) on the Cardiovascular System. *Toxicology* 261 (1–2):1–8.

Sack, K. 2009. Screening Debate Reveals Culture Clash in Medicine. *The New York Times*, November 20. Available at http://www.nytimes.com/2009/11/20/health/20assess.html?_r=1&ref=weekinreview, accessed June 13, 2011.

Sackett, D.L., Straus, S.E., Richardson, W.S., Rosenberg, W., and Haynes, R.B. 2000. *Evidence-Based Medicine: How to Practice and Teach EBM,* 2nd ed. Philadelphia PA: Churchill Livingstone.

Tu, J.V., Nardi, L., Fang, J., Liu, J., Khalid, L., and Johansen, H. 2009. National Trends in Rates of Death and Hospital Admissions Related to Acute Myocardial Infarction, Heart Failure and Stroke, 1994–2004. *CMAJ* 180 (14):E118–E125.

USPSTF (United States Preventive Services Task Force). 2009a. Available at http://www. ahrq.gov/CLINIC/uspstfix.htm#Recommendations, accessed June 13, 2011.

——. 2009b. *Screening for Breast Cancer,* Topic Page. Agency for Healthcare Research and Quality, Rockville, MD. Available at http://www.uspreventiveservicestaskforce. org/uspstf/uspsbrca.htm accessed June 13, 2011.

Weatherly, H., Drummond, M., Claxton, K., Cookson, R., Ferguson, B., Godfrey, C., Rice, N., Sculpher, M., and Sowden, A. 2009. Methods for Assessing the Public Health Effectiveness of Public Health Interventions: Key Challenges and Recommendations. *Health Policy* 93 (2):85–92.

Williams, B.A. 2010. Perils of Evidence-Based Medicine. *Perspectives in Biology and Medicine* 53 (1):106–20.

Wolbers, M., Koller, M.T., Witteman, J.C.M., and Steyerberg, E.W. 2009. Prognostic Models with Competing Risks: Methods and Application to Coronary Risk Prediction. *Epidemiology* 20 (4):555–61.

Wright, J. D., Hirsch, R., and Wang, C. Y. 2009. One-third of U.S adults embraced most heart healthy behaviors in 1999-2002. *NCHS Data Brief.* (17):1–8.

Zhou, W., Pool, V., Iskander, J.K., English-Bullard, R., Ball, R., Wise, R.P., Haber, P., Pless, R.P., Mootrey, G., Ellenberg, S.S., Braun, M.M., and Chen, R.T. 2003. Surveillance for Safety After Immunization: Vaccine Adverse Event Reporting System (VAERS)— United States, 1991–2001. *MMWR* 52 (1):1–24.

5

Prevention and the Science and Politics of Evidence

DIANA B. PETITTI, MD, MPH ■

In the past 15 to 20 years, the paradigm for using scientific evidence to inform policy has shifted from (1) a reliance on statements by experts based on their experience, to (2) the use of expert panels and processes that rely on the consensus of experts, to (3) the use of explicit methods that identify and synthesize evidence and map the results of this synthesis to recommendations that are called "evidence-based." The term "evidence-based" to describe recommendations, the use of a common collection of methods to create evidence-based recommendations, and attempts to use the evidence-based recommendations as input to policy have become accepted not only in medicine and health but in the social sciences, software engineering, criminal justice, and management science.

PREVENTION IN THE EVIDENCE-BASED SCIENCE MOVEMENT

Sackett et al. (1996) are credited with the definition of evidence-based medicine as "the conscientious, explicit and judicious use of current best evidence in making decisions about the care of individual patients." The roots of the evidence-based medicine movement go back much farther and are deeply rooted in prevention.

In the middle 1970s, the value of screening in general and the periodic health examination in particular was an issue of intense interest and controversy.

In Canada, England, and the United States, experts in epidemiology and medicine were at the center of writing and critical thinking on this topic. Leaders in what became recognized as the "evidence-based medicine" movement wrote extensively about screening, the periodic health examination, and evidence criteria to use in evaluating screening tests. Prominent among these leaders were Archie Cochrane (Cochrane et al. 1951; Wilson, Chamberlain, and Cochrane 1971; Cochrane 1971) and David Sackett (Sackett 1972, 1973, 1975a, 1975b; Sackett and Holland 1975).

The role of evidence-based recommendations in policy can be traced to the Canadian Task Force on the Periodic Health Examination (later named the Canadian Task Force on Preventive Health Care). This body was established in 1976 by the Deputy Ministers of Health of the 10 Canadian provinces to describe the preventability of various conditions and to provide guidance about what should be done at a periodic health examination. The Canadian Task Force spent the first 2 years after its establishment developing methods for weighing scientific evidence.[1] Its first report, published in 1979 (Canadian Task Force on the Periodic Health Examination 1979), contained a review of the scientific evidence for the preventability of 78 conditions and made what was then an unprecedented recommendation that undefined "annual check-ups" be replaced with age-specific "health protection packages" to be performed during medical visits made for other purposes.

What is now called the first United States Preventive Services Task Force (USPSTF) convened for the first time in 1984 under the direction of the United States Public Health Service. It patterned itself on the Canadian Task Force and adopted its methodology, with minimal modification, as the framework for its reviews of the evidence on clinical preventive services. The USPSTF issued its first report, "Guide to Clinical Preventive Services," in 1989 (United States Preventive Services Task Force 1989).

The second USPSTF did its work between 1990 and 1995. It used methods for identifying and reviewing evidence similar to those used for the 1988 guide. It developed a comprehensive set of recommendations on 200 preventive services, which were published in 1996 (United States Preventive Services Task Force 1996).

The third USPSTF was established in 1998 by the U.S. Congress as a standing committee under Title IX of the Public Health Service Act (42 USC 299-299c-7 as amended by Public Law 106-129). It was officially charged by Congress to "review the scientific evidence related to the effectiveness, appropriateness, and cost-effectiveness of clinical preventive services for the purpose of developing

1. Available at http://www.canadiantaskforce.ca/_archive/index.html, accessed January 26, 2011.

recommendations for the health care community, and updating previous clinical preventive recommendations."

The USPSTF has been at the forefront of the evidence-based movement in the United States. The work of the USPSTF and clinical prevention has been a focal point for developing standard methods and processes for making evidence-based recommendations. USPSTF recommendations have been pivotal to practice policy about clinical preventive services for primary care physicians.

Over the three decades during which the USPSTF has played this role, prevention has become more technologically based. Screening to detect disease early was done in the 1970s and 1980s using physical examination by a primary care physician, supplemented by simple x-rays and blood tests done with an autoanalyzer. Screening now includes endoscopic visualization done by specialists, computed tomography (CT) and magnetic resonance imaging (MRI) interpreted by radiologists, and tests done in highly sophisticated molecular genetics laboratories. Furthermore, primary prevention, which was mostly related to nutrition, exercise, smoking cessation, hypertension control, and stress management in the 1970s, now increasingly relies on medications, some quite expensive.

In the 1970s and 1980s most clinical prevention was done by primary care physicians. Now involved in prevention are radiologists, cardiologists, endocrinologists, vascular surgeons, and a panoply of nonphysician providers. Over the past three decades, the number of advocacy groups in all areas of health and medicine has increased dramatically. The public has become keenly interested in all things that touch on prevention.

These changes in the technical aspects of prevention, the professionals involved in prevention, and the number of groups and individuals who see themselves as stakeholders in prevention make prevention an increasingly high-stakes game economically, in terms of professional hegemony, and in the large public arena of politics. Recommendations about prevention, whether or not evidence-based, will be increasingly subject to attempts to bring political forces to bear because of these fundamental changes in science and delivery.

STATE OF THE SCIENCE OF EVIDENCE-BASED RECOMMENDATIONS: CONFRONTING THE CHALLENGES AND LIMITS OF "EVIDENCE-BASED"

Evidence-based recommendations strive for objectivity, minimization of bias, and consistency. Many people and groups have contributed to the development of the methods and approaches that are used to accomplish these aims.

Prominent among these are the Cochrane Collaboration, the Campbell Collaboration, the Agency for Healthcare Research and Quality's Effective Health Care Program,[2] and the Grading the Quality of Evidence and Strength of Recommendations (GRADE) working group (Atkins et al. 2004a, 2004b, 2005; Guyatt et al. 2006a, 2006b).

There is a growing field—the science of evidence—informed by a large body of published empirical studies. Considerable methodological work remains uncompleted, and many methodological challenges in making evidence-based recommendations remain unresolved (Teustch and Berger 2005; Helfand 2005).

For example, an especially critical step in making evidence-based recommendations is rating the quality of the individual studies that comprise the evidence. A 2002 comprehensive review identified 121 different approaches to rate the quality of evidence (West et al. 2002). The number of different' rating schemes in use may now be fewer, but agreement on this fundamental methodological issue is still not universal.

Equally important, the simplicity of the term "evidence-based" belies enormous complexity in the multistep process of making evidence-based recommendations. Evidence-based is much more than finding studies and evaluating their quality (Mulrow and Lohr 2001; Teutsch and Berger 2005). As done by USPSTF (and others), the process of making evidence-based recommendations involves five distinct steps. First is formulation of the question or questions to be addressed and delineation of the kinds of evidence to be considered. Second is identification and retrieval of the individual studies that comprise the evidence. Third is critical appraisal of the quality of the individual studies. Fourth is synthesis of the evidence across studies in order to arrive at a conclusion about the body of evidence as it pertains to the question(s) at hand. The fifth step is linkage of the conclusion about the body of evidence to a suggested action. All of these steps contain methodological challenges that make their results imperfect. Policies that flow from this process reach limits when the challenges have not yet been, or cannot be, overcome.

The entities that undertake to make evidence-based recommendations conduct their work based on a set of explicit methods and rules that are made publicly available.[3] The USPSTF attempts to publish these (Barton et al. 2007;

---

2. For further details see, respectively, http://www.cochrane.org/, http://www.campbell collaboration.org/ and http://effectivehealthcare.ahrq.gov/ehc/index.cfm/all, last accessed January 26, 2011.

3. See, for example, http://www.acponline.org/clinical_information/guidelines/process/ceap/ and http://www.ahrq.gov/clinic/uspstf08/methods/procmanual.htm, all accessed on January 26, 2011.

Sawaya et al. 2007; Petitti et al. 2009), as do others. There are past and continuing attempts to standardize methods across entities that provide input to policies that are meant to be evidence-based. But consensus is not complete (nor should it be) and there are inconsistencies in recommendations based on evidence even when made by well-motivated and honest reviewers using acceptable methods and processes.

Evidence-based recommendations, and the policies that flow from them, also suffer from the rapidity with which evidence changes. The fact is that with the involvement of human beings in the processes that turn evidence into recommendations being so complex, changes in the recommendations cannot be made as quickly as the evidence changes.

Finally, evidence-based recommendations are limited by the limitations of the evidence, which is almost never able to address all of the issues that arise when making policy. Almost all evidence-based recommendations rely on indirect evidence based on a chain of reasoning that brings together several distinct bodies of evidence. For example, four different randomized trials of screening for abdominal aortic aneurysm in men reported that screening decreases mortality due to aneurysm rupture in the populations recruited to the trials who had surgery in settings chosen for skill in aneurysm repair. Recommendations made for "real life" settings must consider surgical mortality rates *in the community* to assess whether there would be a net benefit in these settings. All evidence-based recommendations involve judgments and an element of subjectivity (Steinberg and Luce 2005).

A DOUBLE STANDARD FOR PREVENTION?

Why Standards Might Differ

A difference in the evidence standard for preventive services compared with treatment and diagnostic services might be fully justified from the perspective of the physician dealing one-on-one with a patient. A decision about whether to treat or pursue a diagnosis is required for every patient with a disease or a complaint suggesting illness. Prevention is offered to an asymptomatic person as a putative "extra" good. If a test or service existed but there was no evidence of net benefit, a decision not to offer the service is perfectly acceptable, as the patient is healthy and without complaint (Petitti et al. 2009).

From the societal perspective, evidence standards might justifiably differ between preventive services and treatment and diagnostic services because the number of people who would potentially receive a preventive service is often much larger than the number who would receive any particular treatment or diagnostic service. Thus, the societal cost implications of a recommendation to provide a preventive service are often large, even when the unit cost is relatively small. From the societal perspective, where money spent to achieve one good is not available to achieve another, it is reasonable to hold a service that consumes a large amount of goods to a high evidence standard. For something that affects a very large number of people, the implications of even a small probability of harm to an individual could be large on a population basis. Avoiding population harm might demand a higher evidence standard for certainty about the magnitude of any harm. Finally, as with physicians and individual patients, preventive services are provided on a policy basis with the intention of improving the health of the population as a whole. The standard for certainty of a net population benefit—that is, a favorable balance of benefits and harms overall for the population—might be justifiably higher for preventive services because the goal of prevention is a *population* goal.

Standards for Insurance Coverage

The Centers for Medicare and Medicaid Services (CMS) provides payment for more than 50% of all health care services in the United States. In 2010, and prior to passage of the Patient Care and Affordable Care Act of 2010 (PL 111-148), Medicare provided coverage for only 15 preventive services under highly specific conditions (Table 5.1).

This suggests, given the huge number of treatment and diagnostic services covered by Medicare, that the Medicare evidence standard for preventive services has historically been different than the standard for treatment and diagnostic services.

Medicare did not, however, provide coverage for outpatient prescription drugs until 2004. From an evidence perspective, the lack of Medicare coverage of prescription drugs until 2004 could not have been based on the application of any evidence standard. This would imply that there was no evidence to support coverage of any outpatient prescription drug for any condition. The fact that Medicare did not provide coverage of prescription drugs until 2004 illustrates starkly and sadly that Medicare coverage decisions have not historically been evidence-based.

As described by Faust in Chapter 6 of this volume, Medicare coverage of individual prevention modalities, such as vaccines for pneumonia and hepatitis and breast and cervical cancer screening, required individual acts of Congress. Medicare did not permit more comprehensive coverage of preventive services until January 2005.[4] With passage in 2008 of the Medicare Improvements for

---

4. Through the Medicare Modernization Act of 2003, effecting coverage on January 1, 2005.

Table 5.1. Preventive Services Covered for Medicare Beneficiaries
before Passage of the Patient Protection and Health Affordability Act

Preventive Services	Criteria
Abdominal aortic aneurysm screening	When done as based on referral from "Welcome to Medicare" visit in high-risk people: a family history of abdominal aortic aneurysm or men age 65 to 75 who have smoked at least 100 cigarettes in their lifetime
Bone mass measurement	At risk for osteoporosis with a definition of at risk that is broad
Cardiovascular screening: lipids	Every 5 years
Colorectal cancer screening	Age 50 and older
Diabetes screening	Up to twice a year in people at high risk: diabetes, history of abnormal cholesterol, obesity, or a history of high blood sugar
Flu immunization	Yearly in fall or winter
Glaucoma screening test	High risk: diabetes, family history of glaucoma, African American, and age 50 or older
Hepatitis B immunization	Medium or high risk once in a lifetime
Mammogram	Women age 40 and older. Also baseline at age 35–40
Medical nutrition therapy (counseling)	Diabetes or renal disease
Pap test and pelvic examination	All women
Physical examination	In conjunction with "Welcome to Medicare" visit done within 12 months of having Part B
Pneumococcal immunization	Once in a lifetime
Prostate cancer screening	Men age 50 and older
Smoking cessation	In people with smoking-related disease

http://www.medicare.gov/navigation/manage-your-health/preventive-services/preventive-service-overview.aspx.

Patients and Providers Act, the secretary of Health and Human Services was permitted (but not required) to provide Medicare coverage for preventive services that received an A or B grade by the USPSTF. As described in detail in Chapter 1 of this volume, the Patient Protection and Affordable Care Act of 2010 (PL 111-148, PPACA) redressed many of the preventive care exclusions that previously marked Medicare, Medicaid, and private insurance. Most important for this chapter, PPACA permits benefits coverage for "evidence-based items or services that have in effect a rating of 'A' or 'B' in the current recommendations of the United States Preventive Services Task Force and immunizations recommended by the Advisory Committee on Immunization

Practices." As pointed out in both Chapters 1 and 6 of this volume, no similar language defines a mandate for insurance coverage for treatment or diagnostic services, nor a requirement for review by a specific entity as a condition of coverage. For the purposes of insurance coverage, prevention is now clearly subject to a vastly different standard of evidence compared with treatment and diagnosis. Is this standard a higher standard or a lower standard? Is it justified, and is it good?

Many would argue that the USPSTF evidence standards for giving a service an "A" or "B" recommendation are extremely high. The Advisory Committee on Immunization Practices is regarded as making less evidence-based recommendations than the USPSTF, but appears to be attempting to evolve toward methods and standards that are like those of the USPSTF (Smith et al. 2009). The evidence standard for coverage of immunizations is thus also likely to become very high.

A higher evidence standard for coverage of prevention could be viewed negatively as a reflection of a lower value for preventive than for treatment services. The high evidence standard for prevention could also be viewed positively, prevention alone being grounded in rational and objective assessment of evidence as a precondition for using resources. It was possible for the Patient Protection and Affordable Care Act of 2010 to set a minimum coverage mandate for prevention with links to specific entities attempting to adhere to the principles of making evidence-based recommendations precisely because only for preventive services did entities with credible processes and products exist. In 2008, the Institute of Medicine (Institute of Medicine 2008), in its report "Knowing What Works in Health Care: A Roadmap for the Nation," called for the development of "a national clinical effectiveness program to facilitate the development of standards and processes that yield credible, unbiased, and understandable syntheses of the available evidence on clinical effectiveness" (Institute of Medicine 2008, 9) and for "providers, public and private payers, purchasers, performance measurement groups, patients, consumers, and others to preferentially use clinical recommendations developed according to these standards" (Institute of Medicine 2008, 13). Prevention, including clinical preventive services reviewed using the methods and processes of the USPSTF, and immunizations using reconfigured and evidence-based methods of the Advisory Committee on Immunizations Practices (ACIP) are likely to set the standards for use of evidence in policy.

Yes, the standard that is used for prevention is higher. But basing decisions and policy on best-evidence approaches is rational and forward thinking. Prevention should continue to embrace its role as the standard setter even if the standard is different.

MAMMOGRAPHY SCREENING RECOMMENDATIONS: THE RULE OR THE EXCEPTION?

What Happened in 2009

On November 17, 2009, the USPSTF recommendations on screening mammography were released in the *Annals of Internal Medicine* (United States Preventive Services Task Force 2009), accompanied by a summary of the evidence report (Nelson et al. 2009) and the findings from a set of mathematical models (Mandelblatt et al. 2009) that were used by the USPSTF to inform its recommendations. The recommendations were a routine update of recommendations on breast cancer screening that had last been reviewed in 2002.

There were two important changes in the mammography screening recommendations, one related to screening of women in their 40s and one related to screening interval. In 2002, the USPSTF recommended screening women age 40+ years every 1–2 years, which was a B grade recommendation, meaning moderate certainty of moderate benefit. In 2009, the USPSTF recommended biennial screening mammography between 50 and 74 years, which was a B grade recommendation. The USPSTF stated that the decision to start regular screening before the age of 50 should be an individual one and take into account patient context, including values regarding specific benefits and harms, which was a C grade recommendation.

The recommendations received instantaneous and massive attention from the print media, with front-page articles in the *New York Times*, the *Washington Post*, and *USA Today*, among others. They were the subject of broadcasts on National Public Radio, CNN, the McNeill Lehrer report, the NBC Today Show, and CBS Good Morning America. On December 2, 2009, the House Subcommittee on Health of the Energy and Commerce Committee (which oversees legislation related to health) held hearings at which the USPSTF Chair and Vice-Chair were subjected to several hours of hostile and unpleasant questions about the recommendations by members of the committee.

Is Mammography the Exception or the Rule? Is Prevention Different?

Details on the mammography recommendations and how they came to be released in the midst of hearing about health care reform were provided to the House subcommittee in the form of written testimony. An analysis of the mistakes made by the USPSTF and some of the implications about how it needs to work in the future is a topic addressed extensively by others (Woolf 2010;

DiAngelis and Fontanarosa 2010; Woloshin and Schwartz 2010; Thrall 2010; Barbour et al. 2010). Most commentators agree that the extraordinary amount of attention received by the mammography screening recommendations and the degree of vitriol in the attacks on the USPSTF were driven by the coincidence of the timing of the release with key votes on health reform legislation (Editors' note 2010). The mammography recommendations were a pawn in the much larger political game of health care reform. They were conveniently controversial. They spoke to the almost universal experience of adults in the United States as knowing someone with breast cancer or having or wanting to have a mammogram. They had a well-funded, vested interest group, the American College of Radiology, ready and willing to use the situation to take the stage to foster their self-interest.

In fact, the 2009 skirmish between politics and the evidence about mammography screening is not the first one for this topic. As described in detail by Fletcher (1997) and Woolf and Lawrence (1997), a 1997 National Cancer Institute consensus panel concluded, in a 10 2 vote, that evidence was insufficient to support routine mammography in women age 40–49 years. In a virtual repeat of the 2009 mammography affair involving the USPSTF, the topic of screening mammography was taken up by the media and became the subject of a special hearing, at that time in the Senate. In 1997, the National Cancer Institute eventually "repackaged" the evidence in response to the intense external attack and the recommendation was changed to state that women in their 40s should be screened routinely (Woolf and Lawrence 1997).

Mammography seems to be a particular lightning rod for politically motivated attacks on the evidence and on the bodies that describe the evidence. But mammography is not the only topic involving the application of evidence-based principles as the subject of politically motivated attack.

Deyo et al. (1997) and Gray, Gusmano, and Collins (2003) describe the mid-1990s attack by the North American Spine Society on the guidelines for acute care for back pain that were based on state of the science approaches to guideline development. In this case, an evidence-based review done by a highly credible independent group concluded that there was no evidence to support spinal fusion surgery and that the surgery often had complications. A behind-the-scenes effort was organized to lobby congressional representatives not just to repudiate the guidelines but also to terminate funding for the federal agency that had provided support for the guidelines.

Rosenstock and Lee (2002) give several other accounts from the 1990s in which evidence and evidence-based recommendations and policies came under severe attack involving a variety of tactics and strategies. Their case examples include attacks on evidence from many health fields. The common denominator for politicization of these topics identified by Rosenstock and Lee is the existence of vested interests, defined as those who "for whatever reason, are committed to a predetermined outcome independent of the evidence." Although financial interests are the most common reason for an interest being vested, Rosenstock and Lee emphasize that emotional and ideological interests are also important. When the evidence and the policy are not in alignment with the interests of vested interests, attack on the evidence and the policy appears to be unexceptional and in no way particular to prevention.

CONCLUSIONS AND RECOMMENDATIONS

Health policy must consider scientific evidence but also contextual evidence (Lomas et al. 2005; Tilburt 2008). Decision makers appropriately consider a broad array of information when making policies and recommendations for different settings (Steinberg and Luce 2005; Clancy and Cronin 2005; Atkins, Siegel, and Slutsky 2005; Lomas et al. 2005; Tilburt 2008). Policy cannot be made free of politics. Policy is evidence-informed, not evidence-determined.

Legitimate political influences on evidence-informed policy must, however, be distinguished from politicization that threatens to corrupt the evidence, the methods, or the process of making evidence-based recommendations. The common denominator in past instances of corrupt politicization of evidence, evidence-based recommendations, and evidence-based policies is the existence of groups with vested interests and entrenched positions. The goal in evidence for policy must be first and foremost to insulate the process of finding, synthesizing, and interpreting the evidence from the direct intrusion of vested self-interests. Evidence-based recommendations can and should be superseded in circumstances in which society, acting through the political process, places a high moral value on a strategy with a lesser evidence base. The ability of individuals to make informed choices that are not supported by evidence needs to be preserved.

To ensure a continued legitimate place in the policy process, the development of the field of making evidence-based recommendations must ensure that these recommendations are as objective, free of bias, and as consistent as they can be using methods and processes that are rigorously defined. Those doing the work of the science of evidence need to remain cognizant of the limitations of evidence and the challenges of being evidence-based.

With passage of the Patient Care and Affordable Care Act of 2010, insurance coverage for clinical preventive services will be tied to recommendations made by the USPSTF and those for vaccines to the recommendation of ACIP. These coverage policies, and related practice policies, may create, or may be perceived to create, winners and losers. Those who see themselves as losers can be expected to introduce more politics into the discussion about policy.

Recommendations about mammography screening are politicized as a rule and the extreme political nature of the debate about mammography screening appears to be a special case. Politicization is not limited to prevention.

Preventive services often have special features that might justify a higher evidence standard than for treatment and diagnosis. This needs to be recognized and accepted.

The field of prevention has been involved prominently in a leadership role in the evidence-based medicine movement. It has imposed on itself standards of evidence that are higher than those imposed in other fields. In doing this, the standards of evidence have been made high for prevention. Prevention needs to continue to lead the way in defining how to use evidence to inform rational policies that maximize the contributions of health and medicine to the health of the public.

REFERENCES

Atkins, D., Best, D., Briss, P.A., Eccles, M., Falck-Ytter, Y., Flottorp, S., Guyatt, G.H., Harour, R.T., Haugh, M.C., Henry, D., Hill, S., Jaeschke, R., Leng, G., Liberati, A., Magrini, N., Mason, J., Middleton, P., Mrukowicz, J., O"Connell, D., Oxman, A.D., Phillips, B., Schünemann, H.J., Edejer, T.T., Varonen, H., Vist, G.E., Williams, J.W., Jr., Zaza, S.; GRADE Working Group. 2004a. Grading Quality of Evidence and Strength of Recommendations. *British Medical Journal* 328 (7454):1490.

Atkins, D., Eccles, M., Flottorp, S., Guyatt, G.H., Henry, D., Hill, S., Liberati, A., O'Connell, D., Oxman, A.D., Phillips, B., Schünemann, H., Edejer, T.T., Vist, G.E., and Williams, J.W., Jr.; GRADE Working Group. 2004b. Systems for Grading the Quality of Evidence and the Strength of Recommendations I: Critical Appraisal of Existing Approaches. The GRADE Working Group. *BioMed Central Health Services Research* 4 (1):38.

Atkins, D., Briss, P.A., Eccles, M., Flottorp, S., Guyatt, G.H., Harbour, R.T., Hill, S., Jaeschke, R., Liberati, A., Magrini, N., Mason, J., O'Connell, D., Oxman, A.D., Phillips, B., Schünemann, H., Edejer, T.T., Vist, G.E., and Williams, J.W., Jr.; GRADE Working Group. 2005. Systems for Grading the Quality of Evidence and the Strength of Recommendations II: Pilot Study of a New System. *BioMed Central Health Services Research* 5 (1):25.

Atkins, D., Siegel, J., and Slutsky, J. 2005. Making Policy When the Evidence is in Dispute. *Health Affairs (Millwood)* 24 (1):102–13.

Barbour, V., Clark, J., Jones, S., Peiperl, L., Veitch, E., and Yamey, G. 2010. Science Must Be Responsible to Society, Not to Politics. *Public Library of Science Medicine* 7 (1):e1000222.

Barton, M.B., Miller, T., Wolff, T., Petitti, D., LeFevre, M., Sawaya, G., Yawn, B., Guirguis-Blake, J., Calonge, N., and Harris, R. 2007. How to Read the New Recommendation

Statement: Methods Update from the U.S. Preventive Services Task Force. *Annals of Internal Medicine* 147 (2):123–27.

Canadian Task Force on the Periodic Health Examination. 1979. The Periodic Health Examination. *Canadian Medical Association Journal* 121 (9):1193–254.

Clancy, C.M., and Cronin, K. 2005. Evidence-Based Decision Making: Global Evidence, Local Decisions. *Health Affairs (Millwood)* 24 (1):151–62.

Cochrane, A.L., Fletcher, C.M., Gilson, J.C., and Hugh-Jones, P. 1951. The Role of Periodic Examination in the Prevention of Coal Workers' Pneumoconiosis. *British Journal of Industrial Medicine* 8 (2):53–61.

Cochrane, A.L., and Holland, W.W. 1971. Validation of Screening Procedures. *British Medical Bulletin* 27 (1):3–8.

DeAngelis, C.D., and Fontanarosa, P.B. 2010. U.S. Preventive Services Task Force and Breast Cancer Screening. *Journal of the American Medical Association* 303 (2):172–73.

Deyo, R.A., Psaty, B.M., Simon, G., Wagner, E.H., and Omenn, G.S. 1997. The Messenger Under Attack—Intimidation of Researchers by Special-Interest Groups. *New England Journal of Medicine* 336 (16):1176–80.

Editors' note on the USPSTF Recommendation on Screening for Breast Cancer. 2010. *Annals of Internal Medicine* 152 (8):544.

Fletcher, S.W. 1997. Whither Scientific Deliberation in Health Policy Recommendations? Alice in the Wonderland of Breast-Cancer Screening. *New England Journal of Medicine* 336 (16):1180–83.

Gray, B.H., Gusmano, M.K., and Collins, S.R. 2003. AHCPR and the Changing Politics of Health Services Research. *Health Affairs (Millwood)* WebExclusives: W3–283–307.

Guyatt, G., Gutterman, D., Baumann, M.H., Addrizzo-Harris, D., Hylek, E.M., Phillips, B., Raskob, G., Lewis, S.Z., and Schünemann, H. 2006a. Grading Strength of Recommendations and Quality of Evidence in Clinical Guidelines: Report from an American College of Chest Physicians Task Force. *Chest* 129 (1):174–81.

Guyatt, G., Vist, G., Falck-Ytter, Y., Kunz, R., Magrini, N., and Schunemann, H. 2006b. An Emerging Consensus on Grading Recommendations. *American College of Physicians Journal Club* 144 (1):A8–9.

Helfand, M. 2005. Using Evidence Reports: Progress and Challenges in Evidence-Based Decision Making. *Health Affairs (Millwood)* 24 (1):123–27.

Institute of Medicine (IOM). 2008. *Knowing What Works in Health Care: A Roadmap for the Nation.* Washington, DC: The National Academies Press.

Lomas, J., Culyer, T., McCutcheon, C., McAuley, L., and Law, S. 2005. *Conceptualizing and Combining Evidence for Health System Guidance.* Ottawa, Canada: Canadian Health Services Research Foundation.

Mandelblatt, J.S., Cronin, K.A., Bailey, S., Berry, D.A., de Koning, H.J., Draisma, G., Huang, H., Lee, S.J., Munsell, M., Plevritis, S.K., Ravdin, P., Schechter, C.B., Sigal, B., Stoto, M.A., Stout, N.K., van Ravesteyn, N.T., Venier, J., Zelen, M., Feuer, E.J.; Breast Cancer Working Group of the Cancer Intervention and Surveillance Modeling Network. 2009. Effects of Mammography Screening under Different Screening Schedules: Model Estimates of Potential Benefits and Harms. *Annals of Internal Medicine* 151 (10):738–47.

Mulrow, C.D., and Lohr, K.N. 2001. Proof and Policy from Medical Research Evidence. *Journal of Health Politics, Policy and Law* 26 (2):249–66.

Nelson, H.D., Tyne, K., Naik, A., Bougatsos, C., Chan, B.K., and Humphrey, L.; U.S. Preventive Services Task Force. 2009. Screening for Breast Cancer: An Update for the U.S. Preventive Services Task Force. *Annals of Internal Medicine* 151 (10):727–37, W237–42.

Petitti, D.B., Teutsch, S.M., Barton, M.B., Sawaya, G.F., Ockene, J.K., and DeWitt, T.; U.S. Preventive Services Task Force. 2009. Update on the Methods of the U.S. Preventive Services Task Force: Insufficient Evidence. *Annals of Internal Medicine* 150 (3): 199–205.

Rosenstock, L., and Lee, L.J. 2002. Attacks on Science: The Risks to Evidence-Based Policy. *American Journal of Public Health* 92 (1):14–18.

Sackett, D.L. 1972. The Family Physician and the Periodic Health Examination. *Canadian Family* 18 (8):61–65.

———. 1973. The Usefulness of Laboratory Tests in Health-Screening Programs. 1973. *Clinical Chemistry* 19 (4):366–72.

———. 1975a. Laboratory Screening: A Critique. *Federation Proceedings* 34 (12): 2157–61.

———. 1975b. Screening for Early Detection of Disease: To What Purpose? *Bulletin of the New York Academy of Medicine* 51 (1):39–52.

Sackett, D.L., and Holland, W.W. 1975. Controversy in the Detection of Disease. *Lancet* 2 (7930):357–59.

Sackett, D.L., Rosenberg, W.M., Gray, J.A., Haynes, R.B., and Richardson, W.S. 1996. Evidence Based Medicine: What It Is and What It Isn't. *British Medical Journal* 312 (7023):71–72.

Sawaya, G.F., Guirguis-Blake, J., LeFevre, M., Harris, R., and Petitti, D.; U.S. Preventive Services Task Force. 2007. Update on the Methods of the U.S. Preventive Services Task Force: Estimating Certainty and Magnitude of Net Benefit. *Annals of Internal Medicine* 147 (12):871–75.

Smith, J.C., Snider, D.E., and Pickering, L.K.; Advisory Committee on Immunization Practices. 2009. Immunization Policy Development in the United States: The Role of the Advisory Committee on Immunization Practices. *Annals of Internal Medicine* 150 (1):45–49.

Steinberg, E.P., and Luce, B.R. 2005. Evidence Based? Caveat Emptor! *Health Affairs (Millwood)* 24 (1):80–92.

Teutsch, S.M., and Berger, M.L. 2005. Evidence Synthesis and Evidence-Based Decision Making: Related but Distinct Processes. *Medical Decision Making* 25 (5):487–89.

Thrall, J.H. 2010. U.S. Preventive Services Task Force Recommendations for Screening Mammography: Evidence-Based Medicine or the Death of Science? *Journal of the American College of Radiology* 7 (1):2–4.

Tilburt, J.C. 2008. Evidence-Based Medicine Beyond the Bedside: Keeping an Eye on Context. *Journal of Evaluation in Clinical Practice* 14 (5):721–25.

United States Preventive Services Task Force. 1989. *Guide to Clinical Preventive Services: An Assessment of the Effectiveness of 169 Interventions. Report of the U.S. Preventive Services Task Force.* Baltimore, MD: Williams & Wilkins.

————. 1996. *Guide to Clinical Preventive Services*. Baltimore, MD: Williams & Wilkins.

————. 2009. Screening for Breast Cancer: U.S. Preventive Services Task Force Recommendation Statement. *Annals of Internal Medicine* 151 (10):716–26, W-236.

West, S., King, V., Carey, T.S., Lohr, K.N., McCoy, N., Sutton, S.F., and Lux, L. 2002. *Systems to Rate the Strength of Scientific Evidence. Evidence Report/Technology Assessment No. 47*. Rockville, MD: Agency for Healthcare Research and Quality.

Wilson, M., Chamberlain, J., and Cochrane, A.L. 1971. Screening for Cervical Cancer. *Lancet* 1 (7693):297–98.

Woloshin, S., and Schwartz, L.M. 2010. The Benefits and Harms of Mammography Screening: Understanding the Trade-Offs. *Journal of the American Medical Association* 303 (2):164–65.

Woolf, S.H. 2010. The 2009 Breast Cancer Screening Recommendations of the US Preventive Services Task Force. *Journal of the American Medical Association* 303 (2):162–63.

Woolf, S.H., and Lawrence, R.S. 1997. Preserving Scientific Debate and Patient Choice: Lessons from the Consensus Panel on Mammography Screening. National Institutes of Health. *Journal of the American Medical Association* 278 (23):2105–8.

6

Historical Perspectives on Structural Barriers to Prevention

HALLEY S. FAUST, MD, MPH, MA ■

INTRODUCTION

In his 1980 seminal two-volume work *Explorations in Quality Assessment and Monitoring* Avedis Donabedian, the late pioneer of quality improvement in health care, described his conceptualization of health care systems as composed of structure, process, and outcome (Donabedian 1980a, 1980b). *Outcome* is the final product: morbidity and/or mortality from health care-related activities. For example, do we live longer, with less disability? *Process* is what happens in the health care system. Have we vaccinated 95% of children for measles? Have we determined cholesterol levels for the entire adult population? Many of the objectives of the "Healthy People" series from the Department of Health and Human Services have been process oriented. For example, because sun exposure is a precursor to melanoma cancers, as a way to reduce melanoma incidence and deaths *Healthy People 2010* had the following goal: "Increase the proportion of persons who use at least one of the following protective measures that may reduce the risk of skin cancer: avoid the sun between 10 a.m. and 4 p.m., wear sun-protective clothing when exposed to sunlight, use sunscreen with a sun-protective factor (SPF) of 15 or higher, and avoid artificial sources of ultraviolet light" (U.S. Department of Health and Human Services 2000).

The *structure* of health care systems is, generally, the physical component: how many hospitals and hospital beds are available in Albuquerque? Are there available and acceptable sunscreen options that can be purchased for a reasonable amount of money? Are funds available to permit adequate staffing for vaccination clinics?

This chapter presents an historical picture of such structural barriers to prevention services in the United States. A significant part of the structural barriers to prevention can be reduced to financing: the underfunding of public health and the historically limited insurance coverage to reimburse primary care clinicians for providing prevention services. Structural barriers can also be associated with nonfinancial resources; for example, it is questionable as to whether there are adequate medical personnel to handle mammography screening for breast cancer if the frequency of obtaining mammograms were followed (D'Orsi 2004). Similarly, as of 2005 gastroenterologists reported spending 50–80% of their practice time simply performing screening and diagnostic colonoscopies (Ransohoff 2005). But fully 42 million average-risk people aged 50 and older were not screened for colorectal cancer as of 2004. It could take up to 10 years to screen this unscreened population (Seef et al. 2004).

Other nonfinancial structural barriers to prevention are often inadvertent externalities:

- New high schools built on the periphery of towns and along busy roads without sidewalks force students to reduce physical activity because they have to use motor vehicle transportation instead of human-propelled bicycles or walking.
- Putting high fructose sugared fruit juices in vending machines in schools increases students' caloric intakes.
- Treaties with Native American Indian tribes permit untaxed cigarettes to be sold to the public over the internet from sovereign reservations at lower prices, encouraging higher cigarette consumption, particularly in lower socioeconomic groups (Townsend, Roderick, and Cooper 1994; Goolsbee, Lovenheim, and Slemrod 2010).
- In rural areas, or in urban areas with limited transportation (perhaps 20–25% of the U.S. population), there are physical access barriers that make it difficult to get to both health care and health-enhancing services such as physical trainers, nutritionists, or healthy food stores.[1]
- Having fewer fruit and vegetable markets, bakeries, specialty stores, and natural food stores in poorer and nonwhite neighborhoods reduces options for healthier food choices (Moore and Roux 2006).

---

1. Clinical preventive services generally are provided in two environments: primary care practices and public health departments. Some of this care is overlapping, such as with sexually transmitted disease and tuberculosis treatments.

Other market barriers also influence prevention practices in the United States. People eating at fast food restaurants consume more calories, saturated fat, and sugar-containing foods and fewer fruits and vegetables (Paeratakul et al. 2006). The takeover of big agriculture reduces our reliance on farm-fresh, local, more nutritious foods (Nestle 2002). Product placement of higher margin or higher total profitable goods influences consumer choice in grocery stores by placing these items at eye level (Weathington 2011). In recent years some jurisdictions have started addressing these practices through chain restaurant nutrition labeling laws and excise taxes on highly sugared drinks.[2]

Patient convenience and/or untimely physician–patient communications are also barriers to obtaining prevention services. Because most patient visits to primary care physicians are related to acute illnesses, these immediate concerns usually take precedence over future concerns (see Chapter 7 in this volume). Prevention needs of patients can therefore take a back seat to acute care by both patients and physicians; if prevention were better integrated into practices then more prevention services would be provided. To that end, although there is some controversy as to its efficacy, patient and physician reminders have been shown to enhance the uptake of prevention services by patients (Dubey et al. 2006). Timely reminders and "nudges" can increase the relative importance and priority for patients as well. Coordinated availability of prevention services of care delivery teams in one location organized around the chronic care model also enhances improvement of health risk behaviors (Hung et al. 2007). Newer technologies such as WiFi scales and integrated websites to maintain prevention data for individual patients that can be pushed to physicians for regular review and feedback may provide virtual integrated communication and practice models for the future.[3]

Although these nonfinancial issues, as well as environmental pollution concerns, are important, the core questions of this section of this volume are economic: why is so much more spent on treatment rather than prevention,

2. As of November 2009 three jurisdictions—King County, WA; New York City, NY; and Westchester County, NY—had implemented menu-labeling policies. Similarly, at least another 11 jurisdictions had passed such legislation and another 13 had had legislation introduced in 2009. Information is from the Center for Science in the Public Interest available at http://cspinet.org/new/pdf/ml_map.pdf, accessed January 6, 2011. The Patient Protection and Accountable Care Act (PPACA) mandates chain restaurant nutrition labeling (Section 4205), which will supersede state or local laws.

3. Thanks to Kevin Patrick for suggesting this issue of wireless push technologies. For an example of some of the possibilities, see the University of California at San Diego's CitiSense program for environmental monitoring (Kane 2009). The new West Wireless Health Institute was established at Scripps Health with Qualcomm for the purpose of "advancing health and well being through the use of wireless technologies" (Tikka 2009).

and what would be a defensible, optimal balance? The core of these questions is focused on payment through the traditional medical system. Miller et al. in Chapter 2 of this volume primarily use data from the National Health Expenditure Accounts showing that of 8.7% of total annual expenditures on health care in the United States in 2007, fully 61% or $120 billion is for direct medical and dental clinical services. This figure is up from 56% in 1996, and though their data do not provide information from before 1996, I would suspect that the relative share of *clinical* prevention expenditures prior to 1996 was an even smaller percentage of total prevention expenditures because many health insurance plans did not cover prevention services until recently.

I also suspect that because of the deep recession starting in 2008, the relative financial contribution to total U.S. health expenditures of public health services was lower in 2010 than in 2007, the last year of the Miller et al. data. State prevention and public health programs are often quickly cut under budget crunches, yet total health care expenditures continue to go up during recessions.[4] According to the National Association of County and City Health Officials, the 2008 recession caused local health department budget cuts resulting in 27,000 cut public health jobs in 2008–2009. On a base of 155,000 jobs nationwide, 17.4% of local public health positions were lost,[5] resulting in reduced services in public health programs "such as maternal and child health, environmental health, and emergency preparedness" (National Association of County and City Health Officials 2010). The neglect of our public health infrastructure likely results in higher costs for future private and public medical expenditures (Ormond et al. 2011).

The balance of this chapter will concentrate on the history of prevention benefits coverage by health insurance, including the lack of benefits coverage, lack of mechanisms to bill for reimbursement, problems with legislation that

4. From data from 1960–2006; whereas U.S. national health expenditures (NHE) as a percentage of the gross domestic product (GDP) have occasionally flattened or dipped during recession years, total inflation-adjusted expenditures have not—there has been consistent inflation-adjusted percentage growth in NHE during these 45 years, with rates fluctuating from approximately 3.5% in 1995 to as high as close to 10% in 1965. During recession years when there was real negative GDP growth (1974–1975, 1980, 1982, and 1991) NHE was always above positive 3% (Baker 2008).

5. The 155,000 total employed local public health workers figure from 2007 was provided to me by the National Association of County and City Health Officials executive Director, Robert Pestronk, in a personal e-mail on January 14, 2010. His additional comments state the following: "I'm expecting the losses for 2010 to be at least equal to 2008. Across the U.S., the recession has disturbed local, state, and federal government revenues, and therefore local health department budgets and programming, in asynchronous waves. Differences in fiscal years among governmental jurisdictions also prompt recognition, alarm, and action at different points during the year."

prohibited or did not foresee the value of prevention, and personal and health care barriers to obtaining care. At the end I will offer three suggestions for reducing these and other barriers to providing prevention services.

PREVENTION AND THE GROWTH OF INSURANCE COVERAGE

At the time of the establishment of the first European national health insurance programs little was known about how clinical preventive services could help an individual lower risk for, or prevent, disease. Besides the use of the smallpox vaccine, nearly all advances in the health of populations were due to public health measures such as proper human waste disposal, drinking from pure water sources, enhanced availability of food sources, and improved garbage disposal. Clinical preventive efforts were the same as those mentioned in the writings of Hippocrates: diet, exercise, and correct rest "designed to keep the delicate system in balance." In addition to its medical tone, eating, exercising, and resting well had a moral tone (Martin and Howell 1989).

The first nationalized, compulsory health insurance plans were established in Europe for two primary reasons: (1) to provide income replacement and (2) to provide medical care for victims of accidents or illness (Thomasson 2002). These were part of more generalized social insurance reforms for income stabilization in the event of disability, old age, or unemployment.[6] It was an instance of the state taking over from what otherwise were charitable enterprises that couldn't keep up in the increasing industrialization movement (Starr 1982). In some cases it was also for political reasons, such as Germany's Otto von Bismarck using social rights to help him maintain the allegiance of the German population and unify the new German republic (Reid 2009).

At the same time, concepts of disease were changing—the germ theory took hold and individual prevention efforts by clinical physicians started making headway. There was increasing reliance on laboratory and other diagnostic tests related to infectious diseases: the Wasserman test for syphilis, the tine test for tuberculosis, and chest x-rays for both tuberculosis and other lung-related early detections were added to the physicians' armamentarium. As Martin and Howell point out (1989), in 1922 the American Medical Association adopted a

---

6. Germany had the first system developed in 1883. Between 1888 and 1913 Austria, Hungary, Norway, Serbia, Britain, Russia, and the Netherlands also developed nationalized systems. Contrary to popular thinking, Canada and the United Kingdom were not the first or earliest nationalized systems, coming into legislative existence only in 1961 and 1948, respectively (Reid 2009).

resolution endorsing the concept of a periodic health examination for seemingly healthy people who might have asymptomatic disease that could be mitigated by early intervention. The recommendation was for an annual history, physical examination, and specific laboratory studies. However, this wasn't widely adopted by the American public because "[i]t was difficult to convince people...that they actually needed medical care." Politically, after World War I, physicians turned against the annual physical because it too closely resembled the kind of socialistic medicine adopted by Germany (Martin and Howell 1989).

In its individualistic, manifest destiny character, the United States took a different turn. Instead of developing a compulsory nationalized system to develop sickness insurance it relied on the free market. The first plans were for coverage of hospital stays; hence the initiation of the Blue Cross plans by hospitals.[7] The only plans that attempted to incorporate prevention in the early years were those established to keep workers healthy and on the job for difficult construction projects, such as the program started by Sidney Garfield for workers at the Grand Coulee Dam in 1938. Henry J. Kaiser then extended this program to his shipyards and steel mills on the west coast during World War II (Starr 1982).

The medical care system before the 1920s was very low technology, low cost, and not well regarded by the public. In 1850, life expectancy at birth was only about 40 years, and in 1900 it was only about 50 years. There was less worry about developing a chronic disease such as heart disease or cancer than about developing infection-related ailments or significant disabilities due to accidents or occupational exposures. In Britain, chronic bronchitis was considered to be "normal" during the reign of Elizabeth I (Freymann 1975). Rather than worrying about preventing disease per se, the greater perceived threat was income loss due to accidents or the sequelae of infectious illnesses. Visiting the physician to prevent disease did not start until the 1890s, when well-baby checks were initiated by an obstetrician in Paris, and in 1908 in Britain. The United States saw its first prenatal care program at the Boston Lying-In Hospital in 1912. Prenatal care wasn't done in private physician offices, but in welfare and factory clinics (Freymann 1975). Much of prevention was related to screening for venereal diseases and treating tuberculosis in public health clinics. Most physicians considered prevention too dull and routine to want to be involved.

---

7. The first Blue Cross-like plan was established in 1929 by Baylor University Hospital in Dallas. It provided the 1500 school teachers of the county with up to 21 days of hospital coverage. The cost was $6 per year. Although the voluntary hospital plans were slowly increasing, so, too, were private insurance plans by for-profit entities. Blue Shield (physician-established) plans began in 1939 in California (see Starr 1982, 295–334).

In the early days of the twentieth century there were few health insurance policies available because insurance companies did not consider health events to be normal insurable events: "(1) definite and measurable, (2) unexpected and uncontrolled, and (3) widely disbursed and not subject to catastrophic loss" (Thomasson 2002). There was no widespread knowledge of morbidity and mortality data or costs of services. This started changing in the late 1920s, but still *prevention* services were not considered an integral part of most insurance plans for two primary reasons: (1) a lack of appreciation for the value of prevention in individual clinical services, and (2) the predictability of prevention services—they could be budgeted—they were not unexpected catastrophic events for which insurance was designed. Periodic health examinations were touted by life insurance companies, medical societies, health departments, and voluntary health agencies, but not by health insurers or individual physicians, who believed that they were low yield and unnecessary (Rosen 1976). The recognition of the value of keeping a workforce healthy became more apparent when 25% of the second million men drafted for World War I were rejected for military service based on physical examinations and medical histories (Jolissaint et al. 2006).

In the early 1900s and even until the 1970s there was an underappreciation of the value of clinical preventive services. As Freymann (1975) observed, even when there is an appreciation for prevention in relationship to a community's future, the launching of public health programs requires three things: (1) a sufficient knowledge base through epidemiology and demography, (2) an effective method of administering services, and (3) personnel resources trained and qualified for the task. In the early 1900s only immunizations and nutrition were reasonably well accepted by the population at large. Immunizations available before 1930 included smallpox, rabies, plague, cholera, typhoid, diphtheria, pertussis, tuberculosis (BCG), and tetanus (Loughlin and Strathdee 2007), and only smallpox, diphtheria, pertussis, and tetanus were given routinely. Nutrition was primarily appreciated as preventing malnourishment or undernourishment due to micronutrient deficiencies (vitamin and mineral deficiencies), not the excesses like obesity that we counsel against today. Although smoking as a health hazard was identified as an "evil practice" and an addiction going back centuries, the strong epidemiological evidence of its nefarious health effects was not established until the 1950s (Sullum 1998). Once the concept of nutrition and physical activity counseling for future prevention of disease was lost in the 1920s and 1930s, it did not reemerge as a standard part of primary care practice until the mid-1970s.[8] Screening for cancer ("Fight Cancer with a

---

8. Though it may be that the use of nutrition as a preventative came back sooner than physical activity, which, aside from Ken Cooper's "Aerobics" boost, did not become substantially

Checkup and a Check") was the American Cancer Society's slogan beginning in the mid-1950s. The checkup involved a periodic chest x-ray and a routine physical examination, both of which have subsequently been shown to be of little value in the early (presymptomatic) detection of cancer.

Not only are data needed to support the cause and effect of modifiable risk factors for disease, but also studies are needed to show that eliminating the epidemiologically determined cause can indeed reduce the disease effects. For example, we may know that high cholesterol can predict higher rates of cardiovascular diseases, but we may not know if lowering cholesterol can actually reduce the incidence or mortality for those diseases.

Studies to determine cause and effect often take a long time, require large numbers of participants, are expensive and difficult logistically to manage, and can have conflicting results depending on the methods of analysis. Thus it is not uncommon for the public to be cynical of announcements of new "causes" of disease (cyclamates and cancer in 1969), revised schedules for screening (mammography screening in women under 50 years of age and the U.S. Preventive Services Task Force in 2009; see Petitti's chapter in this volume), or concerns about overuse of desirable common foods, such as alcohol (yet a drink a day, and especially certain red wines, may be good for us). Sometimes the public is confused about what to do, such as when different bodies have different recommendations for cancer screening. When the public is confused the default position often is "Do nothing" (Taubes 1995; Thaler and Sunstein 2009).

Clinical preventive services generally are provided in two environments: primary care practices and public health departments. Some of this care is overlapping, such as with sexually transmitted disease and tuberculosis detection and treatment. The public has not been particularly confident that their main source of primary medical care is proficient in preventive medicine. It is not uncommon to hear in normal social discourse that physicians are either not well schooled in preventive medicine or they do not care to emphasize it in their practices. Though primary care physicians (family practitioners, general internists, and pediatricians) are schooled in providing some primary care preventive services, board-certified preventive medicine physicians are the only residency trained doctors in both population medicine (e.g., public health/ insurance/occupational) and clinical medicine. Yet historical funding for residency programs in preventive medicine has been poor to nonexistent from the federal government. In the past 20 years, residency programs have been only one-third filled because of lack of funding. With the exception of pediatric residency training programs, which have their own reliable source of federal

part of primary care until the early 1990s. Thanks to Kevin Patrick for pointing this out to me.

funding separate from Medicare, preventive medicine residencies are the only ones not paid for through Medicare graduate medical education funds. Thus, not surprisingly, there has been a significant deficit of such physicians in the United States for many years. Recently the Institute of Medicine (IOM 2007) determined that the deficit is close to 10,000 physicians in public health and preventive medicine careers. The IOM called for funding for an additional 400 residents per year, a number that likely would need to be increased given the IOM's goal of doubling the number of preventive medicine-trained physicians over the next few years.[9] This deficit of 50% of the need for preventive medicine physicians is greater than any other medical specialty.[10]

BARRIERS TO PREVENTION COVERAGE BY HEALTH INSURERS

Some of the barriers to prevention coverage in health insurance were mentioned above: lack of interest and training by physicians, the nature of insurance related to catastrophic coverage, the predictability of health maintenance, the confusion concerning what is important and what works in prevention, and the sense that most prevention historically was dealt with through nonclinical administrative entities of public health and sanitation: water, sewage, milk, food, insect/rodent control, quarantine, etc.

There was also a problem with employee or insured turnover: if an employer/insurer encourages prevention benefits, and the employee is likely to move to another employer/insurer within 3–5 years (and in any case move into Medicare at 65 for the most expensive years, where prior prevention arguably makes the largest difference), no likely benefit of prevention-related savings in future medical claims would accrue to the particular employer or insurer.[11] Furthermore, the notion of assessing risk for disease and dealing with risk factors, although prominent in life and disability insurance underwriting, was not

9. The IOM report (2007) also recognizes the need to replace 1350 public health physicians annually in addition to doubling the current number; 400 additional residency slots would not accomplish this need.

10. Manpower needs by specialty have not been estimated for many years, but a 2002 article in *Health Affairs* projects a total physician deficit of 20% of projected demand, or approximately 200,000 physicians by 2020 (Cooper et al. 2002). This may be an underestimate given the added demand for prevention services from the Patient Protection and Accountable Care Act of 2010 (see Chapter 1 of this volume).

11. Although gains in externalities such as reduced absenteeism and increased productivity were possible. See the discussion of worksite programs below.

well-developed in health insurance. Additionally, much of clinical preventive services recommendations were for singular services such as breast cancer screening or hypertension and cholesterol screening. Criteria were variable for assessing the evidence-based effectiveness of screening and counseling for prevention. Recommendations were often tainted by conflicts of interest of specialty societies, or conflicts of commitment by advocacy groups.

Often physicians did not know which prevention interventions were of greater priority for any individual patient. Assistance with this issue occurred with the release of Lewis Robbins' and Jack Hall's 1970 text "How to Practice Prospective Medicine," which helped correct this problem. Robbins' manual ushered in the era of chronic disease risk assessment by giving clinicians a tool for appraising individual patients' health risks through a health risk assessment (HRA). This initial approach was very labor intensive until in the late 1970s the U.S. Centers for Disease Control and Prevention released its computerized HRA version, and subsequently a number of HRAs were developed by private and academic entities.[12] To alleviate the conflicts of specialty societies and advocacy groups a scientific and independent approach to determining what maneuvers were useful and effective in clinical preventive services was finally established with the U.S. Preventive Services Task Force (USPSTF), whose first publication was in 1989.[13]

Another problem with the adoption of prevention interventions by health insurers was their skepticism about the effectiveness of prevention interventions when done as individual clinical services in primary care settings. For a long time the dogma was that if a primary care physician can get 5% of his patients who smoke to quit after 1 year of effort that was good, but not very cost effective.[14] Fraud in insurance billing was well known.[15] And insurers had bad experiences with mental health providers and other counselors who were overtreating patients for psychologically related problems such as smoking cessation or eating patterns by (1) billing for maximum benefits for all their patients, and (2) using unproven counseling methods. All of these things had insurers

12. Lew Robbins was a founder of the Society of Prospective Medicine, established in 1974 to promote the use of HRAs in the United States and Canada.

13. The second edition was released in 1996. Now all recommendations are released electronically and are available at http://www.uspreventiveservicestaskforce.org/, accessed June 5, 2011.

14. As an example of results from the 1980s, see Thompson et al. (1988).

15. Insurer fraud units went after large frauds, whereas smaller ones were sometimes detected through individual medical review of cases. Wynia (2000) documented how physicians often manipulate reimbursement rules through up-coding, purposefully inaccurately coding, or unbundling services either to increase their own reimbursement or to assist patients in obtaining reimbursement for otherwise uncovered services.

concerned that if there were coverage for prevention counseling interventions such as nutrition, physical activity, and smoking cessation there would be more fraudulent practices by practitioners.

Once the USPSTF elaborated its first report on what works and therefore is recommended in prevention assessment, at least one insurer, Aetna Life and Casualty, developed a rider for preventive medicine services and counseling based on the USPSTF recommendations. Aetna tried to limit the counseling and reimbursement abuse issues by using a typical indemnity approach: specifying the number of counseling visits and maximum payments for visit per defined services. Before Aetna's activities, prevention services were irregularly covered, depending on how employers requested such coverage and depending on mandated benefits coverage by individual states.[16]

Another structural barrier existed: there were no recognized codes for physicians to bill insurers for prevention services. The Current Procedural Terminology (CPT) codes are established by the American Medical Association and are the basis of billing by physicians. Prior to the late 1980s the only prevention-related CPT codes available were associated with history and physical examinations, immunizations, and newborn/infant care. Counseling codes were for individual psychiatric counseling but not for individual nutrition or tobacco cessation counseling, for example. Most likely this lack of codes was a lack of lobbying for such codes by interested physician groups. To correct this, in 1987 the American College of Preventive Medicine (ACPM) established its Policy Committee with an initial objective of tackling prevention reimbursement. Working within the medical political structure the ACPM Policy Committee chairman was appointed to the AMA's CPT committee to concentrate on the process of getting more CPT codes directly relevant to prevention activities by practitioners. In 1990 there were only a handful of CPT codes that might be used (Davis et al. 1990). Today there are many more codes encompassing nearly all of the possible prevention activities done clinically (Parkinson and Lurie 1996; National Business Group on Health 2010).

FROM CPT CODES TO BENEFITS COVERAGE

The presence of CPT codes does not guarantee benefits *coverage* under insurance plans, but at least the presence of the codes removed one more barrier to reimbursement.

---

16. The first mandated state coverage requirements were primarily for breast and cervical cancer screening. The author chaired the working group at Aetna that put this rider together. Notably in the first 2 years of availability only one employer group purchased the coverage, i.e., the market demand was not high.

Larger employers increasingly have recognized the value of prevention benefits coverage. In 2007 most large employers offered "full coverage" for preventive care, and even 100% preventive services coverage with no deductible, including vaccinations, examinations, and screening for the early diagnosis of breast, colon, and cervical cancer. Additionally, 46% of employers surveyed by Watson Wyatt offered economic incentives for employees to participate in wellness and fitness programs, and they were expecting this number to increase to 72% in 2008 (Emerman and Arnoff 2009). The primary motive for such broad coverage seems to be that employers expect a financial return from these offerings, even though many of them do not cover the lifestyle modification items that would have the largest impact on costs. For example, Bondi et al. (2006) found that among employers there was a large discrepancy between coverage of tobacco cessation and alcohol prevention programs and their potential impact and value on health insurance costs.

Nearly all large U.S. employers are self-insured under the federally authorized Employee Retirement Income Security Act (ERISA), which permits employers to determine benefits covered under their plans and exempts those plans from state law. Smaller employers do not have the same flexibility to determine benefits coverage. The survey of employers done by Mercer and reported on by Bondi et al. (2006) showed that small and medium-sized employers much less frequently covered preventive services: they required coverage of one or more clinical preventive services only 17% and 30% of the time, respectively, and they negotiated or requested additional coverage only 8% and 12% of the time. Table 6.1 shows coverage by employer size for select preventive services as reported by Bondi et al.[17]

Health insurance companies that take full premium risk on policies that are not ERISA-based are regulated primarily by state insurance commissioners. These (mostly) politically appointed people must also work with their political constituencies to deal with the pressures that come to bear from special interest groups, which may exert their influences directly on the insurance commissions, or through state legislatures. The inclusion of preventive services for coverage in insured accounts has slowly been increasing over the years. Most recently the Council for Affordable Health Insurance (Bunce and Wieske 2010) tabulated the states that have mandatory benefits coverage in certain areas, including 14 benefits that are substantively primary or secondary prevention. Table 6.2 shows these benefits and the number of states that mandate them.

Though there are no effective ways to screen for ovarian cancer, one state, Georgia, requires it as well. It is easy to note how different political concerns

17. An original sample of 12,176 extant employers yielded 8956 that offered health benefits. Of the 8956, the numbers in the table are based on 2180 employers that responded to the survey (21% survey response overall).

Table 6.1. PREVENTIVE SERVICES PERCENT COVERAGE BY NUMBER OF EMPLOYEES, 2004 (BUNCE AND WIESKE 2004)

Preventive Service	Percent Coverage by Employer Size (Number of Employees)		
	Small (10–99)	Medium (200–999)	Large (1000+)
Physical examination	81	84	85
Childhood vaccines*	79	88	94
Cholesterol screen*	62	68	77
Chlamydia screen*	39	46	54
Breast cancer screen*	88	91	95
Colorectal cancer screen*	73	78	79
Nutrition counseling*	19	27	21
Weight loss management	17	21	18
Physical activity counseling*	14	23	11
Alcohol problem prevention	21	22	19

*$p < 0.01$ by chi square with two degrees of freedom.

have mandated these: mammography screening is the only prevention mandated in all 50 states. Indeed, no other mandate—prevention or treatment—is established in all 50 states other than mammography. Also of note is a lack of a mandate for tobacco, nutrition, or physical activity counseling, even though tobacco use and obesity/lack of physical activity are two of our nation's largest health problems.

Similarly, prepaid health plans or health maintenance organizations (HMOs) have emphasized prevention benefits coverage for many years. The original

Table 6.2. PREVENTION-RELATED MANDATED BENEFITS IN THE UNITED STATES BY NUMBER OF STATES, 2004

Medical Insurance Required Coverage	Number of States in 2004
Blood lead level screening	6
Cervical cancer screening	26
Chlamydia screening	3
Colorectal cancer screening	21
Contraceptives	29
Diabetes management	22
In vitro fertilization	15
Mammography	50
Maternity	21
Newborn hearing screening	13
Newborn sickle cell screening	2
Phenylketonuria (PKU)	33
Prostate cancer screening	34
Well-child care	31

Nixon 1973 HMO legislation stipulated that to become federally qualified (giving the HMO certain rights and privileges related to employer mandates) certain minimum benefits coverage was required, including (Dorsey 1975):

> (H) preventive health services (including voluntary family planning services, infertility services, preventive dental care for children, and children's eye examinations conducted to determine the need for vision correction).

These requirements were modified over the years, including the removal of dental benefits requirements in 1976 under President Ford. Obviously the looseness of the language left a lot of discretion concerning which benefits to provide by HMOs. As a medical director and general manager of an HMO in the early 1980s (and later regional medical director for about 15 HMOs in the eastern United States), I recall many conversations and memos in which we debated the pros and cons of including different prevention services in standardized benefits packages. Once the U.S. Preventive Services Task Force was established and published its recommendations in 1989, this debate became somewhat easier. At the same time, we had to react to the public's mood and employers' requests based upon political influences. For example, one significant debate occurred on whether we should spend scarce financial resources on covering mammography screening or tobacco cessation programs. The latter would have a greater long-term disease prevention result, whereas the former had a more forceful voice demanding coverage by women's groups.[18]

To their credit, HMOs were in the forefront of attempting to establish performance-based quality criteria for accreditation through the National Committee for Quality Assurance (NCQA). NCQA established the Healthcare Effectiveness Data and Information Set (HEDIS), which, from its inception, used preventive services delivery as some of its quality criteria. As of 2010 the HEDIS measures were very strong on preventive services, and apply to commercial, Medicaid, and Medicare accreditation of health plans.[19]

WORKSITE HEALTH PROMOTION

Medical benefits through health insurance policies are not the only way employees obtain prevention services. Many employers provide worksite health

---

18. This debate had different emphases and political conclusions depending on whether it was being held in tobacco-producing states such as Kentucky or North Carolina, or tobacco-consuming states such as Pennsylvania or Indiana (See also Rothman 2011).

19. See http://www.ncqa.org/Portals/0/HEDISQM/HEDIS2010/2010_Measures.pdf, accessed June 5, 2011, for the "HEDIS 2010 Summary Table of Measures, Product Lines and Changes." The first one and one-half pages are prevention criteria.

promotion programs (WHP) of variable types and emphasis. Some of these programs provide comprehensive risk factor identification and reduction programs such as nutrition and physical activity counseling, stress management, tobacco use cessation, and hypertension control. Others are more limited, or simply provide discounts at local health spas. As Goetzel and Ozminkowski (2008) state, "At their core, WHP programs support primary, secondary, and tertiary prevention efforts." They cite a 1999 survey by the Federal Office of Disease Prevention and Health Promotion showing that "90% of work sites offered workers at least one type of health-promotion activity."

However, some employers do not offer these programs because of ethical considerations for the privacy of their workers or because they are opposed to workplace paternalism. Others think that WHP programs are luxuries, or are not central to the organization's mission, or may distract workers from their duties. Other employers may try to develop programs and find a lack of attendance, or labor union objections (Goetzel and Ozminkowski 2008). Sometimes it is the workers who refuse to participate in worksite health promotion programs out of fear of divulging personal information to their employers. Finally, the case for a positive return on investment (ROI) is complex, and could take years until the ROI is attained with perhaps a workforce that has high turnover. One example is the Go To Health project at Blue Cross and Blue Shield of Michigan in the early 1980s that looked at ROI. This randomized trial found that the costs and benefits were essentially equal. The two large issues that factored into the equation were future pension liabilities and productivity. Participants in the full health promotion program gained an actuarially determined 1.2 additional years of life because of their reduced risk factors. At the same time the trial found that those in the full participation arm statistically significantly increased productivity by ~14% the first year, which would have outweighed the pension liability 10-fold. Unfortunately, because of personnel dropouts related to the recession at the time, the productivity increase for the second year of the study, although maintained in magnitude, was not statistically significant. The modeled breakeven point for productivity versus pension costs was an increase in productivity of <1% (Faust 1983).

More recently many studies have found program effectiveness on par with other investment returns. This was recently reaffirmed in 2010 by the Task Force on Community Preventive Services (2010). There was particularly strong evidence for the effectiveness of tobacco and alcohol use reduction, dietary fat consumption reduction, improved blood pressure control, lower total serum cholesterol levels, increased physical activity counseling, increased seat belt use through health education programs, and reduced days of absenteeism due to illness. At the same time there was insufficient evidence to show improvements in dietary intake of fruits and vegetables, reduced overweight/obesity, or improved physical activity levels (Soler et al. 2010).

In summary, we have seen how the establishment of CPT codes, increased coverage for primary and secondary preventive services through private health insurers, the emphasis of prevention in HMOs, and the increasing provision of worksite health promotion programs have improved the availability of preventive services. At the same time, countervailing this trend is the reduction in services provided by public health departments because of reduced budgets and personnel nationwide.

MEDICARE

As noted by Petitti in Chapter 5 of this volume, the authorizing legislation of Medicare in 1965 was specifically for the *diagnosis and treatment* of disease; there were no provisions for covering prevention. It wasn't until 1981 that the first authorized preventive service was covered by a specific act of Congress; PL 96-611 permitted coverage for pneumococcal vaccination. This was followed by coverage for hepatitis B vaccine (1984), mammography (1988, repealed in 1989 and later reinstated), and Pap smears (1989). As an example of the difficulty of permitting preventive services coverage, because prevention was not included in the original authorizing legislation in 1965 each of these preventive services—pneumococcal vaccine, mammography, and Pap smears—required an act of Congress. Indeed, in 1985 the Omnibus Budget Reconciliation Act (OBRA) mandated that the financing arm of Medicare develop demonstration projects "to assess health outcomes and costs associated with the provision of preventive services to Medicare beneficiaries" (Davis et al. 1990). This was the first time the congress required justification of inclusion of benefits based on cost—a good step forward for all interventions, but one that, notably, was (and is) not required for treatment services.

From 1985 until 2003 mammography, Pap smears, hepatitis vaccine, diabetes management, colorectal screening, medically related nutritional counseling, bone mass density, and glaucoma screening were added one by one. Then in 2003 the congress passed the Medicare Modernization Act (MMA), which authorized coverage for certain preventive services, and in 2008 with the Medicare Improvements for Patients and Providers Act (MIPPA) prevention was based specifically upon U.S. Preventive Services Task Force A or B recommendations. As a result of MMA and MIPPA, Medicare expanded its preventive services coverage to include a one-time initial preventive physical examination (IPPE or "Welcome to Medicare" exam), cardiovascular risk factor screening (blood pressure, cholesterol, high-density lipoprotein, triglycerides), and diabetes screening (fasting blood sugar, postglucose challenge if necessary). For smokers an ultrasound examination of the abdominal aortic artery was approved in 2007. If the practitioner were to obtain full reimbursement the IPPE exam had to include height, weight, blood pressure, screening electrocardiogram, and education counseling and referral as appropriate.

An ongoing, real-time evaluation of new prevention-related technologies is now an important part of Medicare's activities, providing practitioners with timely guidance. For example, Medicare rejected the use of computerized tomography colonoscopy because of the lack of evidence of its equivalence to endoscopic colonoscopy in the elderly population (Dhruva et al. 2009). Practitioners now can get the most recent "Guide to Medicare Preventive Services" on the web and keep up to date on the latest Center for Medicare and Medicaid Services (CMS) rulings (Medicare Learning Network 2009).

Now that Medicare has caught up with the rest of the nation on preventive services coverage, using the most scientifically determined approach to date through the USPSTF it will maintain its currency on prevention as mandated by the 2010 health care reform act (PPACA - see Chapters 1 and 5 in this volume).

MEDICAID

The Medicaid Early and Periodic Screening, Diagnostic and Treatment (EPSDT) program was initiated in 1967 as part of the Social Security Act child health amendments that provided low-income children under age 21 with preventive and curative services. In 2008 CMS oversaw financing of health care services for over 60 million low-income Americans. The Medicaid program under federal law[20] requires that all Medicaid children under age 21 participate in EPSDT, which includes coverage for a comprehensive health and development history, an unclothed physical examination, appropriate immunizations, certain laboratory tests, and health education. Additional services include vision and hearing screenings and dental health maintenance. An annual goal of CMS is that 80% or more of all Medicaid children in every state receive an EPSDT well-child check-up (Cackley 2009). In the GAO assessment from 2000 through 2007 most states do not achieve the CMS goal. For example, in 2007 "on average, 58% of Medicaid children received at least one EPSDT well-child check up for which they were eligible; rates in individual states varied from 25 to 79%" (Cackley 2009).

20. 42 USC §§ 1396a(a)(10)(A), 1396d(a)(4)(B).

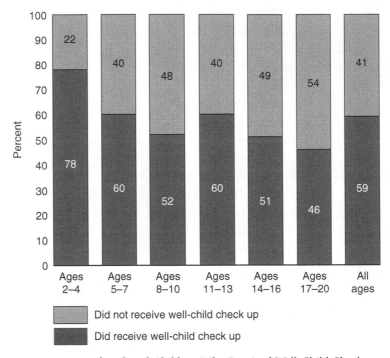

Figure 6.1 Percentage of Medicaid Children Who Received Well-Child Check-ups over a 2-Year Period, by Age (Cackley 2009).

Figure 6.1 from the GAO report (Cackley 2009) illustrates the percentage of Medicaid children that received well-child checkups over a 2-year period, by age.

Medicaid programs do not have to cover preventive services for adults. Prior to PPACA most states did not explicitly cover preventive services, though they could opt to cover services under the optional benefit category subsumed in the "preventive, diagnostic, and screening services." When state Medicaid programs were surveyed about eight prevention services, mammograms, and cervical cancer screenings were provided by almost all states (49 and 48 states, respectively). Additionally, 75% of the states covered diabetes screening, cholesterol testing, colorectal cancer screening, and influenza immunizations. Thirty-nine states covered well-adult checkups (Cackley 2009).

Given that the EPSDT mandate started in 1967, it was far ahead of most other insurance programs, public or private, in the United States. Unfortunately the eligible population is not taking advantage of these covered benefits for both typical health care barrier, and other reasons. Riportella-Muller et al. (1996) found the health care barriers include lack of knowledge of frequency of checkups, lack of available checkup slots by providers, scheduling difficulties, inconvenient clinic hours, and lack or dislike of community providers. Some individuals found themselves with interrupted Medicaid coverage, becoming ineligible before they could make an appointment. Non-health care-related barriers include competing family/personal priorities such as conflicts with family events, a lack of clarity as to who should be taking care of the child, an inability to take time off from work, or the need to handle family crises.

When I was in private practice, although I felt it my duty to see Medicaid patients and never limited the number I would see in my practice, I was often discouraged by the length of time to reimbursement and the low reimbursement rate by the state, typically about 20 or 30 cents per dollar billed. And my clinic's rates were lower than most others in the area. Many physicians have stopped seeing Medicaid patients, or limit the number they will see. For example, a big problem in obtaining adequate dental care for young children is that there are:

> too few dentists willing to accept Medicaid and many who do limit the number of Medicaid patients they see. . .because reimbursement rates are often below the cost of providing the service, paperwork and preauthorization burdens. . . In addition, care-seeking behavior among Medicaid recipients is spotty and the no-show rate for dental appointments is high (Gehshan and Wyatt 2007).

THE PATIENT PROTECTION AND AFFORDABLE CARE ACT OF 2010 (PPACA)

PPACA is the result of the first year of the Obama administration's efforts to reform the health insurance system in the United States. A comprehensive listing of the prevention-related services can be found in Chapter 1 of this volume. From the viewpoint of this chapter, PPACA has redressed many of the preventive care services exclusions that have been neglected components of Medicare, Medicaid, and private health insurance. By eliminating cost-sharing for prevention benefits PPACA removes historical financial barriers. However, the other structural barriers mentioned earlier, such as built environment, transportation, scheduling, and child care, continue, particularly for low-income populations.

Even with PPACA there continue to be at least three differences that show an ongoing division in values between prevention and treatment:

1. The Task Force on Clinical Preventive Services is encouraged to use costs as part of their criteria for assessing Grade A or B *prevention* services. Costs are not explicitly mentioned for treatment coverage.

2. Medicare-covered prevention services are specified individually for certain services, so although the Task Force recommendations are to be the basis for coverage,[21] certain prevention coverage may not be excluded (Section 1305). This is not true for treatment coverage.

3. Preventive medicine residency graduate training programs will still require an annual fight to get the funds authorized.

DISCUSSION

I have reviewed the history of structural barriers to prevention, including the lack of benefits coverage, lack of mechanisms to bill for reimbursement, problems with legislation that prohibited or did not foresee the value of prevention, and personal and health care access barriers to obtaining care. I have also briefly discussed other structural barriers such as the limitation of health manpower resources and the complexity of an environment that often does not encourage more physical activity or sound nutrition choices. I did not discuss negative structures that purposefully were put into place by industries trying to increase their market share: cigarettes available for purchase by minors or unhealthy but profitable foodstuffs arranged to entice higher volume purchases. Some of these have been resolved: in most states tobacco laws require age identification (carding) before purchase. Nutritionists in schools are starting to use market-scientific ways of displaying food options in cafeteria lines to encourage smarter food selections by children (Thaler and Sunstein 2009).

At the same time, most companies that are self-insured, and most states that mandate benefits, now have some coverage of preventive services, though it is not as universal or comprehensive as recommendations made by authoritative bodies such as the U.S. Preventive Services Task Force or the Task Force on Community Preventive Services.[22]

Three things can be done to reduce these ongoing structural barriers to preventive services: (1) provide full and first dollar benefits coverage for

---

21. Except for mammography. Because of the controversy over the mammography guidelines elaborated by the United States Preventive Services Task Force at the end of 2009 (see Petitti's chapter 5 in this volume) the USPSTF's guidelines were exempted by special section 2713 in the PPACA:

(5) for the purposes of this Act, and for the purposes of any other provision of law, the current recommendations of the United States Preventive Service Task Force regarding breast cancer screening, mammography, and prevention shall be considered the most current *other than those issued in or around November 2009.* (italics added)

22. http://www.thecommunityguide.org/index.html, accessed June 5, 2011.

prevention, (2) integrate preventive clinical services into all health care delivery, and (3) reinforce our public health infrastructure.

Provide Full and First Dollar Benefits Coverage for Prevention

As noted above, PPACA takes care of this issue. Medicare has been moving in this direction vigorously since the Medicare Modernization Act. Medicaid has been in the forefront of benefits coverage, at least for children. However, private insurers generally have lagged behind unless states had mandated such coverage. Where coverage was reasonably comprehensive it was not unusual for co-pays and deductibles, among other reasons, to be financial barriers to individuals obtaining preventive care (Okoro et al. 2005). Based upon the new PPACA law, private insurance plans will have to provide first dollar coverage for USPSTF grade A or B recommendations. By 2011 Medicare and Medicaid will also have to comply.

Integrate Preventive Clinical Services into All Health Care Delivery

"Integrate" does not mean only providing preventive services at the same time that treatment services are provided or in a visit available only in a month solely for prevention. Additionally it means thinking prospectively for patients: evaluating their future risks, providing care that mitigates these risks, and taking into account the patient's individualized needs—financially, socially, culturally, and clinically on a fully integrated basis. Snyderman and Dinan (2010) recently called this "taking it personally." As Snyderman and colleagues stated in an earlier editorial: "Personalized health planning to anticipate and minimize each individual's risk for the onset and progression of disease is what our health care future will require" (Williams, Sanders, and Snyderman 2003).

An integrated delivery of health care requires additional personnel to assist patients in changing risk factors for disease. Physicians rarely can spend the time, and often don't have the knowledge, to do individualized risk factor reduction counseling. Although it is true that physicians can help to motivate patients at teachable moments to undergo risk behavior change (Lawson and Flocke 2009), spending the hours of counseling, follow-up, and change management with patients is better left to clinical nutritionists, exercise physiologists, stress management specialists, and others who are integrated into the primary care setting. It takes significant capital to hire personnel, establish offices and testing equipment, and provide computer systems that enhance integrated work among the specialists. Most physicians cannot afford to establish these practices independently, thus larger group practices could provide a structure that can make this type of integrated care feasible. Until primary and preventive care is integrated into our whole system of care, prevention services will continue to be underutilized.

Reinforce Our Public Health Infrastructure

Finally, we need to be sure that our public health infrastructure is not decimated by resource constraints. It cannot be "last in, first out" in government budgets, occupational health worksite settings, or health promotion at the worksite. We need to guard against legislators' desires to raid prevention budgets to satisfy budget deficits in other areas. Once these items are stabilized we need a closer working relationship among the local and state health departments, private practitioners, retailers, manufacturers, and developers in order to preserve healthy lifestyle activity and nutritional and environmental choices.

ACKNOWLEDGMENTS

Thanks to Paul Menzel, Kevin Patrick, and Robert Wallace for their reviews and comments on earlier drafts of this chapter.

REFERENCES

Baker, S.L. 2008. *U.S. National Health Spending 2006.* University of South Carolina, Arnold School of Public Health. Available at http://hadm.sph.sc.edu/Courses/Econ/Classes/nhe06/ accessed, June 5, 2011.

Bondi, M.A., Harris, J.R., Atkins, D., French, M.E., and Umland, B. 2006. Employer Coverage of Clinical Preventive Services in the United States. *American Journal of Health Promotion* 20 (3):214–22.

Bunce, V.C., and Wieske, J.P. 2004. *Health Insurance Mandates in the States.* Alexandria, VA: Council for Affordable Health Insurance.

———. 2010. *Health Insurance Mandates in the States 2010.* Alexandria, VA: Council for Affordable Health Insurance.

Cackley, A.P. 2009. Medicaid Preventive Services: *Concerted Efforts Needed to Ensure Beneficiaries Receive Services.* U.S.G.A. Office, Ed. Washington, DC: GAO.

Cooper, R.A., Getzen, T.E., McKee, H.J., and Laud, P. 2002. Economic and Demographic Trends Signal an Impending Physician Shortage. *Health Affairs* 21 (1):140–54.

Davis, K., Bialek, R., Parkinson, M., Smith, J., and Vellozzi, C. 1990. Paying for Preventive Care; Moving the Debate Forward. *American Journal of Preventive Medicine* 6 (4 Supplement):27.

Dhruva, S.S., Phurrough, S.E., Salive, M.E., and Redberg, R.F. 2009. CMS's Landmark Decision on CT Colonography—Examining the Relevant Data. *New England Journal of Medicine* 360 (26):2699–701.

Donabedian, A. 1980a. *Explorations in Quality Assessment and Monitoring Volume I: The Definitions of Quality and Approaches to Its Assessment.* Ann Arbor, MI: Health Administration Press.

———. 1980b. *Explorations in Quality Assessment and Monitoring Volume II: The Criteria and Standards of Quality.* Ann Arbor, MI: Health Administration Press.

Dorsey, J.L. 1975. The Health Maintenance Organization Act of 1973 (P.L. 93–222) and Prepaid Group Practice Plans. *Medical Care* 13 (1):1–9.

D'Orsi, C. 2004. Mammography: Will Adequate Manpower Exist? *Radiologic Clinics of North America* 42:4.

Dubey, V., Mathew, R., Iglar, K., Moineddin, R., and Glazier, R. 2006. Improving Preventive Service Delivery at Adult Complete Health Check-Ups: The Preventive Health Evidence-Based Recommendation Form (PERFORM) Cluster Randomized Controlled Trial. *BMC Family Practice* 7:44–56.

Emerman, E., and Arnoff, S. 2009. *Watson Wyatt Identifies Major Benefit Trends During Open Enrollment Season.* Washington, DC: Watson Wyatt.

Faust, H.S. 1983. The Pension Costs of Worksite Health Promotion Programs. In *Priorities in Health Statistics: Proceedings of the 19th National Meeting of the Public Health Conference on Records and Statistics.* Hyattsville, MD: U.S. Department of Health and Human Services.

Freymann, J.G. 1975. Medicine's Great Schism: Prevention vs. Cure: An Historical Interpretation. *Medical Care* 8 (7):11.

Gehshan, S., and Wyatt, M. 2007. *Improving Oral Health Care for Young Children.* Washington, DC: National Academy for State Health Policy.

Goetzel, R.Z., and Ozminkowski, R.J. 2008. The Health and Cost Benefits of Work Site Health-Promotion Programs. *Annual Review of Public Health* 29:303–23.

Goolsbee, A., Lovenheim, M.F., and Slemrod, J. 2010. Playing with Fire: Cigarettes, Taxes, and Competition from the Internet. *American Economic Journal: Economic Policy* 2 (1):131–54.

Hung, D.Y., Rundall, T.G., Tallia, A.F., Cohen, D.J., Halpin, H.A., and Crabtree, B.F. 2007. Rethinking Prevention in Primary Care: Applying the Chronic Care Model to Address Health Risk Behaviors. *Milbank Quarterly* 85 (1):69–91.

Institute of Medicine (IOM). 2007. *Training Physicians for Public Health Careers.* Committee on Training Physicians for Public Health Practice Careers, Board on Population Health. Washington, DC: Author. Available at: http://www.nap.edu/openbook.php?record_id=11915

Jolissaint, J.G., Swiatkowski, S.A., Mangalmurti, S.S., and Gutke, G.D. 2006. History of Recruit Medicine in the United States Military Service. In B.L. Koning, Ed., *Recruit Medicine.* Washington, DC: Borden Institute, Walter Reed Army Medical Center.

Kane, D. 2009. *San Diegans—and Their Cell Phones—Will Help Computer Scientists Monitor Air Pollution.* UC San Diego, December 4. Available at http://ucsdnews.ucsd.edu/newsrel/science/12-09CellAirPollution.asp, accessed January 6, 2011.

Lawson, P.J., and Flocke, S.A. 2009. Teachable Moments for Health Behavior Change: A Concept Analysis. *Patient Education and Counseling* 76 (1):25–30.

Loughlin, A.M., and Strathdee, S.A. 2007. Vaccines: Past, Present, and Future. In K.E. Nelson and C.F.M. Williams, Eds., *Infectious Disease Epidemiology; Theory and Practice* (pp. 345–82). Boston, MA: Jones and Bartlett.

Martin, S.C, and Howell, J.D. 1989. One Hundred Years of Clinical Preventive Medicine in America. *Primary Care* 16 (1):6.

Medicare Learning Network. 2009. In Center for Medicare and Medicaid Services, Ed., *The Guide to Medicare Preventive Services*. Baltimore, MD: Department of Health and Human Services.

Moore, L.V., and Roux, A.V.D. 2006. Associations of Neighborhood Characteristics with the Location and Type of Food Stores. *American Journal of Public Health* 96 (2):325–31.

National Association of County and City Health Officials. 2010. *Survey of Local Health Department Job Losses and Program Cuts*. National Association of County and City Health Officials 2009. Available at http://www.naccho.org/advocacy/upload/JobLossProgramCuts_ResearchBrief_final.pdf, accessed June 5, 2011.

National Business Group on Health. 2010. *Understanding Evidence Statements, Summary Plan Descriptions (SPDs) and CPT Codes*. National Business Group on Health 2010. Available at http://www.businessgrouphealth.org/preventive/topics/understanding. cfm, accessed June 5, 2011.

Nestle, M. 2002. *Food Politics: How the Food Industry Influences Nutrition and Health*. Berkeley, CA: University of California Press.

Okoro, C.A., Strine, T.W., Young, S.L., Balluz, L.S., and Mokdad, A.H. 2005. Access to Health Care Among Older Adults and Receipt of Preventive Services. Results from the Behavioral Risk Factor Surveillance System, 2002. *Preventive Medicine* 40 (3):337–43.

Ormond, B.A., Spillman, B.C., Waidmann, T.A., Caswell, K.J., and Tereshchenko, B. 2011. Potential National and State Medical Care Savings from Primary Disease Prevention. *American Journal of Public Health* 101 (1):157–64.

Paeratakul, S., Ferdinand, D., Champagne, C., Ryan, D., and Bray, G. 2006. Fast-Food Consumption Among U.S. Adults and Children: Dietary and Nutrient Intake Profile. *Journal of the American Dietetic Association* 103:6.

Parkinson, M.D., and Lurie, P. 1996. Reimbursement for Preventive Services. In S.H. Woolf, S. Jonas, and R.S. Lawrence, Eds., *Health Promotion and Disease Prevention in Clinical Practice* (pp. 525–42). Baltimore, MD: Williams & Wilkins.

Ransohoff, D. 2005. Colon Cancer Screening in 2005: Status and Challenges. *Gastroenterology* 128:10.

Reid, T.R. 2009. *The Healing of America— A Global Quest for Better, Cheaper, and Fairer Health Care*. New York: Penguin Press.

Riportella-Muller, R., Selby-Harington, M.L., Richardson, L.A., Donat, P.L.N., Luchok, K.J., and Quade, D. 1996. Barriers to the Use of Preventive Health Care Services for Children. *Public Health Reports* 111 (1):71–77.

Robbins, L.C., and Hall, J.H. 1970. How to Practice Prospective Medicine. Indianapolis, IN: Methodist Hospital of Indiana.

Rosen, G. 1976. *Preventive Medicine in the United States 1900–1975*. New York: Prodist.

Rothman, S.M. Health Advocacy Organizations and Evidence-Based Medicine. *Journal of the American Medical Association* 305 (24):2569–570.

Seef, L.C., Manninen, D.L., Dong, F.B., Cattopadhyay, S.K., Nadel, M.R., Tangka, F.K., and Molinari, N.A. 2004. Is There Endoscopic Capacity to Provide Colorectal Cancer Screening to the Unscreened Population in the United States? *Gastroenterology* 127 (6):3.

Snyderman, R., and Dinan, M.A. 2010. Improving Health by Taking It Personally. *Journal of the American Medical Association* 303 (4):363–64.

Soler, R.E., Leeks, K.D., Razi, S., Hopkins, D.P., Griffith, M., Aten, A., Chattopadhyay, S.K., Smith, S.C., Habarta, N., Goetzel, R.Z., Pronk, N.P., Richling, D.E., Bauer, D.R., Buchanan, L.R., Florence, C.S., Koonin, L., MacLean, D., Rosenthal, A., Koffman, D.M., Grizzell, J.V., Walker, A.M., and Task Force on Community Preventive Services. 2010. A Systematic Review of Selected Interventions for Worksite Health Promotion: The Assessment of Health Risks with Feedback. *American Journal of Preventive Medicine* 38 (2S):S237–S262.

Starr, P. 1982. *The Social Transformation of American Medicine*. New York: Basic Books.

Sullum, J. 1998. *For Your Own Good—The Anti-Smoking Crusade and the Tyranny of Public Health*. New York: The Free Press.

Task Force on Community Preventive Services. 2010. Recommendations for Worksite-Based Interventions to Improve Workers' Health. *American Journal of Preventive Medicine* 38 (2S):S232–S236.

Taubes, G. 1995. Epidemiology Faces Its Limits. *Science* 269 (5221):5.

Thaler, R.H., and Sunstein, C.R. 2009. *Nudge—Improving Decisions about Health, Wealth, and Happiness*. New York: Penguin Books.

Thomasson, M.A. 2002. From Sickness to Health: The Twentieth Century Development of U.S. Health Insurance. *Explorations in Economic History* 39:20.

Thompson, R.S., Michnich, M.E., Friedlander, L., Gilson, B., Grothaus, L.C., and Storer, B. 1988. Effectiveness of Smoking Cessation Interventions Integrated into Primary Care Practice. *Medical Care* 26:14.

Tikka, J.P. 2009. *West Wireless Health Institute Established with $45M Donation*. Xconomy, San Diego, March 30. Available at http://www.xconomy.com/san-diego/2009/03/30/west-wireless-health-institute-established-with-45m-donation/, accessed June 5, 2011.

Townsend, J., Roderick, P., and Cooper, J. 1994. Cigarette Smoking by Socioeconomic Group, Sex, and Age: Effects of Price, Income, and Health Publicity. *BMJ or British Medical Journal* 309 (6959):923–27.

U.S. Department of Health and Human Services. 2000. *Healthy People 2010*. Washington, DC: Government Printing Office.

Weathington, S. 2011. What is Product Placement? http://www.helium.com/items/868427-what-is-product-placement, accessed June 5, 2011.

Williams, R., Sanders, H.F.W., and Snyderman, R. 2003. Editorial: Personalized Health Planning. *Science* 300 (5619):549.

Wynia, M.K., Cummins, D.S., VanGeest, J.B., and Wilson, I.B. 2000. Physician Manipulation of Reimbursement Rules for Patients: Between a Rock and a Hard Place. *Journal of the American Medical Association* 283(14): 1858–65.

PART TWO

Philosophical and Legal Analysis

7

Our Alleviation Bias

Why Do We Value Alleviating Harm More than Preventing Harm?

HALLEY S. FAUST, MD, MPH, MA ∎

INTRODUCTION

One of the questions posed to the contributors of this volume at first seems to concern the moral and professional priorities associated with an individual practitioner—what should I do when faced with making a professional decision to see one of two patients or fulfill a community obligation? The thought experiment constructed to illustrate this question (see Chapter 1 of this volume) begins, "You are a versatile and accomplished solo primary care physician working in a backwater rural area." You have to make a decision among three competing obligations: the needs of a patient in acute distress, the needs of a patient who wants to prevent acute disease in the future, and the needs of a community—a group of seemingly faceless individuals who may benefit from your actions.

This thought experiment originally was devised to determine how ethical theories can be used to explore and justify ethical decisions at the microlevel, during the daily practice of a physician. A subtext of the thought experiment asks why the demands for justification of prevention interventions appear to be higher than those for treatment. In the introduction of this book, Menzel and I illustrate a number of the ways in which society indicates it values treatment over prevention. We also note how the Patient Protection and Affordable Care Act of 2010 has mitigated some of this discrepancy. Broadly the fact that the amount we spend on treatment is 14 times more than the amount we spend on prevention is an accumulation of many small and specific decisions: how patients choose to enter and make demands on the health care system, how physicians choose to use their time with patients, including making decisions about prescribing diagnostic tests and treatments, and how insurers and employers provide incentives for the attention of practitioners and insureds/ employees.

Some might say that part of the cause of this prevention lag may have been that prior to the mid-1970s few studies proved the effectiveness of prevention. This can hardly be the only reason, or a reason at all—there were similarly few studies on the effectiveness of most treatments of the day. Indeed, even for something as simple as treating strep throat the original 10-day treatment with penicillin was not confirmed with randomized trials until the mid-1980s (Gerber et al. 1987), and the controversy continues (Zwart et al. 2000).

How physicians choose to use their time when seeing a patient and how they make spending decisions for diagnostic tests and treatment involve a subtext as well: physicians have traditionally been poorly trained in preventive medicine, and are less confident in their abilities to help patients prevent disease. Other than in some primary care residency training programs, where there is usually an emphasis on prevention, physicians often assume that they are relatively ineffective when it comes to helping a patient quit smoking, lose weight, increase exercise, or eat more nutritious meals. When pushed for time physicians tend to ignore prevention items to address the acute needs of patients (Cogswell and Eggert 1993). Part of the reason for this attention to acute needs derives from an historical lack of payment for preventive services. But there also is the general feeling by physicians (and patients) that prevention can be addressed in the future when "I (or others) can get around to it."

This "when I can get around to it" point is important. When the Bill/John/Public's Health thought experiment (the thought experiment, or BJPH) is presented to groups, one of the most common early responses, even though it violates the rules of the thought experiment, is, "We can see John at another time; he can make another appointment." The implication is that waiting to start prevention activities is both effective and satisfactory for most patients. We clearly know that this is not the case with effective secondary prevention activities—if we wait too long between screening intervals we may miss significant amounts of treatable, often curable, disease. Take just one example: colorectal cancer. Computed tomography (CT) colonography and colonoscopy have sensitivities of 87–96% (smaller adenomas being 71–85%), meaning that 4–13% of cancers will be missed with the first screening (Whitlock et al. 2008). Furthermore, it is believed that most colorectal malignancies arise from adenomas over long periods of time ranging from 5 to perhaps 20 years (Peipins and Sandler 1994).

Missing the transition time from adenoma to malignancy, which may involve critical timing of screening intervals, may make treatment more complex and/or less successful.

What we don't know is whether there are similar timing thresholds for the *primary* prevention of disease. Might we prevent more heart disease if we begin prevention programs in our 20s rather than our 50s? Is there a time between childhood and mid-adulthood when coronary disease reaches a threshold beyond which we cannot prevent or reverse certain types of future harm? Might our lives be enhanced with less disease if prevention interventions were to take precedence over, or at least be given equal weight with, treatment interventions?

The American Academy of Pediatrics seems to think so. In 2008 it issued a report urging more proactive work for reducing childhood obesity and risk factors for cardiovascular disease (Daniels, Greer, and Committee on Nutrition 2008). Shonkoff, Boyce, and McEwen (2009) argue that early childhood experiences can affect adult health either because of cumulative damage over time or "biological embedding of adversities during sensitive developmental periods" causing lags of years or decades before the adverse effects of physical or mental illnesses become manifested. It is likely that similar thresholds or "biological embeddings" continue to take place as we age.

The questions and problems raised here, as well as those raised in the introduction to this book, generally deal with two kinds of ethical elements: (1) a utilitarian analysis of cost-effectiveness, and (2) nonutilitarian values harbored within our cultural propensity to help the needy—ones who are suffering *now*. There are problems with how we treat prevention (and treatment) in utilitarian methods such as cost-effectiveness and cost–benefit analyses. It is worthwhile to attend to these problems, as have Russell (Chapter 3) and Menzel (Chapter 11) in this volume, and others elsewhere (Nord 1999; Harvard Program in Ethics and Health 2009).

In this Chapter I address the second element: all outcomes being equal, how do we account ethically for the much greater preference for harm alleviation over harm prevention despite a common desire of the U.S. population to have an increasing emphasis on prevention (Cogswell and Eggert 1993)? I believe the answer is found in the concept of compassion and its driving force, vividness of suffering. Vividness in turn is driven by spatial and temporal proximity. Vividness is diluted by the need for the imagination to reach beyond our experiences. When something confronts us at the moment, we move to attend to it *at the moment*.

My claim, though it is ethically and psychologically related, is fundamentally an empirical/descriptive claim, not a normative one—compassion is an overwhelming moral emotion that causes us to ignore cost–benefit analyses, cost-effectiveness analyses, public opinion polls taken in calm times (outside of crises), epidemiological data, and careful health policy and economic analyses. Why? *Because what evokes compassion is suffering.* Because of Bill's current suffering, which is vivid to us in both time and space, we are more likely to act for Bill– "we can't let Bill suffer now"—than we are for John—"we can't let John get heart disease sometime in the future."

In this Chapter I begin with a discussion of some medical professional ethics issues. Then, after defining terms, I discuss the doing vs. allowing literature and where it is and is not helpful in analyzing the prevention vs. treatment debate. I then analyze the harm alleviation (treatment) bias through brief thought experiments that vary the underlying components of compassion and vividness, illustrating why compassion and vividness are so critical in our intuitions about the BJPH thought experiment. Finally, I comment on the difference between this empirical claim and what could be a normative claim of the priority of treatment over prevention.[1]

PROFESSIONAL OBLIGATIONS AND THE THOUGHT EXPERIMENT

Should I see Bill or John, or should I take the health department's call? The outcomes are hypothesized to be the same in utilitarian terms: 12 person-years of life saved over what the alternative scenarios would be. Bill, who is 62, would live to age 75 if treated, and only to age 63 if not treated. John, Bill's brother and therefore of similar genetic heritage, with prevention would live to age 75 relatively disease free, and otherwise die at age 63 from heart disease if not seen for prevention. The local health department/public health (LHD or PH) option would enact a previously proven effective program that would save 12 years of life in some unknown individual. The cost for all three is the same. Concurrently I would feel the same satisfaction no matter which course of action is taken.

Let us assume that there is no utilitarian escape in the thought experiment (BJPH)—that each of the three scenarios is crafted to entail that the outcomes are identical, just with different individuals achieving them through different means: Bill's outcome through immediate treatment and John's outcome through immediate prevention, and the unknown health department's effects through a community-wide outreach effort. If you are a strict consequentialist you should be indifferent to which of the three options you would exercise. If you are a deontologist you might think of other issues: do I have a greater duty to John, Bill, or the local health department? We can categorize the deontological

---

1. Throughout this chapter I will use "prevention" and "treatment" to mean the same thing as "preventing harm" and "alleviating harm respectively."

choice as either one related to patients (John and Bill) or a community commitment (LHD). A common claim is that a physician's duty to a patient takes precedence over a duty to the community.

Duty to Care

If John were our long-established patient and Bill just came along hoping to see the doctor because of his epigastric discomfort, then the duty to care for a long-standing patient might guide us to see John. Otherwise we would be shirking our duty of care to someone with whom we have an established relationship. In the eyes of the law, this relationship is even considered an implied contract, obligating physicians to a type of "continuing attention" to a patient until the doctor–patient relationship is formally terminated (Furrow et al. 2000). Morally it is part of the trust relationship with a physician, particularly a primary care physician, with whom patients expect to maintain long-term relationships over multiple encounters. If only John were my established patient and Bill were not, then based on this duty to care principle alone I'd be obligated to see John.

Promise-Keeping

On the other hand, if both were long-established patients and Bill had the appointment whereas John did not, then a promise-keeping duty in the opposite direction is involved. Promise-keeping and promise-breaking could apply to the justification for seeing Bill (Beauchamp and Childress 2001, 312–19). It could also apply to taking the PH phone call; taking on the obligation of a board position as a fiduciary of the public's health entails a duty of care and loyalty. Though for some reason it seems that we don't weigh our moral priority as highly when our obligation is to an organization rather than to an individual. This is evident to anyone who has been on hospital committees or public health boards and observed how physician members of the committees and boards tend to prioritize their attendance at meetings as secondary to their obligations to individual patients. One reason may be financial—most of these committees and boards do not provide remuneration for service. However, I think the majority of the time physicians will argue, correctly or not, that they have an obligation to their established patients first, and to an organization or a community second.[2]

2. Though some codes of ethics for physicians could be confusing in this regard, stating that the physician's primary responsibility is solely and inviolately to the patient, but that

Some might argue that you should take the public health department tele-conference because if the grant reduces heart attacks, it could be the beginning of a larger activity in the long run that would benefit many more people—its results would be persuasive for future added funding and save many more lives, whereas seeing either Bill or John would impact only that particular individual without a likely future gain for other patients. Although this argument is rea-sonable, it violates the rules of the thought experiment, which postulated equiv-alent outcomes.

Personal Relationships vs. Unknown Beneficiaries

The involvement with Bill and John would be a more personal one than the PH option, evoking a direct caring relationship for individuals. PH good works are associated with a broader group of unknown individuals that is diffused throughout a population. Even so, if each human life is given equal weight in our moral deliberations, then in a consequentialist mode it shouldn't matter if those lives (or life-years) are from known and existing patients, or from anony-mous folks out in the community.[3]

Even with these variations on BJPH, most health care and bioethics audiences confronted with this thought experiment overwhelmingly proclaim that we should see Bill. Occasional quotes, aside from the postponement approach for prevention mentioned in the introduction, include, "He is the most in need at the moment" or "We have to see Bill, he has the most suffering." This preference is expressed even if Bill doesn't have an appointment or isn't an established patient. On rare occasions someone will opt for seeing John because he is showing the most responsible behavior, or choose the local health department option because of a communitarian orientation to obligation. But these are truly rare responses that tend to come from community medicine/public health workers.

physicians also have an ethical responsibility to be involved in serving the health care needs of all members of society and the formation of health policy. With guidance like this, how does a physician know the right balance? (Council of Medical Specialty Societies 1999)

3. I am assuming that our moral obligations are equivalent in considering either individual lives or life-years. We could also consider the quality of the life-years, but again I am assum-ing they are identical, though given a successful prevention program I believe John's quality would be greater than Bill's. John's suffering would be in how he viewed and endured reason-able physical activity and nutrition lifestyle changes. Bill's would be related to the discomfort of bypass surgery or interventional radiology (e.g., stent placement) and cardiac rehabilita-tion, which has endurance issues similar to John's prevention programs.

Personal Responsibility

There is a broad literature on how our own actions might have an impact on our ability to have priorities for the use of health care resources. Usually this literature compares two people with existing harm, in which limited resources means using resources for one person would diminish the resources available for the other (a zero sum game). I have not seen any literature that compares using prevention vs. treatment resources. The relevant criteria considered usually include voluntariness, competence in choice, foreknowledge of the effects of actions, and reasonable certainty that the effects were caused by the individual's actions (Walker 2010). Should we deem that someone is more responsible and praiseworthy, and therefore less culpable for the costs of future actions, by working conscientiously to prevent future disease? If that is the case, then clearly we should see John. This criterion is rarely weighted as strongly in our resource decision making, though as we will see in the next section, compassion usually means that an individual's misfortune is undeserved, i.e., not self-inflicted.

On a more visceral level, think of yourself as a patient, and then reflect on the way you would feel if you were sitting in a waiting room for your physician who is running 60 minutes behind schedule. You will more readily excuse his lateness because of a life-threatening emergency than for a phone call counseling a patient on an exercise program, or taking a board of health conference call.

So clearly something more than the duty to the patient, promise-keeping, or the praiseworthy behavior of someone who wants to prevent disease is involved among those who would argue to see Bill. I claim this is our bias toward compassion.

DEFINING TERMS—COMPASSION AND VIVIDNESS

To explain why compassion is such a motivating force we need to understand what it is. I use "compassion" in this chapter as Martha Nussbaum defines it deriving from Aristotle: "a painful emotion occasioned by the awareness of another person's undeserved misfortune" (Nussbaum 2001, 301). There are five components to this definition. The first three are related to our judgment of the sufferer: the suffering (misfortune) must be (1) serious (nontrivial), (2) not purposefully self-inflicted, and (3) adverse to the well-being of the sufferer— what Nussbaum calls the observer's ability to make a *eudaimonistic* judgment about the sufferer's well-being.[4] The fourth component of compassion is that

---

4. This notion of a eudaimonistic judgment is Nussbaum's way of modifying Aristotle's criterion of the perceived vulnerability of the observer: that the suffering of the one experiencing misfortune could "befall us soon." See Aristotle's *Rhetoric*, Book 2 1385b12–1386a3.

the observer (i.e., the one feeling compassion) must have "a painful emotion." Perhaps this painful emotion is something akin to a feeling of empathy.[5] It must be sufficiently strong to motivate the observer into wanting to alleviate the suffering, this "wellspring to action" being the fifth and final requirement of compassion. Without the action motivator we would be indifferent to which option to choose in BJPH.

Simply from this definition it is easy to see how treatment would take priority over prevention. For if suffering is present in party A (needing treatment) but not in party B (needing prevention) by definition we cannot have compassion for B. Unless we can conceive of the suffering that may be in the future for B, or relate to B's current angst about his own future, there would be no reason to have compassion for B in B's current state. For us to have compassion for B requires imagination of two sorts: understanding what B's condition may be like in the future and envisioning B in that condition. Both of these are animated by how vivid B's condition can be imagined, by how well we know B and his likely reaction to a future condition, and by the links of that vividness to arousal of our own feelings. As noted by Kogut and Ritov (2005), "vividness exerts great influence on feelings." One series of studies (Jenni and Loewenstein 1997) seemed to indicate that vividness does not readily affect our decisions in choosing between known and unknown victims (or statistical vs. identified lives), whereas other studies show that vivid information often produces more impact on decision making than empirical evidence. (Kogut and Ritov 2005; Rottenstreich and Hsee 2001; Slovic, Monahan, and MacGregor 2000).[6] Slovic et al. (2007) term this "the affect heuristic," defined as

> images, marked by positive and negative affective feelings, guide judgment and decision making. . .That is, representations of objects and events in people's minds are tagged to varying degrees with affect. In the process of making a judgment or decision, people consult or refer to an "affect pool" containing all the positive and negative tags consciously or unconsciously associated with the representations. . . [These representations] serve as a cue for many important judgments.

5. For further elaboration see Nussbaum (2001) and Faust (2009). Crisp (2008) argues that contemporary common usage of the term eliminates the cognitive component and is the painful emotion where "Compassion is a feeling or emotion analogous to fear or anger." I don't agree—Crisp's description of a feeling devoid of external criteria is better termed *empathy*.

6. This study showed that people were more willing to take action (contribute funds toward an expensive treatment for a 2-year-old child) when single victims were identified by age, name, and a picture than if only age or age and name were given. Ratings of empathic distress were significantly correlated with willingness to contribute.

For current, proximate sufferers we can reach into the affect pool relatively easily. The image is in front of us—we can see and touch the one suffering. But for future sufferers we need to construct an image, and such construction takes imagination. In BJPH we can see Bill with discomfort, whereas we have to imagine John's suffering 12 years from now. Can we have compassion for John? To do so would require a moral emotional imagination based upon prior experience ("I would never want to have that happen to anyone again") or vivid description that can be internally understood as serious ("That's repugnant and should not be allowed to happen"). This is more difficult to inculcate into others than their experiencing an extant suffering they can understand in someone in front of them. Preventing harm requires not just a statistical analysis of lives saved or morbidity reduced. It also requires an emotional judgment of the impact of the preventive intervention.

What makes something vivid? Generally information that is "(a) emotionally interesting, (b) concrete and imagery-provoking, and (c) proximate in a sensory, temporal, or spatial way" (Nisbett and Ross 1980). And so, direct experience—requiring proximity in time and space—more vividly impacts how we form judgments and react to circumstances. As I will show later with various thought experiments, these influences are important in how we evaluate specific prevention vs. treatment situations.[7]

---

7. Admittedly thought experiments have intrinsic problems as a form of explanation or justification for action: they rely on intuition, and intuition is a controversial form of philosophical inquiry. How do we access and arrive at our intuitions? What biases, prejudices, experiences, natural behavior, and values do we already possess that influence our intuitive conclusions and may lead us astray? One of the main psychological problems of philosophical intuitions is that philosophers consider propositions in a comprehensive, contemplative way. Meanwhile most people don't make decisions the way philosophers think they might; instead of considering propositions or circumstances comprehensively, most people consider propositions one by one as they are faced with them–i.e., in isolation. As Shafir (1998) states, "Intuitions about importance, worth, gravity, as well as ethical propriety are often obtained in comparative settings. . .In life, we often encounter the relevant scenarios one at a time." Because of this, "Simple principles of merit, entitlement, worth, or maximization, which can play a decisive role in comparative settings, often prove difficult to apply in isolated settings." This is why political forces often displace policy development in health care—policy is developed using aggregated information and stepwise reasoning whereas politics causes a focus on issues and solutions posed in isolated situations from constituent to constituent. Similarly, other factors such as uncertainty (Savage 1954) and abnormal events (Miller and Solomon 2003) cause most people to make decisions that otherwise might seem irrational.Meanwhile, as Audi (2008) asserts, "philosophy, like any theoretical enterprise, must have data, and intuitions are crucial philosophical data." Thought experiments can be valuable; until we can establish a science of values based on solid empirical evidence we must start somewhere. As Jamieson (1999) states, "if a moral principle conflicts with a deeply held, reflective moral judgement, it is far from clear why the judgement should defer to the principle rather than

SORTING OUT RELEVANT TERMS: DOING, ALLOWING, PREVENTING, ALLEVIATING

It is important to examine and sort out some of the various terms that could be used in understanding the prevention vs. treatment issue. There is a spectrum of nuance among terms such as preventing harm, not preventing harm (where no harm occurs), allowing harm, not treating harm, treating harm, not doing harm, and doing harm.

A great deal has been written comparing our intuitions regarding "doing" vs. "allowing." We get trolley experiments (Foot 1967) and their broad extensions (Unger 1996), life preserver experiments (Kagan 1998), cutting up healthy Chuck for organ transplants (Kagan 1998), wife poisoning (Thomson 1971), and more. Our intuitions are taxed to decide if allowing a runaway trolley to continue on its way and kill five people is less concerning than flipping a switch to divert the trolley (at no risk to ourselves) and saving the five lives but knowing that we will kill one person who is on the diverted track. These thought experiments evoke our intuitions to ask which is worse: *allowing* harm to be done or *doing* harm.

The seeming simplicity of the doing vs. allowing paradigm doesn't quite address our question about the relationship between prevention and treatment, however, because the dilemma illustrated by the runaway trolley problem, doing harm (by diverting the trolley) vs. allowing harm (by doing nothing), is different from alleviating harm (treating any survivors) vs. preventing harm (stopping the trolley before it hits anyone, or ensuring its construction and maintenance such that it could never become runaway).

This is a complicated analysis that is worthy of further detail, which I shall not pursue here except for a few comments. First, the variables involved in each of these actions are complex. Allowing or doing may be intentional or unintentional, active or passive. They may be harm-inducing, harm-preventing, risk-inducing, risk-alleviating, or harm-alleviating actions.[8] Furthermore, they may be proximately causal or only contributory (probabilistic). In these terms, to *prevent* is to inhibit disease or injury development for a period sufficiently lengthy as to avoid foreseeable harm. This is usually considered an action that is intentional and active (except for primordial prevention) and causally contributory

the principle to the judgement...whatever approach we take must equilibrate between our principles and our considered moral judgements."

8. Granted, placing someone "at risk" (i.e., at higher probability of harm, even if direct harm does not result) could be considered harm inducing, but I think it is something different. This requires further study.

(but not proximate).[9] To *treat* is similarly to correct existing harm actively and intentionally, but contra-prevention, treatment is also usually considered a proximate cause of the alleviation of the harm.

In other words, the analysis for allowing vs. doing needs to include situations in which not doing, preventing, not preventing, alleviating, and not alleviating fit in. As Shelly Kagan (1998) says, "it is more important not to *do* harm to one than it is to *save* five." But this is incomplete for our purposes, as "not doing harm" is not the same thing as preventing harm or not treating when harm exists.

CONDITIONS OF PREVENTING AND ALLEVIATING HARM

This is my understanding of the logic of the *primary prevention of* harm:

1. In person Z disease (or injury) D does not exist.
2. There is a (reasonable) risk that D could manifest itself in Z, i.e., Z is susceptible to getting D.
3. Some (in)action or series of (in)actions P can be taken by Z (or done to Z) that causes D not to manifest itself (at this time and for some relevant ongoing time period).
4. P must be done temporally *before* D could manifest itself.

There are a number of issues that arise in understanding this set of conditions and causal inferences. Regarding the first statement, we must be sure D does not exist in Z. But for some diseases such as very early stage cancers this is a challenge because sensitivity of detection is low, meaning there are many false negatives.

Regarding the second statement, we can have all the presumed components for disease and yet disease does not develop. Strep throat carriers are examples; having *Streptococcus pneumoniae* in one's nasopharynx does not guarantee the development of strep throat. In other words, the right set of conditions for disease does not guarantee the development of disease, but simply increases the *risk* of disease. There is a large causal field associated with human biology—many factors can increase or decrease the chances that exposure to harmful

---

9. Though some might argue it is proximately causal, except for certain discrete prevention interventions such as vaccinations, I don't agree; there are many factors that cause disease and injury and certain types of prevention, particularly related to chronic diseases such as coronary heart disease and diabetes, contribute to a reduction of the disease probabilistically, but reliably can't be said to be proximately causal.

influences will indeed cause harm. Thus the uncertainty of the actual development of disease means that in any individual Z we don't know if D would have occurred without intervention P. *Not preventing* (i.e., not doing P or not consciously choosing to avoid risk factors) may indeed not lead to disease. And because there is often a significant lag between action P and the likely manifestation (or prevention) of D, it is often hard to know if P indeed had an effect, or if Z simply never would have had D anyhow.

Regarding the third statement, by preventing D we might be creating a set of circumstances in which a different disease, call it D', may become more likely. In this case I don't mean a side effect of P, but a competing disease that may not have developed in someone with D. For example, studies seem to indicate that being a carrier for sickle cell disease may reduce susceptibility for malaria (Williams et al. 2005). If we took action P to reduce the number of carriers for sickle cell (D), then we may be increasing malaria (D') within the same population. Similarly, by reducing the development or deaths from heart disease we permit individuals to live longer and therefore increase the likelihood of developing diseases of aging or cancers (Mackenbach et al. 1995). Would we then say that P *caused* malaria or cancer? I don't think so. P simply allowed a barrier to malaria or cancer to be removed for the purpose of reducing the risk of sickle cell transmission or heart disease. Would we then say that P *allowed* or *didn't prevent* malaria in Z?[10] Perhaps the former—it is a bit like throwing the switch to divert the trolley; although one harm is averted, another harm is permitted, even if at a substantially later point in time.

Which brings us to the second part of statement 3 above, "that causes D not to manifest itself (at this time and for some relevant ongoing time period)." If P postpones D for *1 week* is it prevention? Yes. Is it relevant? Unlikely. The *fact* of prevention does not dictate its *value* or relevance. Furthermore, the fact of no-D does not immediately tell us that P was effective, which is partly an epistemic question—if we quit smoking we know statistically that Z's risk will come down dramatically, but, as noted earlier in this chapter, we don't know if that reduction for Z actually occurred, or if the disease was already set up with an invariable progression. We can determine such effects for populations. For individuals we can only infer effect. Thus we need a fifth condition to have prevention:

5. P must not cause another condition Q such that the intensity of Q > D.

It's not that P is ineffective in preventing D, just that if it causes more harm in other ways than preventing harm of D, then we wouldn't use P clinically. This is not a causal link, but a values-relevant one.

10. I am conflating allowing with not preventing. There may be relevant distinctions between the two.

What about alleviating harm? To *alleviate* harm means that:

1. Disease (injury) D exists in person Z.
2. Some action (or series of actions) T can be taken to (or by) Z such that D will (one of the following)[11]:
    a. be eliminated
    b. slowly regress, but not to elimination
    c. be rendered steady state (not progress)
    d. have its inevitable progression slowed
    e. progress at its normal pace but have diminished symptoms

For T to be advocated for a patient or a population of patients, statement 5 from above also likely would attain: T must not cause another condition Q such that the intensity of Q > D. Whether T gets used for any person Z with D depends on how Z (and his physician) assesses and values the type of outcome in 2.a–2.e. compared with any potential side effects of the treatment. *Treating* harm can have components of *allowing* harm because of the risk of side effects of T.

As Pearl (2000, 25) points out, "causal relationships are *ontological*, describing objective physical constraints in our world, whereas probabilistic relationships are *epistemic*, reflecting what we know or believe about the world." When we give a treatment to alleviate harm we often see the improvement of the patient in quick/real time. We infer proximate causation (ontology) of the effect of the treatment even though there are other possibilities: the patient would have gotten better on his or her own in the normal course of the self-limited disease, or the patient would have gotten better *faster* without the treatment, i.e., the treatment could have retarded the speed of self-healing. What actually happens to the patient we can only infer, and determine epistemically, from probabilistic inference.

As Pearl further states, "people prefer to encode knowledge in causal rather than probabilistic structures" (2000). Assessing the effectiveness of P is a probabilistic assessment, working against the causal heuristic Pearl claims most people like to use. So is assessing the effectiveness of a treatment once disease develops, even though people think they can infer the causal response as opposed to the probabilistic response.

So although there may be some relevance to the allowing vs. doing philosophical literature, clearly, we can conclude that the comparison between doing and allowing is not sufficiently analogous to the comparison between preventing

---

11. T could also have no effect, or indeed cause more harm than currently exists, but then we couldn't argue that T is *alleviating* harm.

and alleviating, and therefore any arguably different, justified responses to doing as compared to allowing require substantially more work. To permit a harmful act, or to actively partake in a harmful act, is not the same comparison as to prevent something harmful or to cure the harm present.

Next let us look at some scenarios that isolate prevent and treat specifically and that attempt to evaluate the critical factors of vividness—image, immediacy, proximity, and suffering. Throughout all of these the question of imagination is important as well.

IMAGE AND VIVIDNESS

The cases I use in this chapter are derived and modified from the common cases used by Singer (1972) and Kamm's variants of those (2000). Consider the following two cases:

> **Pond Now** (PN): I alone see an anonymous drowning child in a pond.[12] I cannot save the child myself. On my left is Machine PN that can safely save the child if activated by my putting my credit card into it. It will cost me $500. If I don't put my credit card into the machine I will witness the child's death.

> **Pond Hidden** (PH): To my right is a brick wall through which I cannot see or hear anything on the other side, nor can I walk around it. I know[13] that on the other side of the wall is a pond in which an anonymous child is drowning. If I put my credit card into Machine PH it will safely retrieve the child. It will cost me $500. If I don't put my credit card into the machine the child will die. No one else is available to save the child.

If you were put in the situation such that you had to choose between putting your credit card into Machine PN or Machine PH, which would you choose? A strict act consequentialist would be indifferent—the outcomes of PN and PH are identical.[14] But most of us are not strict act consequentialists; the image of the child sputtering, gasping, and crying for help in PN would more likely evoke emotions that would move us to put our credit card into Machine PN. In seemingly equal outcome situations we likely would take into account our

12. I use an anonymous child because the issue of special obligations to those we know (relatives or friends) would add an additional dimension.

13. By "know" here and hereafter I mean that I am told and believe this to be true.

14. Though, as Kelly Sorensen points out to me, this might be unfair to the act consequentialist who acknowledges the general utility value of emotions, even if they do not promote the maximal good.

emotional judgments when we make decisions. In fact, an act consequentialist would also have to take into account the effect on us of watching a helpless child die in PN were we to choose to put our money into Machine PH.[15] PN and PH illustrate how alleviating harm at the time harm is being inflicted may be influenced by the vividness of the harm as related to both visual and auditory images.

Now let's alter the case to include prevention:

Pond Barrier (PB): I alone see a pond with an anonymous child happily playing around it. I know that the child will be drowning in the pond within the next 10 minutes. The only way to save the child (with no sequelae) is, if in the next 10 minutes, I put my credit card in Machine PB, which will create a barrier that prevents the child from drowning.[16] It will cost me $500. If I don't put my credit card into the machine I will witness the child's death.

Will you put your credit card into Machine PN or Machine PB? If you put your card into PB, there will be no drowning process, no image of drowning, no regrets of not having saved the child, but you will witness the child drown in PN. If you put your money in PN you will witness the child drown in PB in 10 minutes, and you will witness the child engaged in the drowning process in PN, but also the child's complete recovery. To choose Machine PB means the need to ignore the gasping of the child in PN, but it also means you only have to transfer the existing image of the child in PN to the one that will occur in PB. There is, in essence, no substantive distance between PN and PB.

Now let us alter PB to PB* and have it stand alone:

If I don't put my credit card into Machine PB* within the next 10 minutes I can still do so when the child is drowning (like PN), and the child will be rescued. If the child is rescued from drowning the child will recover completely.

Turning PB into PB* creates the option of contrasting preventing harm with alleviating harm, and we withdraw the need for imagining the future because

---

15. Some people may claim that knowing that the child in PH drowned because of our inaction could be as traumatic, even though not witnessing the event. If true it would equally hold for either witnessed event, then, resulting in indifference to PN or PH.

16. In all of the "B"—barrier cases—assume that the barrier is placed just when the child would fall into the pond and begin to drown, not sooner or later, so that the child can still enjoy the pond in all ways children enjoy ponds.

we can act at any time. But choosing when to act is what makes the distinction between preventing and alleviating. If we wait to alleviate we remove any uncertainty that the child might not drown, but we also permit the child to experience the harmful sensation of drowning and then having the harm alleviated. Intuitively we shudder at the thought of a child feeling helpless, panicked, and uncomfortable in a drowning situation; we commonly consider it irresponsible behavior to *put* someone in harm's way, or in this case to *allow* a child to encounter harm's way. Similarly, it seems irresponsible to *permit* someone, particularly a child, to get into harm's way when it is avoidable. Although changing PB to PB* does not contrast doing vs. allowing, it does contrast *doing now to prevent* with the ability to *do later to alleviate* a harmful event. However, it also mitigates our concern for uncertainty—we can observe the child first so that we don't have to commit the resources until we are sure harm is occurring. If I don't act now I can still act in 11 minutes to save the child, and the child's outcome and my costs will be the same: $500 and complete recovery, respectively.

PB* puts us into the common attitude that "if we don't prevent we can treat/cure."[17] Often this is the position of society when it comes to health care; our values imply that we believe our treatments are as (or are more) effective than our preventions and therefore we don't put the effort into preventing—we'd rather wait to see what happens and then activate whatever machines we have to alleviate the disease. Of course the PB* scenario is unrealistic—most of the time our alleviation techniques may be effective at reducing the impact of the health harms befalling us, but not as effective as preventing the harms in the first place. There are almost always sequelae to treating most preventable illnesses: coronary bypass surgery leaves us with scars, pain, and substantial rehabilitation requirements. Diabetes, even when well-controlled with treatment, still produces up to 6.2% of all-cause mortality and 9% of mortality from cardiovascular disease in the United States (Narayan et al. 1999).

This is not to say that we should ignore the sequelae of prevention, for example: sports-related injuries in long-term vigorous exercisers (Waller et al. 2010), the many vaccinated to develop herd immunity while some will have temporary adverse reactions to the vaccine,[18] the less than one person per hundred thousand who will develop rhabdomyolysis from statin therapy (Chang et al. 2004), the false-positive mammography (Fletcher and Elmore 2003), and prostate-specific antigen results culminating in unnecessary biopsies for breast and prostate cancer (Wolf et al. 2010).

17. Thanks to Paul Menzel for pointing this out.

18. See the Vaccine Adverse Event Reporting System, for example: http://vaers.hhs.gov/data/, accessed June 2, 2011.

Vulnerability

In the PB* case the cost for preventing or treating is the same. So why not put our money into Machine PB* now and prevent the drowning process? One reason may be the uncertainty issue mentioned. Another reason may be disbelief about the likelihood of harm at a time when we (or others) do not feel vulnerable. Because vulnerability (either to ourselves or the *eudaimonia* of others) is a necessary component of compassion, its absence produces less emotion, and therefore we are less likely to be moved to action.

PROXIMITY AND VIVIDNESS

Now let us examine some of the proximity-related time and space issues in prevention vs. treatment and how they affect vividness. There are many similarities in the ways we consider space and time separately, and almost invariably we end up conflating them. We can be very close geographically, but distant temporally (1 mile as the crow flies, but 3 hours through winding mountainous roads to get there). Similarly, we can be very distant geographically, but close temporally (access to a jet plane can make the 706 mile trip from Albuquerque to Austin only a couple of hours). Space and time are physically interchangeable elements. The concept of near and far are "intuitive measures of proximity" (Kamm 2000).

PB*—being able to pay by credit card to either prevent or treat with full recovery—is unrealistic; it assumes complete recovery and normalization of the child's life. It does not consider any residual effects such as posttraumatic stress disorder, pneumonia, and fear of water later by the child saved. It also does not isolate the prevention component for which there is no obvious treatment option. Furthermore, it assumes that there is a reliable sensor that never fails to rescue. Let us try another Pond scenario that isolates the action from the future harm:

> Pond Barrier 2-hour (PB2H): I alone see a pond with an anonymous child playing around it. I know that this child will be drowning in the pond 2 hours from now. If I put $500 into the machine now it will put a barrier between the child and drowning just at the right time, preventing the child from drowning. I have to get to a meeting and can't hang around, so I need to make a decision now.

PB2H does not permit me to see the effects of my act (as I can in Pond Now and Pond Hidden). But it has also introduced a new element as compared with PB*: PB2H does not permit me to hedge my bets—I am unable to save the drowning child if I do not act now, even though it is 2 hours before the actual event will occur. If I can foresee a child's drowning and if I can prevent the drowning through a fail-proof mechanism, is it not worth my $500 to prevent the drowning? In this case I think the term "foresee" is the key issue. Often we don't or we can't imagine the implications of future events even if we can foresee their occurrence; for example, we can foresee that we will die, yet 53% of Americans don't have a will (Findlaw. com 2010). Denial can be one reason for the lack of a will, but so might a lack of emotional imagination on our part to appreciate the consequences of *not* having a will.

In PB2H the "distant" is not a geographic distance, but the 2-hour time delay effect of our action—a type of time distance. Kamm (2000, 663) acknowledges this temporal element by recognizing that time impacts our ability "to traverse a distance, someone who moves very slowly can still be near and someone who has a very fast vehicle can still be far." For Kamm the moral relevance of distance is related to time to action. In all of the Pond cases in this chapter distance is near and actions are effective and timely. The difference is in our willingness to take action based upon when we think the action will take effect and how long it is from now until then. The moral relevance, similar to Kamm's reasoning, is the relationship of time and action.

The true test of the priority of preventing or treating harm comes then in a *comparison* of two pond cases:

> Pond Comparison (PC): I am walking between two ponds. In pond 1 is the Pond Hidden (PH) scenario, in which I will not witness the child's drowning or death, but will be told it is happening in real time. In pond 2 is the Pond Barrier 2-Hour (PB2H) scenario, in which I will prevent the same child from drowning 2 hours from now. My credit card is limited to $500 of expenditure. Do I put my credit card into the machine at Pond 1 (PH) or Pond 2 (PB2H)?

Empirically most of us likely would put our money into the PH scenario even though PB2H would actually create more net well-being—the child in PB2H would not experience any of the "process of drowning" sequelae that he might in PH. The only conceivable reason to choose PH and not PB2H is because we know harm is happening *right now*, and this somehow moves us to act *right now*. Otherwise we could simply flip a coin to choose, or we could make the argument that preventing harm is more important than alleviating harm, and choose PB2H.[19]

---

19. We could also do the comparison, call it PC*: should we choose to save a child drowning now or to save (not prevent) a child from drowning in 2 hours. This asks, "Do we owe an equal moral effort toward those who will have *future harm* (for treatment) than toward those

Here is one last set of scenarios to which I will refer in my further analysis. Assume you have only $500 total to give to the Famine *Now* Charity, or the Famine *Later* Charity:

Famine Now (FN): I know that there are 500 people on the other side of the world who are starving. A $500 contribution will completely alleviate the problem for these 500 currently starving folks for the foreseeable future.

Famine Later (FL): I know that there are 500 well-nourished people on the other side of the world who will be starving in 1 month if I don't *now* give $500 to the Famine Later Charity to prevent their upcoming famine. If I contribute, the beneficiaries will maintain their well-nourished status for the foreseeable future.

This is similar to the PC case, but there are a couple of differences. First, more lives are involved for the same cost than in the Pond cases. Second, I cannot witness any of the pain and consequences of the harm currently being inflicted (FN) or that will be inflicted in the future (FL). Third, the spatial proximity variable is neutralized—both scenarios are "on the other side of the world." In addition, though, in FL I am restricted by the lack of both spatial and temporal proximity variables. In both cases my imagination must be used to understand, sympathize for, and judge how I should act with my limited resources.

Recognizing these differences, how many people would give $500 to the FL group that is currently healthy even with foreseeable future harm? A quick review of the various organizations that exist related to nutrition are labeled "Hunger Relief" and include organizations with names such as "Save the Children" or "Action Against Hunger" or "Americans for Famine Relief" or "Empty Bowls" or "Stop Hunger Now." These are self-described humanitarian "relief" organizations, meaning they emphasize Famine Now scenarios. Our overwhelming desire to help those in nutritional need goes to those with current need. There is something in our moral awareness to help the needy that directs us to help the needy *now*.

Alternatively, it could be argued that *development* assistance programs are those that deal with Famine Later scenarios; these organizations work to

---

with harm today (for treatment)?" This question would invoke both temporal issues and issues involving resources: if we were to use up all of our resources in treatment today, we would have none for future treatment. If we reserved some resources from today's treatment allocations for future treatment allocations, then we'd have to determine how to prioritize today's needy, i.e., those undergoing current harm.

improve infrastructures such as clean drinking water, proper sanitation, crop development, and food transport. Because of various marketing activities designed to raise money by aid organizations, and because of the lack of uniform reporting requirements for these organizations, it is difficult to know the relative allocations between relief aid and development aid. A recent *Wall Street Journal* article (Maxey 2010) states:

> The economic turmoil of recent years has helped drive the trend toward a longer-term focus among philanthropists. . .With less to give, donors want to be certain that what they do give goes as far as possible, and many are deciding that means helping people improve their lives and their prospects, not just relieving their immediate suffering.

Because, as the Maxey article points out, many governments don't have the funds to maintain long-term projects, some philanthropies "are requiring aid recipients to develop their own sustainability plans." Whether this ends up being a long-term trend remains to be seen. Even so, does it mean philanthropy would go so far as to attend to healthy individuals per FL? Certainly some of the sustainability projects do just that, though the donors may not think in terms of healthy individuals or groups, so much as not having to relieve future harms.

Another issue with Famine Now vs. Famine Later: in addition to our inability to imagine as well how healthy-looking people might suffer, we also have less ability to sympathize with the plight of larger numbers of people as compared with individuals.[20] Images of large groups of starving people are less vivid than of the poor individual starving child with a large belly, flies crawling on his or her brow, and an empty bowl.

I recognize that all the cases noted above, including the original thought experiment of BJPH, ask us to evaluate our actions related to death and prolonging life. This notion of extending life is deeply ingrained in both health care and moral decision making, partially because death is an easily measured endpoint. However, the reality is that a child who almost drowns, or an adult who is treated for a disease that could have been prevented, will have diminished

---

20. This is true even though it may take less energy intellectually to "love humanity," for it may distance us from our emotions, as well as cause us to make fewer efforts because we feel the futility of trying to impact humanity as a whole. As Fyodor Dostoevsky (2009/1880) points out in *The Brothers Karamazov*: "'I love humanity,' he [an anonymous doctor] said, 'but I wonder at myself. The more I love humanity in general, the less I love man in particular.'" Hume (1740/2001, Part 1, Book II, Chapter 4) recognized this as well in his *Treatise*: "When a quality becomes very general, and is common to a great many individuals, it leads not the mind directly to any one of them; but by presenting at once too great a choice, does thereby prevent the imagination from fixing on any single object."

health for some time period. We could modify various scenarios further by changing the possible outcomes; once the child is rescued she will. . .

- recover only partially, leaving her with some neurological damage that will diminish her ability to do arithmetic;
- recover fully physically, but have ongoing nightmares and require psychotherapy for 5 years related to her heightened fear of minimally risky situations, such as walking around bodies of water;
- recover only partially and have a significant inability to ambulate without a walker and handicapped assistance;
- eventually recover physically fully, but only after postdrowning pneumonia, sepsis, renal dialysis, time in the intensive care unit, etc.

Each of these may modify our willingness to deposit $500 in advance of the event depending on our own previous encounters with and understandings of the severity of these outcomes. Were we to modify the Pond cases by determining the nondeath impact of our actions, we might then clearly prefer the PB and P2H over the PN and PB* cases because our net impact would be more positive—we would not only be saving or extending lives, but also saving the morbidity-associated concerns surrounding the drowning activity and its sequelae, such as those mentioned above. The children's lives would be substantially enhanced by what they did not experience: the drowning sensations before rescue.

Spatial Proximity

Spatial proximity is important in vividness as a component of compassion for two reasons: the ability to imagine (1) the suffering of the individual and (2) the effectiveness of an act. Hidden behind a wall (PH) we don't witness the drowning child, nor do we witness the effect of our act of putting a credit card into the PH Machine. Perhaps we don't *believe* the child is actually drowning, or we don't think our payment for an occurrent barrier will be effective at the time. Either way, we can't imagine as vividly the child or the act.

When looking at the question of effectiveness Kamm (2000) notes that we have an obligation to bring things that are far and effective closer to help someone near, but that we don't necessarily have the same obligation to move things that are near to a far distance to alleviate suffering. Similarly, when we see a patient such as Bill in our office we see the pain or discomfort, evoking our compassion, which includes a drive for action to alleviate the pain. When we don't see a patient, but, say, hear about a fellow physician's patient who also has Bill's symptoms, we may be able to relate to the problem and imagine the discomfort of the fellow-physician's patient because we have treated many people such as Bill. But because we do not have contact with the patient directly we may not feel the drive to help the other physician's patient.[21]

As mentioned above, time to help may be more important than distance to help because we can be effective if we can get to the patient "in time." Similarly, distance may be compromised as a barrier through electronic means: if I am Skyping with a patient my sense of nearness may be just as strong as if I am in the same room, even if the patient is around the world. I may be motivated to seek out help for the patient by contacting colleagues in India who could treat the patient, even if I cannot affect the patient directly. At the same time, because of temporal need, such lack of spatial proximity can evoke great anxiety in physicians – they want to help a patient but being so far from the health care system in which the patient would need to obtain help they don't know how to access the proper resources during this temporal need.

Temporal Proximity

A vivid image is more forceful in some modes than others. Seeing a black and white grainy photograph of a suffering person in 1880s dress is less likely to evoke an emotional response than seeing a color video of a woman writhing in pain in an auto accident in 2011. Similarly, seeing the color video is less emotionally evocative than actually being at the auto accident and experiencing the woman writhing in real time. Being at the auto accident in real time is more evocative than seeing a life-like dramatization of a woman suffering in a future auto accident ("imagine this. . .").

Loewenstein et al. (2001) have differentiated anticipat_ory_ from anticipat_ed_ emotions; the former are "immediate visceral reactions (e.g., fear, anxiety, dread)" whereas the latter are "typically not experienced in the immediate present but are expected to be experienced in the future." *Anticipatory* emotions are those used in evaluating the suffering person, whereas *anticipated* emotions are those used in considering future outcomes in more deliberative decision-making models. This difference in how emotions are in play during treatment or

---

21. Here I mean specifically the lesser compassion (or simply empathy) we may feel for the patient, not because we don't have the professional obligation to act for that patient at that time. Of course, we may want to help the physician think through the best way to treat the patient out of our fellowship with our physician colleague. Alternatively, because of compassion fatigue, we may have no feelings related to the patient at all, but simply hear the story and offer advice dispassionately. Similarly, if I am not on call for tonight I can turn off my pager/cell phone even for my own patients – by eliminating spatial proximity through telephone access I am not reminded of their needs and can put their suffering out of my mind.

preventive actions would bias us toward treatment—we should see Bill because we are having anticipatory emotional responses to him, whereas our understanding of John's concerns are merely anticipated responses.

Partially because of this difference between anticipatory and anticipated responses we alleviate those in immediate harm either in purposeful or oblivious disregard for the future health of others, or perhaps even accounting for the fact that we will be providing fewer resources to prevent future disease and disability. Our emotions as judgments (Loewenstein et al. 2001) are simply revealing our considered value judgment that it is worth more to alleviate today's distress now than it is to prevent tomorrow's distress; we value alleviation efforts for today's pain more than tomorrow's pain, today's dysfunction more than tomorrow's dysfunction, today's threat to life more than tomorrow's threat to life. *Anticipated* responses lack the temporal proximity vividness that *anticipatory* responses provide.

Williams (1985, 185–86) considers this not just an emotional judgment, but a deliberative priority that constitutes an obligation:

> One type of obligation. . .[a] positive sort, involves the obligations of immediacy. Here, a high deliberative priority is imposed by an emergency, such as the rescue case we considered before. A general ethical recognition of people's vital interests is focused into a deliberative priority of immediacy, and it is immediacy to *me* that generates *my* obligation, one I cannot ignore without blame. . .In the positive kind of case. . .the underlying disposition is a general concern, which is not always expressed in deliberative priority, and what produces an obligation from it is, precisely, the emergency.

This orientation to immediacy, although directly linked to vividness, also has other rational purposes. For example, metaphysically our lives are time linear. If we do not survive this moment we will not experience the next moment. If we are just discussing mortality/survival we should help people survive this moment without using resources now for future moments.[22] If we are discussing

22. Admittedly we do not *mentally* live linearly. Indeed, it is rare that we "live" in the present. Although we experience qualia through our senses, we are constantly filtering such perceptions through our thoughts, including memories and anticipations. Desires, beliefs, and intentions related to our future intermingle with "reliving" and/or "revising" the past. Our imagination ". . .corrects reality, it enhances colors, and the habitual greyness of life, composed of both light and somber tones, is intensified by imagination to the pitch of black and white" (Tatarkiewicz 1966). Because we may value different memories and expectations differently, we might then value different times of our lives differently as well. In this sense our preferences for when and how we live our lives may change from time to time, even revaluing what we have done or experienced or what we wish to do in our coming moments. We revise and self-justify (rationalize) the past ("gaining perspective"). From our prior physical

suffering that does not lead to death, though, the question is current and future well-being, not an existential threat of mortality.

Time and Well-Being

In analyzing well-being Derek Parfit (1984, 185–86) takes up our various attitudes toward time from the agent's perspective.[23] Parfit addresses the question, "How should I act as an agent related to fulfilling *my own* desires, satisfactions, or preferences?" In the cases presented earlier in this chapter the question has been, "What should be my decision on how to act to benefit *others*?" Generally it is difficult to separate these questions, because often our intuition derives from how we would want to be treated (a "golden rule" type of deliberation); personal preferences are relevant. A component of our definition of compassion can include the observer's sense of vulnerability. So it might be instructional to consider how Parfit looks at time.

Parfit's second part of *Reasons and Persons* concerns how time is involved in the "Self-Interest" and "Present-aim" theories (S-theory and P-theory, respectively). The former should be the guiding principle for someone who wishes to "make his life go, for him, as well as possible" (1984, 3). The latter should be the guiding principle for someone who wishes to best achieve his present aim(s). As part of his critique of these two theories Parfit looks at various attitudes to time (1984, Chap. 8). He discusses whether the S-theorist and the P-theorist would prefer past, present, or future desires. The S-theorist "can rationally ignore desires that are not mine." The P-theorist would claim "I can rationally now ignore desires that are not mine now." Thus the P-theorist does not worry about past desires, nor need he or she strive to fulfill such desires; the only desires that count are those that should be fulfilled to achieve his or her current aims.

The S-theorist and P-theorist would agree that I "should give equal weight to all of my present and future desires." *Now* my future desire is not my present aim, but *then* it will be. Assuming I am not falling into a senile dementia, I am likely to be wiser in the future than I am now. This means that my judgments in the future will be better than those now. If so, then even *now* I should give more weight to my "future evaluative desires" than to my present ones. But this is not

experiences we alter our priorities for the future, all while consciously or subconsciously absorbing what is happening in the present. And as we revise the past we alter how we perceive reality in space and time.

23. The dominant discussion about present, past, and future occurs from Parfit (1984, 145–95).

how we usually think and act. Parfit claims that though rationally it doesn't make sense (at least according to the P and S theories), we act consistently with a "bias toward the near." This is not because of uncertainty, but because of the way we think about nearer and later. Parfit (1984, 159) quotes Jeremy Bentham: "although we should be rationally concerned about the future, we should be less concerned about it according as it is more remote—and this quite independently of any doubt which attaches to the more remote." Rationally we are willing to endure something bad now for a future good, but as the bad gets closer in time, we generally choose something good now, even though it means we are less likely to achieve our more distant goal. Furthermore, we care less about the *further* future than the *nearer* future.

This bias toward the near is not exclusive and absolute. There are times when we exhibit a bias toward the future (Parfit 1984, 160):

> we bring pains into the nearer future, and postpone pleasures. The bias towards the future provides the explanation. We want to get the pains behind us and to keep the pleasures before us. Since the second bias [towards the future] counteracts the first [toward the present], our tendency to act in these two ways cannot show that we have no bias towards the near. Our bias towards the near may be always outweighed by our bias towards the future.

This bias toward the future is exhibited by, for example, saving money for our child's education or our own retirement. We are postponing gratification, or perhaps in some ways not even experiencing the pleasures of gratification if, for example, we provide a trust for our great-grandchild's education, with the unlikely possibility of ever seeing the child actually enjoy those funds when going to college.

On the other hand, as Parfit notes, we have a significant bias to the near when we think about pain: an hour of pain today may not be preferable to 5 hours of pain in the future.[24] Should we care about pains that are in the nearer future more than those that are in the more distant future? Perhaps, particularly if we believe that we can reduce or eliminate the more distant future pains in some way. This is the causative question: if we can affect pains in the future by reducing them somehow, then most likely if we know they are coming sooner rather than later then rationally we would want to work harder at reducing sooner pains than worrying about (being distracted by) future pains. But, at the same

---

24. Of course, we would much prefer that all of the pain be in the past, but this is not relevant to the inquiry at hand. As Parfit says, "If we did not know whether we have suffered for several hours, or shall later suffer for one hour, most of us would strongly prefer the first to be true" (1984, 167).

time, "Since we can affect both the near and the distant future, our bias towards the near often makes us act against our own interest [related to the distant]" (1984, 169). Although this may be true, it still may be rational—we have a more urgent need to deal with what is happening now or in the nearer future than with what will be happening in the more distant future.

Parfit claims that most of us have a third attitude toward time, an *intrinsic* bias toward the present. Pains are important because they are *now*. *Risks* of pains (or harm) are important only insofar as they *become* pains (or harm), and that can happen only in the becoming present, not in the future. If pains/harms are inevitable they will become the "now" and they will become the priority, even if their current alleviation may cause us greater pains/harms in the future.

As I noted at the beginning of this section, how we act to benefit ourselves is not necessarily how we do or should act toward others. But it seems reasonable to believe that our view of beneficence is clearly colored by our views of what our personal preferences would be. Even though it would be rational to be "equally concerned to all parts of [our] future" (Parfit 1982) we are not. And though it would be rational to be equally concerned about all parts of our patients' futures, we are not—precisely because, at least partly, we act for others on the basis of how we would act for ourselves. The affirmative "golden rule" is at work in our decisions as to whom we would see. Thus we choose Bill over John or Famine Now over Famine Later on a "present" vs. "future" choice, and we would choose Pond Now (and Pond Hidden) over Pond Barrier 2 Hour on a near-future over a distant-future choice because we choose for ourselves based on a bias toward the present, even if not always specifically vividness related.

Now it may well be that in the future, *physical* life will not need to be lived consecutively. Although physically reliving the past is unlikely, physically altering our ability as to when we will live in the future may be possible. The idea that we might be able to place ourselves in a type of suspended animation or hibernation may not be long off.[25] This could mean that in a physical sense we could choose when we want our future lives to be. Suppose I know that I am happier in the presence of my children than in their absence, but I also know that my children are not likely to be in my presence for the next 5 years, because, for example, they are off to college, or starting their careers across the country. If I had the option to take those 5 years and use them when I have grandchildren,

---

25. See, for example (Bakalar 2005): "Researchers have succeeded in putting mice, without harming them, into a state of suspended animation that looks suspiciously like that of a hibernating bear. If the technique can be applied to humans, the scientists say, it may eventually offer new ways to treat hypothermia, slow down bleeding in traumatic injuries, quickly reduce high fevers, or even help heart attack patients in emergencies by slowing their breathing and heart rates."

perhaps I might choose to live discontinuously—take the next 5 years "in hibernation" and append them on to what otherwise would have been the end of my life. Or alternatively, if we have the (unlikely) option of reliving several years that were particularly happy ones, thereby cutting short future years, would we choose to do so? *Should* we choose to do so?

I raise these issues because inherent in how we view life and the flow of time related to life is how we value our lives within the flow of time. And how we value our lives within the flow of time is complex, uneven, and fraught with memory, circumstance, and commitments. Can we say that those who value the immediate treatment for current illness are more or less rational about the view of their lives related to the flow of time than those who value the prevention of future harm? As Heyd (1983) says,

> we do have preferences (of a utilitarian kind) about our lives—both past ("I don't regret it," "I wish I was never born") and future ("I wish I could live longer," "let me die—such a life is not worth it"). . .we sometimes examine our present and expected future and decide whether it is worth living or not. Most of us strive hard to prolong life, *on the assumption that almost any kind of life is worth living.*

Because we assume that "almost any kind of life is worth living" at least in the context of life vs. no life, we strive to maintain a life over all other priorities.

Some might argue that we have an imbalance between alleviating current harm and preventing future harm because the former conforms to a symbolic belief that life has no price—we must preserve it at all costs. However, as Menzel (1983, Chap. 7) points out, there is an inherent paradox in making such claims. By devoting valuable resources to alleviating current harm we are implicitly stating that we put less value on preventing future harm; in other words, life may be essentially priceless (or have an extremely high price) if it is threatened today, but will have a price (or a substantially lesser price) if it is threatened tomorrow. Yet for *life itself,* it would seem odd to believe that this is the case.

And so, at any rate, we choose to emphasize our use of resources for the present. Our priorities seem to be in the order of (1) ensuring the physical continuity of life now, (2) alleviating current harm now, and then (3) preventing future harm. There is even a priority that often comes before preventing future harm: (2') *alleviating future* harm. We devote tremendous resources to "being prepared" for future harm. Our military medicine in times of peace is devoted to keeping the fighting force fit, and being prepared for battlefield injuries and illnesses if a war develops. Our U.S. hospital system is overbedded and supplied for increased need. We are supplying airplanes, apartment buildings, and public facilities with automated electronic defibrillators. Our emergency preparedness system holds community-wide disaster drills. In the past few years we have seen significant resources devoted to pandemic emergency preparedness planning. Whether these activities exceed or equal our "pure" prevention activities is difficult to assess, but nevertheless they are a significant priority in the U.S. health care system.

The notion that we must preserve present life and near-future life in order to have the option of preserving distant-future life has a pragmatic rationale to it, but it doesn't explain our alleviation bias entirely. The proof of this is in the moral distinctions we often make between preserving a life now and preserving a life in the future that would sacrifice the present life for the future life. For if present life were *always* preferable to future life then *all* of our resources would be devoted to providing for alleviating current harm and *no* resources would be devoted to preventing future harm. If our priorities were always those derived in the prior paragraph in the order of 1 > 2 > 3 then we (in theory) might never get to 3 because there is always more harm, suffering, and near-death situations in the world than we possibly have resources to alleviate.[26] We see ourselves shift to 3 when we combine the probabilities of being effective with the size of the threatened risk based on the malady that's at stake, and make some trade-offs into prevention when the gains there are noticeably larger than the gains from 1 and 2. If we never came to think in such statistical fashion, we might never limit 1 and 2. But we do limit 1 and 2, because there is some threshold that permits us to overcome our bias toward 1 and 2, even if spatial and temporal vividness are diminished and compassion through imagination is limited. The big question is, why don't we do it more often, i.e., what is the limit of that threshold?

What Is a Temporal Proximity Threshold?

If Pond Barrier 2 Hour (PB2H) is a foreseeable event in 2 hours, would we think differently if we were preventing an event in 2 days (PB2D)? In 2 weeks (PB2W)? In 2 Years (PB2Y)? How far ahead are we willing to look when there is (theoretical) certainty of outcomes? Would/should PB2H have priority over PB2D or PB2Y? With identical outcomes utilitarians most likely would say they are indifferent—putting our $500 in either circumstance is praiseworthy (and obligatory). But as we've seen above, "vividness imagination" diminishes with

---

26. In fact, we might not even get to 2, *always* attending to 1 in the world. If someone philosophically takes the consecutive view of life as a faith belief, then 2 may be viewed as being instrumental only in achieving 1, and of no value in itself.

time, and therefore also our ability to develop compassion diminishes with time.

It is possible that if I put my $500 in the PB2H slot now I might have the chance to make another $500 to put into the PB2D or PB2W slot later. This violates the thought experiment rules, but also raises the realistic objection to the BJPH case that our choices rarely are so limited in time—we could see John for prevention at another time, even if it means we have to bump another patient with a more minor concern to do so. I took this up earlier with the response that we may have lost the critical opportunity to prevent a disease if we postpone our intervention. There are other responses as well: despite our best efforts we may not gain the additional $500 for PB2D or PB2W. In this case the child in PB2H will be advantaged over those in PB2D/W/Y. Is this fair? Must those who benefit from our largesse always be those who come to our attention first, or who first come down with disease? As noted above, if we are to attend to the most disadvantaged (in time) then, given our limited resources, there will be nothing left for the future disadvantaged. Yet we do decide to store food for the winter and medicines and water for catastrophic events. We choose to pay life insurance premiums instead of sending those funds to our loved ones for current use. There is some threshold of use of funds for the future that is considered beneficial and necessary. We have some level and balance of imagination and rational consideration that spur us to invest some resources in prevention. This says that we *do* give preventing harm priority over alleviating harm *sometimes*—that is, that the vast priority alleviation has over prevention is sometimes limited.

THE "OVERWHELMING EVIDENCE" HYPOTHESIS

If we accept the simple fact that our spending *some* resources on preventing future harm means we sometimes do value prevention over alleviating current harm, then if we could determine why this occurs we might better understand how our moral decision making is impacted by time. Why do we *sometimes* choose PB2Y over PB2H? There may be two reasons: first, because we want to preserve a single life *where there is still a lot of potential life left*—where time remaining seems significant. This is the "potential problem"—a complex element without a clear or consistent claim on preferences for harm alleviation or harm prevention. Thus I shall not discuss it here.

The second reason we might claim a priority for prevention over treatment is when the effectiveness of the prevention effort is overwhelming, either in comparison with the alternative treatments, or just in the bulk force of preventing what would be substantive aggregate (social) harm. Let us call this the

"overwhelming evidence" hypothesis. Our conclusions here may differ depending on our viewpoint; an individual's assessment of evidence may have a different meaning than a social assessment. For example, take the Alar pesticide issue
in 1989. Alar may cause five cancers per million regular apple eaters. Some
individuals may consider this risk intolerable, and politicians acted when
enough constituents in some jurisdictions viewed the risk too high for society
as a whole. Some consumers panicked, discarding millions of apples. On the
other hand, others found the benefits of apple eating, whether for taste or nutritional value, easily overwhelmed the Alar risk, especially after washing apples
carefully.

Tengs et al. (1995) published an analysis of the cost-effectiveness of 587 lifesaving interventions. They reviewed the literature and developed a comparison
of prevention-related costs per life saved. They found that medical intervention
costs per life-year saved were $5,000 for primary prevention, $23,000 for secondary prevention, and $22,000 for tertiary prevention (disease rehabilitation).
Some interventions, such as childhood immunizations, colorectal screening
using the stool guaiac test for those age 55+, drug and alcohol treatment in
select cases, and prenatal care all cost ≤$0 per life saved. In other words, they
save more resources than they consume. However, most medical interventions
have substantially higher costs than any resources they may save, ranging from
the thousands to the millions of dollars per life saved. (See Russell, Chapter 3 of
this volume.) In looking down this long list of tertiary interventions, essentially
all are covered by insurance in the United States, including coverage by
Medicare. Yet, if an "overwhelming evidence" argument is to be made, then
many of those in the list at the upper ends of the cost per life saved would be
replaced by more effective means.

For example, an exercise stress test for asymptomatic men aged 60 costs $40
per life saved, whereas coronary angiography in men aged 45–64 with angina
costs marginally $28,000 (compared with medical therapy). This secondary
prevention (exercise stress test) vs. intervention (angiography) ratio is 1:700 at
the margin (over medical therapy). Yet in the United States the exercise stress
test for asymptomatic men is not a covered benefit in most insurance plans,
whereas both angiography and medical therapy are.[27] Perhaps "overwhelming
evidence" is still feasible, but we'd need to exceed the 1:700 ratio, which may not
be a sufficient threshold to require coverage.

It is not empirically obvious to see how in the United States we choose certain "overwhelming evidence" prevention activities to have preference over

27. As with my earlier stated assumption that how we spend our money is a function of our
values, I am also assuming that those benefits that are typically covered by insurance are a
surrogate for values as well.

harm alleviation. Other nations (e.g., Britain, Australia, and Canada) have started to use "evidence" more transparently. More research is needed in the United States to see if an "overwhelming evidence" factor pushes for harm prevention more than it does for harm alleviation.

COMPASSION, OBLIGATION, SUPEREROGATION, AND REWARDS

Although I have treated the BJPH and Pond cases similarly, there is one significant difference that may be important: in the BJPH cases both Bill and John have arrived looking for care from the physician agent. In the Pond cases the agent must initiate action without a request from the drowning (or future drowning) child. In BJPH, as a physician, I am given certain privileges in society in return for my accepting responsibilities that are not required of a nonphysician. It is expected (and required) that I respond to my established patients. In the Pond or Famine cases I am a citizen without prior-established obligations. I am praised for voluntarily responding to and assisting others to whom I do not have a special relationship. The former is obligatory; the latter is supererogatory.

But in both cases—as a physician with a dilemma of which patient to see between two established patients, or as a citizen faced with Pond Now or Pond Barrier 2 Hour (for example) permitted to act in a supererogatory manner—I still need to make a choice between alleviating current harm or preventing future harm. So this distinction between obligation and supererogation does not help us make a decision in either the BJPH or Pond/Famine cases. The only difference might be that in the supererogation position I do not have to act at all. The simple fact that it is considered supererogatory means that it is optional behavior. Thus I might be less likely to act in the Pond or Famine cases, but does this reluctance or hesitation mean I will make a different decision if I do act? Because I don't feel the same moral pressure to act, might I choose to do so only on the basis of alleviating harm, with an underlying assumption that preventing harm does not offer as much satisfaction or as many rewards?

Quite possibly. Though society purportedly values rational action, it tends not to reward those who act logically and responsibly in the cool hour of reflection. There seems to be a sense that there is less risk in acting to prevent than in acting to alleviate. Consequently there typically is less praise provided as well. The physical act of putting $500 into a machine in Pond Now or Pond Barrier 2 Hour is the same. The motivation of helping a child who is or will be drowning is the same. The desire and intention are similar. But society and the child's parents are more likely to respond with great relief and praise to the one

who acts at the time of despair (Pond Now/Bill/Famine Now) than at the time
in advance of despair (Pond Barrier 2H/John/Famine Later). Awards for heroism are given to the citizen who plucks the drowning child out of the pond long
before recognition is given to those who build fences around the pond. Thus,
might a conscious or subconscious sense of reward be skewing our inclination
toward alleviation over prevention?

This is, of course, a circular argument. If we alleviate because we know (consciously or subconsciously) there will be greater rewards, then somehow we
have learned that our acts of alleviation are more praiseworthy, and, therefore,
when faced with the choice, we will do more alleviation and less prevention. At
the same time we reinforce the value of alleviation, which means we will be
more likely to praise alleviation, which means those who act on the motivation
of praise will do more alleviation, etc. But we are still left with the fundamental
question, "Why are we rewarded more for alleviation? From where did this
greater valuing arise?"[28] The circular nature of the "rewards" argument does
not help us explain our alleviation bias. It may very well be that we reward
action in hectic times because we can better use our imaginations to consider
the consequences were we not to have acted (alleviating harm).

CONCLUSIONS

I have argued that our alleviation bias is a function of our compassion, which is
animated by spatial and temporal vividness. Additionally, physicians have obligations that skew us toward alleviation bias—helping those in immediate need
based upon our professional social contract. These are empirical claims, bol-
stered by psychological studies (Loewenstein et al. 2001; Slovic et al. 2007) and
other philosophical musings (Solomon 1977, 1993).

Hume (1740/2001, Book 2, Part 3, Section 7, §1-3) stated in his *A Treatise on
Human Nature*:

> There is an easy reason, why every thing contiguous to us, either in space
> or time, shou'd be conceiv'd with a peculiar force and vivacity, and excel
> every other object, in its influence on the imagination. Ourself is intimately
> present to us, and whatever is related to self must partake of that quality.
> But where an object is so far remov'd as to have lost the advantage of this

---

28. If there is any question about the value of alleviation vs. prevention in the United States,
just look at the payment for physician services. Surgical and diagnostic procedures are
reimbursed at considerably higher levels than nonprocedure services, such as prevention-
oriented lifestyle behavior counseling.

relation, why, as it is farther remov'd, its idea becomes still fainter and more obscure, wou'd, perhaps, require a more particular examination.

'Tis obvious, that the imagination can never totally forget the points of space and time, in which we are existent; but receives such frequent advertisements of them from the passions and senses, that however it may turn its attention to foreign and remote objects, it is necessitated every moment to reflect on the present. . .

. . .Contiguous objects must have an influence much superior to the distant and remote. . .that men are principally concern'd about those objects, which are not much remov'd either in space or time, enjoying the present, and leaving what is afar off to the care of chance and fortune.

If, as Solomon (1977, 1993) asserts, emotions are deliberative, then perhaps this empirical finding of compassion driving our values is correct. We know that cognitive understanding is only one driver in policy-making, and it often is not how we tend to respond to daily concerns. In human motivation and behavior, it just seems to be that alleviating vivid, immediate suffering evokes our compassion as a value that exceeds our rational design, a value that outweighs calculated utility.

Tatarkiewicz (1966) may say it best: "The present? It is, after all, only a moment—and I can endure even the most dreadful moment, provided I know that things will be better soon." And, thus, we are quite content with doing more to fix the current "dreadful moment" so as to "know that things will be better soon."

As a caregiver, I follow the same sympathetic responses to my patients as I would want for myself. I would want my current "dreadful moment" alleviated as soon as possible, and so I will alleviate one patient's current "dreadful moment" as a priority over another patient's future "dreadful moment." I will work to prevent future "dreadful moments" as a priority for patients only if I know that "the most dreadful [current] moment" is fleeting and not enduring; if it is not a portent of some fatal or debilitating illness that will make our lives unhappy for the future.

This empirical claim does not, of course, mean this is how things should be. Recall that earlier in this chapter my acceptance of the term compassion was based on Nussbaum's five components, including being associated with "a painful emotion." Vividness is a strong influence of this component. Perhaps normatively we can say that it provides *undue* influence, minimizing our ability to consider the future. It clouds our judgments as evidenced by its not providing us with a clear delineation of where the threshold should be between alleviating and preventing.

A common public health sector cry for more prevention resources is often based on a combination of cognitive reasoning and philosophical claims that incorporate a form of compassion that minimizes the vividness component and maximizes the *eudaimonia* component for a population. It is a greater abstraction of the future than a vivid animation of today. It is a claim that the empathic component of compassion weighs too heavily on our policy decision making.

Is it right to claim that we should rebalance the influence of various components of compassion? Perhaps. But if we do, we have to show how we can psychologically dampen our affect heuristic, or retrain how we form judgments from our passions. And we need to do it for whole populations, which in democratic societies determine resource allocation through the political process.

If you asked me, I'd tell you that I'd see John because of my prevention bias. My internal development toward a prevention bias was made early in my career. A deeper probing of the motivation behind my prevention bias might find my rebellion at the wastefulness of the medical establishment, my delight in looking at the economic and political processes of health policy formation, or my enjoyment of running. Certainly within all of these there were judgments formed *from* emotions and *as* emotions. How might I tease them all apart? That is the mystery of rational man (Searle 2001). At the same time, as Hume (1740/2001) reminds us in his *Treatise*, "Whatever supports and fills the passions is agreeable to us; as on the contrary, what weakens and infeebles them is uneasy."

ACKNOWLEDGMENTS

Thanks to Kelly Sorensen, Miller Brown, and Frances Kamm, for their reviews and comments on earlier drafts of this chapter. Special thanks goes to Paul Menzel, who gave me great counsel on revising the organization of this chapter and improving my arguments. Thanks also to the members of the Hartford Ethics Group and the Santa Fe Ethics Group for discussions of initial drafts.

REFERENCES

Audi, R. 2008. Intuition, Inference, and Rational Disagreement in Ethics. *Ethical Theory and Moral Practice* 11:475–92.

Bakalar, N. 2005. Hibernating Mice May Someday Save Humans. *New York Times*, April 26: 1.

Beauchamp, T.L., and Childress, J.F. 2001. *Principles of Biomedical Ethics*, 5th ed. New York: Oxford University Press.

Chang, J.T., Staffa, J.A., Parks, M., and Green, L. 2004. Rhabdomyolysis with HMG-CoA Reductase Inhibitors and Gemfibrozil Combination Therapy. *Pharmacoepidemiology and Drug Safety* 13 (7):417–26.

Cogswell, B., and Eggert, M.S. 1993. People Want Doctors to Give More Preventive Care—A Qualitative Study of Health Care Consumers. *Archives of Family Medicine* 2:611–19.

Council of Medical Specialty Societies. 1999. Ethics Statement. Available at http://www.cmss.org/DefaultTwoColumn.aspx?id=79, accessed June 2, 2011.

Crisp, R. 2008. Compassion and Beyond. *Ethical Theory and Moral Practice* 11:233–46.

Daniels, S.R., Greer, F.R., and Committee on Nutrition. 2008. Lipid Screening and Cardiovascular Health in Childhood. *Pediatrics* 122 (1):198–208.

Dostoyevsky, F. 2009. *The Brothers Karamazov* [1880]. Available at http://www.readprint.com/work-612/The-Brothers-Karamazov-Fyodor-Dostoevsky, accessed June 2, 2011.

Faust, H.S. 2009. Kindness, Not Compassion, in Healthcare. *Cambridge Quarterly of Healthcare Ethics* 18 (3):287–99.

Findlaw.com. 2010. *Most Americans Still Don't Have a Will, Says New Survey by Findlaw* 2009. Available at http://company.findlaw.com/pr/2002/081902.will.html, accessed June 2, 2011.

Fletcher, S.W., and Elmore, J.G. 2003. Mammographic Screening for Breast Cancer. *New England Journal of Medicine* 349 (6):1672–80.

Foot, P. 1967. The Problem of Abortion and the Doctrine of Double Effect. *Oxford Review* 5:5–15.

Furrow, B.R., Greaney, T.L., Johnson, S.H., Jost, T.S., and Schwartz, R.L. 2000. *Health Law*. St. Paul, MN: West Group.

Gerber, M.A., Randolph, M.F., Chanatry, J., Wright, L.L, De Meo, K., and Kaplan, E.L. 1987. Five vs Ten Days of Penicillin V Therapy for Streptococcal Pharyngitis. *American Journal of Diseases of Children* 141 (2):224–27.

Harvard Program in Ethics and Health. 2009. *Fourth Annual International Conference on Ethical Issues in Prioritization of Health Resources*. Available at http://peh.harvard.edu/events/2009/priority_resources/day1.html; http://peh.harvard.edu/events/2009/priority_resources/day2.html, accessed July 29, 2011.

Heyd, D. 1983. Is Life Worth Reliving? *Mind* 92 (365):21–37.

Hume, D. 1740/2001. In D.F. Norton and M.J. Norton, Eds., *A Treatise of Human Nature*. New York: Oxford University Press.

Jamieson, D. 1999. Singer and the Practical Ethics Movement. In D. Jamieson, Ed., *Singer and His Critics* (pp. 1–17). Malden, MA: Blackwell.

Jenni, K.E., and Loewenstein, G. 1997. Explaining the "Identifiable Victim Effect." *Journal of Risk and Uncertainty* 14:235–57.

Kagan, S. 1998. *Normative Ethics*. In N. Daniels and K. Lehrer, Eds., *Dimensions of Philosophy*. Boulder, CO: Westview Press.

Kamm, F.M. 2000. Does Distance Matter Morally to the Duty to Rescue? *Law and Philosophy* 19:655–81.

Kogut, T., and Ritov, I. 2005. The "Identified Victim" Effect: An Identified Group, or Just a Single Individual? *Journal of Behavioral Decision Making* 18:157–67.

Loewenstein, G.F., Weber, E.U., Hsee, C.K., and Welch, N. 2001. Risk as Feelings. *Psychological Bulletin* 127 (2):267–86.

Mackenbach, J.P., Kunst, A.E., Lautenbach, H., Bijlsma, F., and Oei, Y.B. 1995. Competing Causes of Death: An Analysis Using Multiple-Cause-of-Death Data from The Netherlands. *American Journal of Epidemiology* 141 (5):466–75.

Maxey, D. 2010. Gifts That Keep on Giving. *Wall Street Journal*, April 12: 1.

Menzel, P.T. 1983. *Medical Costs, Moral Choices—A Philosophy of Health Care Economics in America*. New Haven, CT: Yale University Press.

Miller, M., and Solomon, G. 2003. Environmental Risk Communication for the Clinician. *Pediatrics* 112:211–17.

Narayan, K.M., Thompson, T.J., Boyle, J.P., Beckles, G.L., Engelgau, M.M., Vinicor, F., and Williamson, D.F. 1999. The Use of Population Attributable Risk to Estimate the Impact of Prevention and Early Detection of Type 2 Diabetes on Population-Wide Mortality Risk in U.S. Males. *Health Care Management Science* 2 (4):223–27.

Nisbett, R.E., and Ross, L. 1980. *Human Inference: Strategies and Shortcomings of Social Judgment*. Englewood Cliffs, NJ: Prentice-Hall.

Nord, E. 1999. *Cost-Value Analysis in Health Care*. New York: Cambridge University Press.

Nussbaum, M. 2001. *Upheavals of Thought, The Intelligence of Emotions*. New York: Cambridge University Press.

Parfit, D. 1982. Personal Identity and Rationality. *Synthese* 53:227–41.

———. 1984. *Reasons and Persons*. New York: Oxford University Press.

Pearl, J. 2000. *Causality-Models, Reasoning, and Inference*. New York: Cambridge University Press.

Peipins, L.A., and Sandler, R.S. 1994. Epidemiology of Colorectal Adenomas. *Epidemiologic Reviews* 6:273–97.

RottenstreichY., and Hsee, C. 2001. Money, Kisses, and Electric Shocks: On the Affective Psychology of Risk. *Psychological Science* 12 (3):185–90.

Savage, L.J. 1954. *The Foundations of Statistics*. New York: Wiley and Sons.

Searle, J.R. 2001. *Rationality in Action*. Boston, MA: MIT Press.

Shafir, E. 1998. Philosophical Intuitions and Cognitive Mechanisms. In M.R. DePaul and W. Ramsey, Eds., *Rethinking Intuition: The Psychology of Intuition and Its Role in Philosophical Inquiry* (pp. 59–73). New York: Rowan and Littlefield.

Shonkoff, J.P., Boyce, W.T., and McEwen, B.S. 2009. Neuroscience, Molecular Biology, and the Childhood Roots of Health Disparities. *Journal of the American Medical Association* 301 (21):2252–59.

Singer, P. 1972. Famine, Affluence, and Morality. *Philosophy and Public Affairs* 1 (3): 229–43.

Slovic, P., Finucane, M., Peters, E., and MacGregor, D.G. 2007. The Affect Heuristic. *European Journal of Operational Research* 177 (3):1333–52.

Slovic, P., Monahan, J., and MacGregor, D.G. 2000. Violence Risk Assessment and Risk Communication: The Effects of Using Actual Cases, Providing Instruction, and Employing Probability Versus Frequency Formats. *Law and Human Behavior* 24 (3):271–96.

Solomon, R. 1977. The Logic of Emotion. *Nous* 11 (1):41–49.

———. 1993. *The Passions—Emotions and the Meaning of Life*. Indianapolis, IN: Hacking Publishing.

Tatarkiewicz, W. 1966. Happiness and Time. *Philosophy and Phenomenological Research* 27 (1):1–10.

Tengs, T.O., Adams, M.E., Pliskin, J.S., Safran, D.G., Siegel, J.E., Weinstein, M.C., and Graham, J.D. 1995. Five-Hundred Life-Saving Interventions and Their Cost-Effectiveness. *Risk Analysis* 15 (3):369–90.

Thomson, J.J. 1971. A Defense of Abortion. *Philosophy and Public Affairs* 1 (1):47–66.

Unger, P. 1996. *Living High and Letting Die, Our Illusion of Innocence*. New York: Oxford University Press.

Walker, T. 2010. Who Do We Treat First When Resources Are Scarce? *Journal of Applied Philosophy* 27 (2):200–11.

Waller, K., Kujala, U.M., Kaprio, J., Koskenvuo, M., and Rantanen, T. 2010. Effect of Physical Activity on Health in Twins: A 30-yr Longitudinal Study. *Medicine and Science in Sports and Exercise* 42 (4):658–64.

Whitlock, E.P., Lin, J.S., Beil, T.K., and Fu, R. 2008. *Screening for Colorectal Cancer: A Targeted, Updated Systematic Review for the U.S. Preventive Services Task Force*. Agency for Healthcare Research and Quality. Available at http://www.ahrq.gov/clinic/uspstf08/colocancer/coloartwhit.htm, accessed June 2, 2011.

Williams, B. 1985. *Ethics and the Limits of Philosophy*. Cambridge, MA: Harvard University Press.

Williams, T.N., Mwangi, T.W., Wambua, S., Alexander, N.D., Kortok, M., Snow, R.W., and Marsh, K. 2005. Sickle Cell Trait and the Risk of *Plasmodium falciparum* Malaria and Other Childhood Diseases. *Journal of Infectious Diseases* 192:178–86.

Wolf, A.M.D., Wender, R.C., Etzioni, R.B., Thompson, I.M., D'Amico, A.V., Volk, R.J., Brooks, D.D., Dash, C., Guessous, I., Andrews, K., DeSantis, C., and Smith, R.A. 2010. American Cancer Society Guideline for the Early Detection of Prostate Cancer: Update 2010. *CA: A Cancer Journal for Clinicians* 60:70–98.

Zwart, S., Sachs, A.P.E., Ruijs, G.J.H.M., Gubbels, J.W., Hoes, A.W., and de Melker, R.A. 2000. Penicillin for Acute Sore Throat: Randomised Double Blind Trial of Seven Days versus Three Days Treatment or Placebo in Adults. *BMJ* 320:150–54.

8

Treatment and Prevention

What Do We Owe Each Other?

NORMAN DANIELS, PhD ■

OVERVIEW

The fragmented insurance schemes that form the U.S. health care system have been criticized for overemphasizing treatment as opposed to prevention. The claim is that any one insurance plan has no incentive to prevent an illness when saving the cost of treating that prevented illness is likely to benefit another private insurance scheme, for example, if workers change jobs or enter Medicare as they age. In effect, there is little profit in prevention if the savings fatten another bottom line. In what follows, I shall not assess this alleged pattern of missing care. Rather, I shall step back from the specifics of the U.S. system and ask a broader ethical question: what do we owe each other by way of promoting and restoring health, and what does this mean about the balance between prevention and treatment? The answer I give would support the criticism, assuming the empirical claims on which it is based are correct.

I shall argue that we have a robust social obligation to protect and promote health and that this obligation means we owe each other a reasonable array of both preventive and curative interventions. I shall, of course, have to say something about what counts as a reasonable array. The issue is even more complicated than it seems because these preventive efforts must be broader than just the public health and medical services that most people may have in mind. Fair distributions of other important goods—basic liberties, education, job opportunities, income, and wealth—have a significant impact on health, protecting it and distributing it more fairly. Social justice prevents ill health in more ways than through health care alone.

To clarify the scope and content of these social obligations, in the next section I shall briefly sketch answers to three questions of social justice, and in the following (third) section I shall draw some inferences about what those answers mean for both prevention and treatment. After arguing that we have these robust obligations and suggesting something about their scope, I consider a challenge to my view and a possible qualification that may be needed. The challenge arises from a question about the limits to our social obligations or responsibility to promote healthy behavior, since many preventive measures involve altering behavior and thus the choices people make. Specifically, in my view we have a social responsibility to provide incentives that promote health behavior, but so-called "luck egalitarian" views (Anderson 1999) provide no basis for doing so.

I then address this challenge in detail in its own section, and in a further section I consider the qualification: do we sometimes have more pressing obligations to treat people in peril—where the risk is concentrated in them—rather than to prevent the less concentrated risk of that peril in some larger group in which the expected loss of life is the same? Reasonable people may disagree about this, as in the general case of deciding what treatments and preventions we owe each other. We must then rely on a fair, deliberative process to resolve such disagreements, which was my answer to one of the three questions of justice addressed initially.

THREE QUESTIONS ABOUT JUSTICE AND HEALTH

In this section, I sketch a view developed in far greater detail elsewhere (Daniels 2008); my intention is to focus on the implications of this view for treatment and prevention in this chapter rather than to support the view itself. Still, the sketch is needed so that we can be clear that if the view is justifiable, then the implications are as well.

Arguably, three questions are central to concerns about justice and health. Is health of special moral importance, and, if so, why? When are health inequalities unjust? And, how can we meet health needs fairly if we cannot meet them all? These may not be all the key questions a theory of justice and health must address, but it must address these.

Health is of special moral importance because of its limited, but significant contribution to the range of exercisable opportunities people should enjoy. By health, I mean (somewhat controversially) normal functioning. This narrow conception of health [as compared with the WHO definition (WHO 1946)] is intended to distinguish health from the broader notion of well-being and to capture what is really measured when, for example, epidemiologists aggregate departures from normal functioning in order to quantify the level of health (or the burden of disease) in a population. In any case, departures from normal functioning limit the range of opportunities open to people—shortening their lives, reducing their levels of functioning, and thus making it harder or impossible to exercise the opportunities they would have were they healthy.[1] If we have social obligations to protect opportunity, as some theories of justice claim [notably Rawls's 1971 theory, but also some views critical of his, such as Sen's focus on capabilities (1980, 1992) and Arneson's (1988), and Cohen's (1989) defense of equal opportunity for welfare or advantage], then we have derivative obligations to protect and promote health. [I argue elsewhere (Daniels 2010) that my account of exercisable opportunities is very similar to Sen's notion of capabilities.] Accordingly, health is of special moral importance, from the perspective of justice, because of the contribution health makes to opportunity, though it is not, of course, the only social good that contributes to opportunity.

If health care, even broadly construed to include traditional public health measures, were the main determinant of health and its distribution in a population, we might think that we have a ready answer to the following question: when are health inequalities unjust? They would be unjust if different groups have unequal access to health care. What we know, however, from many studies in social epidemiology is that levels of population health and its distribution in a population are determined by a much broader range of social factors (Berkman and Kawachi 2000). For example, the Whitehall studies of British civil servants, all of whom have universal access to health care, have high basic levels of education, and are not impoverished, show that significant health inequalities persist by occupational status; in effect, the higher your occupational status in the British civil service then the longer and healthier your life. These findings are robust across many countries, where we see a socioeconomic status (SES) gradient of health—often compounded by race or ethnicity, depending on local social history; the findings have long historical roots (Krieger 2001).

Producing an equitable distribution of health in a society, then, requires more than universal coverage. It requires much more robust forms of social justice that focus on non-health-sector goods. What we observe from the social

---

1. Opportunities count as exercisable; in my view, if they are part of the plans of life it is reasonable for people to pursue, given their talents and skills and health state. Obviously, other individual factors (e.g., income, wealth, education) and societal factors (technological level, cultural factors) affect the range of opportunities exercisable for individuals. Health makes a significant but limited contribution to an individual's fair share of the range of plans of life it is reasonable to pursue in a given society (the normal opportunity range). See Daniels (1985, 2008).

epidemiology literature is that many factors seem to correlate with higher levels of health, and their inequalities in a society seem to contribute to the gradients of health we observe. Among these factors are levels of education, levels of parental family income and wealth, effective political participation, and broader measures of opportunity. Social status—including a possible impact of relative status—is viewed by some leading social epidemiologists as a crucial contributing factor (Marmot 2004). The fair distribution of many of these determinants of health is the subject of general theories of distributive justice, and I have argued elsewhere (Daniels, Kennedy, and Kawachi 1999; Daniels, Kennedy, and Kawachi 2000) that if we take Rawls's principles of justice as fairness as an illustration, conformance with them would capture key determinants of health, and thus flatten SES gradients of health more than we observe in any real-world setting. (Rawls's theory is particularly interesting in this regard since he allows some inequalities in other goods, such as income and wealth, and these very inequalities may contribute to inequalities in health.) This flattening of the SES gradient is the basis for saying that social justice is good for our health because compliance with principles of justice provides us with preventive health protections that go beyond the health sector.

Because resources are relatively scarce, even in richer countries, we cannot meet every health need. But how can we then meet needs fairly? We might think, as I did years ago, that we should simply determine which health needs have the greatest impact on opportunity, and we should give priority to meeting them. I later realized that we encounter a family of "unsolved rationing problems" (Daniels 1993) that made such an approach inadequate. For example, we might identify a health condition that had the most serious impact on opportunity range, whether it was some form of very early death or persistent coma ("persistent vegetative state"). But if we can do little to cure it, then we could pour resources into a bottomless pit with little gain for anyone. We must balance potential benefit against seriousness of a condition to arrive at a plausible approach, yet we have no principled way of describing how to make that trade-off among goals. Similar problems face us when we aggregate benefits across individuals (which aggregations are morally acceptable?) and when we have to weigh the pursuit of best outcomes against giving people fair chances at some benefit.

In short, we lack prior agreement on principles adequate to resolve disagreements about how to face these distributive problems, just as we lack agreement on a variety of other moral disagreements in health policy (such as how to weigh compassion against stewardship in the case of "last chance" but not fully proven therapies). In the absence of a consensus on principles, we should rely on a form of procedural justice. Specifically, James Sabin and I (Daniels and Sabin 2002) have specified the conditions such a fair deliberative process should meet if decision makers are to be "accountable for the reasonableness" of their decisions. Not only does such a process enhance the legitimacy of decisions, but also arguably it provides us with a "defeasible" fair outcome. The outcome is defeasible because we can conceive of later arriving at a consensus on a distributive principle that might disagree with the outcome of the fair process; the outcome would count as (unfeasibly) fair in the absence of a new consensus.

IMPLICATIONS FOR PREVENTION

In the previous section I argued as follows. First, health is of special moral importance because protecting normal functioning makes a limited but significant contribution to protecting the range of exercisable opportunities open to people and because various theories of justice support the idea that we have obligations to protect opportunity, and thus health. Second, a health inequality is unjust when it results from an unjust distribution of the socially controllable determinants of population health, as illustrated by Rawls's (1971) principles of justice as fairness. In effect, we cannot have optimal promotion of population health along with equity in health across groups without the broader achievement of social justice. Finally, to meet health needs fairly, we must supplement the principles of justice that emerge in answering the first two questions with a fair deliberative process. Clearly this is a "results-oriented" account that focuses on health benefits, for it is concerned with both the level of population health and its distribution.

These answers imply that we owe each other universal promotion and protection of health—not only through universal coverage for medical services, but also in equitable protection against health risks through public health and through non-health-sector measures that have an impact on health. First, meeting the health needs of all persons, viewed as free and equal citizens, is of comparable and special moral importance. Second, just health requires that we protect people's shares of the normal opportunity range by treating illness when it occurs, by reducing the risk of disease and disability before they occur, and by distributing those risks equitably. Obviously, how we allocate resources among these goals is an important issue to which I shall return. Within the medical system, this means we must give all people access to services that promote and restore normal functioning; accordingly, we must not neglect preventive medicine in favor of curative interventions. It means that we must look beyond the medical system to traditional public health measures that profoundly affect risk levels and their distribution. We must also look beyond the health sector to the broader social determinants of health and their distribution. Because we cannot meet all the health needs that arise inside or outside the health sector, we must be accountable for the reasonableness of the resource allocation decisions we make (Daniels and Sabin 2002).

Justice in prevention thus requires (1) reducing the risk of disease and (2) seeking an equitable distribution of the remaining risks [which does not mean "leveling risks upward," which would ignore (1)]. The first requirement is obvious. It is often more effective to prevent disease and disability than it is to cure them when they occur (or to compensate individuals for loss of function, where cure is not possible). Cost-effectiveness arguments will have some bearing on claims about the appropriate distribution of acute versus preventive measures (Russell 1986). Arguably, it is better in general to avoid the burdens of disease than to reduce them once they occur: for an individual, it is better not to become ill rather than to become ill and be treated, even if the cure is complete; it is clearly better to prevent an illness, including chronic illnesses, which may have sequelae that are not eliminated by treatment. Consequently, many types of preventive measures will be given prominence in a system governed by my account of just health.

The second requirement should also seem obvious, given our earlier reference to the social determinants of health. Our ability to determine when a significant health inequality between different groups is unjust depends on knowing something about the fair distribution of the socially controllable determinants of health. Consider the point from the perspective of occupational health. Suppose a health care system is heavily weighted toward acute care and that it provides equal access to its services. Thus anyone with severe respiratory ailments—black lung, brown lung, asbestosis, emphysema, and so on—is given adequate comprehensive medical services as needed, but little is done to reduce exposures to risk in the workplace. Does the system meet the demands of justice?

My account of just health says that such a system is incomplete and unjust. If some groups in the population are differentially at risk of getting ill, it is not sufficient merely to attend to their illnesses. Where risk of illness differs systematically in ways that are avoidable, guaranteeing equal opportunity requires that we try to eliminate the differential risks and to prevent the excess illness experienced by those at avoidable, greater risk (of course subject to resource limits and fair process in setting limits, including a consideration of the relative cost-effectiveness of preventive and curative measures). Otherwise the burdens and risks of illness will fall differently on different groups, and the risk of impaired opportunity for those groups will remain, despite the efforts to provide acute care. Care is not equivalent to prevention. Some disease will not be detected in time for it to be cured. Some is not curable, even if it is preventable, and treatments will vary in efficacy. *We protect equal opportunity best by reducing and equalizing the risk of these conditions arising.* The fact that we have an equal chance of being cured once ill because of equitable access to care does not compensate us for our unequal chances of becoming ill.

For these reasons, *the fair equality of opportunity account not only emphasizes overall risk reduction, but also places special importance on measures aimed at the equitable distribution of the risks of disease.* Some public-health measures, such as water and waste treatment, have the general effect of reducing risk. But historically, they have also had the effect of equalizing risk between socioeconomic classes and between groups living in different geographic areas. Many other environmental measures, such as recent clean air laws and pesticide regulations, have both general effects on risk reduction and specific effects on the distribution of risks. For example, pollutants emitted from smokestacks have a different effect on people who live downwind than on those who live upwind. Gasoline lead emissions have a greater effect on urban than on rural populations. But other health-protection measures primarily have an effect on the distribution of risks: the regulation of workplace health hazards is perhaps the clearest example. Only some groups of workers are at risk from workplace hazards, though many workers face some risk or other, especially in manufacturing settings. Just health requires that stringent regulation in all of these ways must be part of the health care system.[2]

What other sorts of social policies should governments pursue in order to reduce inequalities in health risks, especially in light of what we now know about the social determinants of health? The menu of options should include policies aimed at equalizing individual life opportunities, such as investment in basic education and other early childhood interventions, affordable housing, income security, and other forms of antipoverty policy. We know, for example, that early interventions aimed at child development, such as the Perry High/Scope Project (Schweinhart, Barnes, and Weikart 1993), have lasting effects on educational achievement, employment, marriage, and the reduction of mental illness. The War on Poverty Program Head Start produced lasting effects on educational achievement; educational achievement, in turn, has a direct influence on health behavior in adulthood, including diet, smoking, and physical activity (Acheson 1998). Other policies that might reduce differential risk could explore changes in the degree of control and authority workers have in the workplace (Marmot et al. 1997). Though the connection between these broad, intersectional social policies and health may seem somewhat remote, and they

2. In Daniels (1985: Chap. 7–8, and 2008: Chap. 7) I discuss the normative issues surrounding the very stringent "technological feasibility" standard that is supposed to govern U.S. safety and health standards in the workplace. I also note the limited way in which costs enter into the standard.

are rarely linked to issues of health in our public policy discussions, growing evidence suggests that they should be so linked.

One central implication of this view about health for all is that there should be universal access, based on health needs, to whatever array of public health and personal medical services provides support for fair equality of opportunity under reasonable resource constraints. Nevertheless, however much we can reduce risks to population health and do so in an equitable fashion, some people will still become ill or disabled and require personal medical services or other forms of social support that compensate for the effects of loss of function. Even if the proper arrangement of the social determinants of health and adequate attention to public health greatly reduce the burden of disease and disability in a society (Sreenivasan 2007), most people will still need medical care at various points in their lives, especially as they age. To protect the range of opportunities for those whose loss of normal functioning we cannot prevent, or should have but did not, we will have to devote some significant resources to such medical and social support services (Daniels 2007), even if the amount we devote is reduced by the fact that other measures may have more impact. Obviously, careful deliberation in a fair process will be needed to determine the proper allocation of resources to prevention versus cure and social support.

Personal medical services that are deemed essential to promoting fair opportunity for all must be accessible to all. Specifically, this will generally mean "universal coverage" through some form of public or private insurance for services deemed to be a "decent" or "adequate" array, as required by the appeal to the underlying concept of protecting fair equality of opportunity. There should be no obstacles—financial, racial, geographic, and so on—to access the basic tier of the system. Determining what is in that basic tier must be clarified in light of arguments about how to protect fair equality of opportunity under reasonable resource constraints, and these arguments require a fair process (accountability for reasonableness) in which appropriate democratic deliberation can take place (Daniels 2008; Daniels and Sabin 2002). The theory rules out arbitrary exclusions of whole categories of kinds of services that meet types of needs that should be met in the basic tier. Historically, for example, preventive services, mental health care, rehabilitative, and long-term care services have been excluded from both public and private insurance schemes, for various cultural and economic reasons. Most of these "categorical" exclusions are unjustifiable from the perspective of protecting normal functioning, but specific limit-setting choices can be made only through a fair, deliberative process.

Just what forms of organization—public or private administration and financing—are implied is not a question to which just health provides a unique answer. There is probably an array of "just-enough" institutional structures that can provide the needed protection of opportunity. Similarly, just what kinds of "tiering" or inequalities in services above the basic tier are compatible with protecting opportunity for all may not get specific answers from the general theory, though it will clearly supply constraints. Reasonable disagreements about these questions should be addressed in a fair deliberative process.

I conclude this section with a brief remark on the content of a right to health or health care and specifically what this means about right claims to preventive services. If we have a social obligation to promote fair equality of opportunity, as in Rawls's principles of justice as fairness, then we can look at a right to health as a special case of the right to fair equality of opportunity implied by that principle of justice. Specifically, this means we have a right to have our health protected by a fair distribution of the socially controllable factors affecting health. This includes a right to health care, but clearly goes beyond it since other goods that are the focus of social justice, such as education, income, wealth, and social status, count as social determinants of health and they actually fall outside the health sector, as it is usually defined. Our right to health then means we have rights claims on many public health and medical measures that count as prevention, but also on the fair distribution of the social determinants of health.

As I suggested earlier, however, reasonable people will disagree about how to promote population health fairly through the priorities they set for resource allocation. These disagreements will focus on both treatments and preventive efforts. Our actual entitlements to health care—the actual content of our right to health care—are the array of services that it is reasonable to provide given resource constraints. What counts as reasonable to provide is what emerges from the fair deliberative process that holds health-policy decision makers accountable for making reasonable decisions. A right to health or health care, then, is not a right to any intervention that might produce some benefit to an individual; it is a right to a reasonable array of services, as determined by the process I described, and so is system relative.

RESPONSIBILITY FOR PREVENTION

Elsewhere (Daniels 2008, 2011), I argue that our social responsibilities to promote and protect health have priority over our individual responsibilities regarding our health.[3] We can and should specify what we owe each other

3. Our social obligations to protect health are primary in an epistemic sense: we can specify them independently of knowing just what individual choices people have made that might damage their health. (On the luck egalitarian view discussed above, our social obligations cannot be specified until we subtract the consequences of individual choices, and so there is no epistemic primacy to social obligations.) They are also primary in a normative sense: we must design institutions that protect health through prevention and treatment in order

regarding health promotion and protection independently of assessing the consequences of individual choices that affect their health. Still, *our social responsibilities regarding health include encouraging, even through incentives, individually responsible choices of healthy lifestyles.* This is commonly referred to as "health promotion." Attributing responsibility to individuals for such choices must be distinguished from deciding what we owe them by way of prevention and treatment (Scanlon 1998).

There is an important challenge to this view about the primacy of our social obligations to protect health. Some "luck egalitarian" theorists argue that we cannot specify what we owe each other until we are clear about what individuals have brought on themselves with their own choices. Arneson (1988) and Cohen (1989) thus rejected the plausibility of egalitarians pursuing equality of welfare by saying (initially) that what matters to egalitarians is equal opportunity for welfare (Arneson) or advantage (Cohen) (there is a "welfarist" component in Cohen's concept of advantage).[4] Both theorists later abandon egalitarian concerns in favor of prioritarian ones. This "foregrounding of choice" (Cohen 1989) eliminates the possibility of determining what we owe each other independently of knowing what deficits in welfare or advantage derive from the choices people make. We owe people assistance whenever they lack, as a result of bad, brute luck, equal opportunity for welfare, but if they bring deficits on themselves through their own choices ("option luck"), then they lose their claim on us for assistance. [This formulation of the "but" clause about choices is close to what Scanlon (1998) refers to as the Forfeiture View; the initial clause about compensation for bad, brute luck led Anderson (1999) to label this family of views "luck egalitarianism," presumably because all forms of cosmic bad luck give rise to claims on others for compensation, which is highly egalitarian in its implications.[5]] So before we can determine what we owe each other (our social responsibilities), we must be clear about what people brought on themselves. Obviously, this is a rejection of the view that our social responsibilities are epistemically primary and individual responsibilities secondary (see note 3).[6]

to meet the health needs of free and equal citizens. We allow individual choices to overrule those obligations only under special conditions (Scanlon 1988, 1998). See also note 6 and Daniels 2011.

4. In contrast, Dworkin (1981a, 1981b) rejected equality of welfare in favor of equality of resources.

5. More recently Anderson (2008) qualifies the label so that the family still includes Arneson's "responsibility-catering prioritarianism."

6. The Rawlsian account of a division between social and individual responsibility is a deep feature of his view, one I do not do justice to when I (Daniels 2011) portray it as a response to the worry about expensive tastes. Blake and Risse (2004) divide theories of justice into "direct"

Nevertheless, luck egalitarian (responsibility catering) views emphasize that they are capturing something central in our thinking about justice, namely that prominence ought to be given to individual choice or responsibility for what happens to us.

It might seem these views should then encourage individual responsibility for healthy lifestyle choices, at least as emphatically as the social responsibility view I am defending. I believe these accounts have no grounds of justice for doing so, however. Why should there be such an effort at health promotion, given the limits individual responsibility sets to what we owe each other? If people behave irresponsibly or imprudently, despite not being hampered from making good choices by bad, brute luck, we do not owe them assistance for the problems they create. Whether they act imprudently or not, we do not owe them assistance for what results. Rather, we owe them assistance only for what they are not responsible for producing. A peculiar consequence of the theory, then, seems to be that it is hard to see why a proponent would want to make people act more responsibly with regard to their health. *Rather than there being more support for health promotion because of the emphasis put at the core of the luck egalitarian theory on individual responsibility, there is no reason for promoting it as a matter of justice.*[7]

Consider an example. Florida's Medicaid plan[8] gives people incentives in the form of opportunities to obtain some "over-the-counter" health-related products free if they comply with medically responsible practices, such as keeping

accounts of how equality follows from respect for persons or similar notions and "indirect" theories, such as Rawls's, in which other facts about the relations among people, such as that they seek fair terms of cooperation among free and equal citizens, play an important role in justifying concerns about equality. Individual responsibility then plays very different roles in these types of theories. It is used to define the space of what we owe each other—corrections for bad luck—in direct theories, such as those of the luck egalitarians. In Rawls, as soon as we aim for fair terms of cooperation, distributing all purpose means, the primary social goods, to meet the needs of free and equal citizens, then individual responsibility does not define the domain of what we owe each other (correction for whatever disadvantage we are not responsible for) but rather is what people must be accountable for if terms of fair cooperation are to be achievable.

7. A more precise statement of my case would acknowledge that some health promotion that aims at making people act more responsibly is simply removing the unlucky factors that interfere with people making responsible choices, such as lack of access to information or other things that interfere with the voluntariness of their choices. The luck egalitarian can also say, as some do about the possibility of avoiding medical abandonment, that health promotion campaigns are not matters of distributive fairness but are the result of other values coming into play. My claim is that health promotion is a matter of justice, and these two views of justice differ in a way that casts some doubt on the luck egalitarian account. I thank Nir Eyal for pointing out these qualifications.

8. For details about the plan, see http://ahca.myflorida.com/Medicaid/Enhanced_Benefits/approved_credit_amounts_090106.pdf, accessed January 9, 2008.

appointments and complying with medication regimens. These incentives are untested, but let us suppose (contrary to my actual expectation) they can contribute to more responsible behavior. (With this supposition, I ignore the obvious possibility that the incentives are inadequate, given other inequalities in society, to have a significant impact on practices such as weight loss or compliance with medical regimens. I also ignore the risk that they increase stigmatization of less compliant parts of the population and that it is the most vulnerable groups among the eligible poor that are most likely to fail to benefit from these incentives, whereas better-off groups will take advantage of them, but not because they have modified their behaviors.) Because promoting healthy behaviors is a requirement of justice, the social responsibility view would support efforts—such as incentives—to change behaviors as in Florida. In principle (again assuming the risks noted parenthetically do not materialize), there is nothing wrong with the Florida effort and it may be justifiable on grounds of justice.

In contrast, on the luck egalitarian family of views, especially those tracking responsibility closely, there is no justice-based rationale for promoting healthy behaviors. *As a matter of justice we do not owe people assistance for what they bring on themselves as a result of their choices of imprudent behavior, so we do not owe them any effort at making them act more prudently.* I find no support for Florida's experiment in the luck egalitarian framework, and this is a problem for the framework. My conclusion is that we get a better account of why, on grounds of justice, we have social obligations to engage in health promotion, including the provision of incentives to people to make healthier choices, from the account I have sketched than from the luck egalitarian challenge to that view.

TREATMENT VS. PREVENTION: A QUALIFICATION

Could we ever have moral justification for thinking we have a greater obligation to save through treatment a person who will die without it and who will live if treated, than to save, with the same degree of probability through taking a preventive action, one life among some group of people? I shall argue that the concentration of risk is morally relevant and thus that there is some justification for thinking we sometimes ought to treat rather than prevent. If I am right about this, I should then qualify my strong defense of prevention previously articulated in this chapter.

Many will recognize this issue as pointing to the problem of identified versus statistical victims, especially if Jenni and Lowenstein (1997) are right that the main cause of the identified victim bias many people share is the concern about a concentration of risk. Now, I agree with Menzel (1983, pp. 159-63, and in

Chapter 9 of this volume) that the distinction between identified and statistical victims is in general broken-backed with regard to treatment and prevention: sometimes identified people are only statistically likely to need treatment; similarly, some preventive efforts are aimed only at identified individuals. Despite this general point, however, if we focus on the concentration of risk, we may find that some treatments should have priority over some preventive efforts. The "identified victim" in need of treatment concentrates all risk in one person and forms its own reference group; statistical victims are part of a group in which the risk is spread over some number of people.

> Suppose, then, we consider "fully equalized cases" (Kamm 2007, 347-52) in which only the concentration of risk varies to see if it might matter morally. Suppose we have only five tablets of a medicine that can be used either as an effective treatment for a disease, provided that all five tablets are given, or that can be given in one tablet doses to people exposed to the disease, where it acts as an effective vaccination. Without vaccination, there is a 20% chance of contracting the disease once exposed.
>
> Treatment: Cory has the disease. We can give her the whole dose.
>
> Vaccination: Dolly, Ellie, Fannie, Gert, and Hannah have been exposed to Cory. We can vaccinate each one of them with one-fifth of the whole dose we can give to Cory.

One expected life is saved in either case. (Note that the people at risk in the Vaccination case are identified with regard to who will receive preventive treatment, though we do not know which of them will get the disease if they are not vaccinated.) Does the concentration of risk in the Treatment case morally matter? Do we have a greater obligation to treat or to vaccinate?

I believe that we have a stronger obligation to treat Cory than to vaccinate the five others. Some others, I know, do not share my intuitive judgment about this case—a disagreement I return to shortly. There is a relevant contextual fact— the scarcity of the medicine. Given that context, the concentration of risk matters morally. To see that it does, suppose we modify the Vaccination case so that there are 100 named individuals, friends and relatives of Cory, all of whom have been exposed to her, and that there is a 1% chance of infection followed by death, and suppose we need give them only one-hundredth the treatment dose as a vaccination. Again, one expected life is saved in either case. It seems less plausible to reduce the 1/100 chance of contagion and death for each of 100 persons rather than to save the one person already infected. (Assume successful quarantine so there is no further transmission.) If changing the example to 100 people at 1% risk doesn't shift the intuition, then suppose it is 1000 people at 0.1% risk. At some point, the concentration of risks matters.

Some may dismiss a 1% risk (or 0.1% risk) as "insignificant," whereas a 20% risk matters and gives rise to a real claim for assistance; that is, the level of risk must cross some threshold of significance, and then we should attend to it. So the concentration of risk matters, especially if the competing risks fall below that threshold. Still, as the cases with different reference classes show, the concentration of risk matters at some point or other to the belief about duty to treat rather than prevent, despite the equivalence in expected lives lost. Perhaps there will be some disagreement about when different risks give rise to equal claims; we might then have to flip coins or, better, flip weighted die to decide (as in Brock's 1988 and Kamm's 1993 proposals for how to address the "best outcomes/fair chances" problem). To be sure, the issue changes if more expected lives are lost when we forego vaccination of her friends than are gained by favoring treatment of Cory. That again makes it clear that context matters. In effect, we modify the problem into a different kind of aggregation problem, one in which more and fewer lives are at stake (and thus we no longer have Kamm's fully equalized cases). Risk concentration may matter in breaking ties but does not do more: this conclusion would need careful examination.

My intuition depends on Cory having the stronger claim on assistance since she is, ex ante, clearly worse off than the other five. She faces certain death if nothing is done or if the others get a vaccination, whereas they face "only" a 20% chance of death if nothing is done or if Cory is rescued. If her claim on assistance is stronger, it would be unfair to her to favor the others, who have weaker claims. (People with opposing intuitions may complain that Cory is not worse off than the one of her five friends who will become ill and die if she is not vaccinated. Arguably, the complaint turns on the fact that this friend now faces the same concentrated risk as Cory; the disagreement may be about whether this focus on the friend who will die changes the case.) If some think that a 20% chance should count equally with a 100% chance of death, then some version of the treatment versus vaccination case, closer to the 100 or the 1000 pill version, should clarify that not all chances are to be treated as giving rise to equal claims.[9]

There is disagreement at the intuitive level about the strength of our obligations in the original two cases, and the disagreement may be backed by an appeal to reasons. If we cannot resolve such a disagreement by using our intuitions about hypothetical cases, because we find new disagreements about cases,

9. As Kamm has suggested to me (personal communication) we take the concentration of risk into account in other contexts, for example, when workers face risks of death on a project we may rule out higher risks to fewer people in favor of lower risks to larger numbers, even when the expected lives lost are equal. Perhaps, however, in these contexts we are imagining who would consent to the relevant levels of risk and that affects our intuition about the case. If so, such cases may not strengthen my argument above.

then we may need to find another way to arrive at a fair choice about what to do. I believe this is often the case and have proposed accountability for reasonableness as such a way.[10] But even if we all agree at the intuitive level that concentration of risk matters morally in some contexts, I agree with Kamm (2007) that we still need to explain why there may be other, more theoretical, moral considerations that make it plausible to think that the concentration of risk matters.[11]

In my earlier remarks about what we owe each other, I took the following view. In general it seems better to prevent a departure from normal functioning rather than to wait to treat it if the condition occurs. This generalization is open to obvious qualifications: sometimes we can treat a condition but do not know how to prevent it, and sometimes we can treat it more cost-effectively than we know how to prevent it. In those cases, some treatments will seem preferable to the corresponding preventive efforts. A separate qualification is that we know that a very broad set of social determinants of health places considerable emphasis on prevention rather than treatment, though these measures generally fall outside the health sector. In this section, I considered one line of argument that would support giving priority to some cases of treatment rather than prevention because of the way in which some people needing treatment have concentrated risks as compared to the broader group that lowers risks through prevention. Still, even in this case, as in many others, reasonable people may disagree about where priorities lie.

I do not at all consider my intuitions about concentrated risks a conclusive defense of their moral relevance. Rather, I am content to suggest that there may be reasonable disagreement about the matter, which is my main point. Reasonable people might think it matters morally, even if others disagree.

---

10. Daniels and Sabin (2002).

11. Kamm suggests that what happens near an agent may matter morally, in light of the importance of granting such agent-relative space to them, so that agents may be more accountable for what happens near them (Kamm 2007, 179–80). Similarly, we might suggest, agents may be more accountable for addressing the concentrated risks (perils) encountered by those people around them than they are for more dispersed ones. We know from various studies that people treat losses as more important than comparable gains. This judgment ends up mattering morally because it affects how people evaluate their projects in life. Being committed to avoiding significant losses (Cory's life) rather than gaining comparable expected benefits (the safety of five people at less risk) thus is compatible with granting people agent relative prerogatives. Although I suggest the parallel to Kamm's argument here, I am not in fact persuaded of the relevance of Kamm's suggestion about agent-relevant prerogatives; I think the concentration of risk case needs stronger theoretical backing.

RESOLVING DISAGREEMENTS ABOUT WHAT TREATMENTS AND PREVENTIONS WE OWE EACH OTHER

Because reasonable people may disagree in cases in which there is no consensus on principles adequate to resolve their dispute, we have to rely on a fair deliberative process as a form of procedural justice, as I argued previously (for more detail see Daniels and Sabin 2002). I shall say a bit more, albeit briefly, about what conditions such a process should satisfy if it is to hold decision makers accountable for the reasonableness of their priority-setting decisions.

A fair process requires *publicity* about the reasons and rationales that play a role in decisions. There must be no secrets where justice is involved, for people should not be expected to accept decisions that fundamentally affect their well-being unless they are aware of the grounds for those decisions. Fair process also involves constraints on reasons. Fair minded people—those who seek mutually justifiable grounds for cooperation—must agree that the reasons, evidence, and rationales are *relevant* to meeting population health needs fairly, the shared goal of deliberation. Fair process also requires the opportunity to challenge and revise decisions in light of the kinds of considerations all stakeholders may raise.

It is worth noting that accountability for reasonableness occupies a middle ground in the debate between those calling for "explicit" and "implicit" rationing (Klein and Williams 2000). Like implicit approaches, it does not require that principles for rationing be made explicit ahead of time. Like explicit approaches, it does call for transparency about the reasoning that all can eventually agree is relevant. Because, however, we may not be able to construct principles that yield all fair decisions ahead of time, we need a process that allows us to develop those reasons over time as we face real cases. The social learning that this approach facilitates provides our best prospect of achieving a cultural prerequisite for sharing medical and broader health care resources fairly.[12]

My conclusion is that we cannot resolve the questions about an acceptable allocation of resources to treatment as opposed to prevention without such

---

12. Some international efforts at priority setting capture important elements of this process—e.g., in the United Kingdom the broad airing of social issues through Citizen's Councils that are supported by the National Institute for Health and Clinical Excellence (NICE), or the broad consultation with stakeholders in Sweden's efforts to revamp the benefit package in its health system. Though U.S. administrative law captures elements of this approach—consultations with some stakeholders, transparency—many U.S. commissions charged with improving the evidence base for medicine are barred from addressing issues of cost, cost-effectiveness, or other ethical considerations that they should address. The level of public vitriol about "rationing" in the United States, exhibited in the ongoing debate about health reform, shows the need for mechanisms that can broaden public understanding.

a process. I have argued that we have social obligations to promote health through prevention and that these often have some priority in resource allocation. However, I then suggested, more tentatively, that some cases of treating a person in peril might take priority over some cases of preventing comparable harms. Both conclusions should be inputs into such a deliberative process.

REFERENCES

Acheson, D. 1998. *Report of the Independent Inquiry into Inequalities in Health*. London: The Stationary Office.

Anderson, E. 1999. What Is the Point of Equality? *Ethics* 109:287–337.

———. 2008. How Should Egalitarians Cope with Market Risks? *Theoretical Inquiries in Law* 9 (1):239–70.

Arneson, R. 1988. Equality and Equal Opportunity for Welfare. *Philosophical Studies* 54:79–95.

Berkman, L.F., and Kawachi, I. Eds. 2000. *Social Epidemiology*. New York: Oxford University Press.

Blake, M., and Risse, M. 2004. Two Models of Equality and Responsibility. *KSF Faculty Research Working Paper Series*, RWP04–032.

Brock, D. 1988. Ethical Issues in Recipient Selection for Organ Transplantation. In D. Matheiu, Ed., *Organ Substitution Technology: Ethical, Legal and Public Policy Issue* (pp. 86–99). Boulder, CO: Westview Press.

Cohen, G.A. 1989. On the Currency of Egalitarian Justice. *Ethics* 99:906–44.

Daniels, N. 1985. *Just Health Care*. New York: Cambridge University Press.

———. 1993. Rationing Fairly: Programmatic Considerations. *Bioethics* 7 (2/3): 224–33.

———. 2007. Rescuing Universal Health Care. *Hastings Center Report* 37 (2):3.

———. 2008. *Just Health: Meeting Health Needs Fairly*. New York: Cambridge University Press.

———. 2010. Capabilities, Opportunity, and Health. In I. Robeyns and H. Brighouse, Eds., *Measuring Justice: Primary Goods and Capabilities* (pp. 131–149). Cambridge: Cambridge University Press.

———. 2011. Social and Individual Responsibility for Health. In C. Knight and Z. Stemplowska, Eds., *Responsibility and Distributive Justice* (pp. 266–86). New York: Oxford University Press.

Daniels, N., Kennedy, B., and Kawachi, I. 1999. Why Justice Is Good for Our Health: The Social Determinants of Health Inequalities. *Daedalus* 128 (4):215–51.

———. 2000. *Is Inequality Bad for Our Health?* Boston: Beacon Press.

Daniels, N., and Sabin, J.E. 2002. *Setting Limits Fairly: Learning to Share Resources for Health*. New York: Oxford University Press.

Dworkin, R. 1981a. What Is Equality? Part 1: Equality of Welfare. *Philosophy and Public Affairs* 10:185–246.

———. 1981b. What Is Equality? Part 2: Equality of Resources. *Philosophy and Public Affairs* 10:283–345.

Jenni, K.E., and Loewenstein, G. 1997. Explaining the "Identifiable Victim." *Journal of Risk and Uncertainty* 14 (3):235–57.

Kamm, F.M. 1993. The Choice Between People, Commonsense Morality, and Doctors. *Bioethics* 1:255–71.

———. 2007. *Intricate Ethics: Rights, Responsibilities, and Permissible Harm.* New York: Oxford University Press.

Klein, R., and Williams, A. 2000. Setting Priorities: What Is Holding Us Back—Inadequate Information or Inadequate Institutions. In A. Coulter and C. Ham, Eds., *The Global Challenge of Health Care Rationing* (pp. 15–26). Buckingham: Open University Press.

Krieger, N. 2001. Historical Roots of Social Epidemiology: Socioeconomic Gradients in Health and Contextual Analysis. *International Journal of Epidemiology* 30:899–900.

Marmot, M. 2004. *The Status Syndrome: How Social Standing Affects Our Health and Longevity.* New York: Times Books.

Marmot, M.G., Hemingway, B.H., Brunner, E., and Stansfield, S. 1997. Contribution of Job Control and Other Risk Factors to Social Variations in Coronary Heart Disease Incidence. *The Lancet* 350:235–39.

Menzel, P.T. 1983. *Medical Costs, Moral Choices: A Philosophy of Health Care Economics in America.* New Haven: Yale University Press.

Rawls, J. 1971. *A Theory of Justice.* Cambridge, MA: Harvard University Press.

Russell, L. 1986. *Is Prevention Better Than Cure?* Washington, DC: Brookings Institution.

Scanlon, T.M. 1988. The Significance of Choice. In S. McMurrin, Ed., *The Tanner Lectures on Human Values* (Vol. 8, pp. 149–216). Salt Lake City: University of Utah Press.

Scanlon, T. M. 1998. *What Do We Owe Each Other?* Cambridge, MA: Belknap Press of Harvard University Press.

Schweinhart, L.J., Barnes, H.V., and Weikart, D.P. 1993. *Significant Benefits: High/Scope Project Perry Preschool Study Through Age 27.* Ypsilanti, MI: High/Scope Press.

Sen, A.K. 1980. Equality of What? In S. McMurrin, Ed., *The Tanner Lectures on Human Values* (pp. 197–220). Salt Lake City: University of Utah Press.

———. 1992. *Inequality Reexamined.* Cambridge, MA: Harvard University Press.

Sreenivasan, G. 2007. Health Care and Equality of Opportunity. *Hastings Center Report* 37 (2):21–31.

World Health Organization. 1946. Preamble to the Constitution of the World Health Organization. Adopted by the International Health Conference held in New York, June 19–July 22, 1946, and signed on July 22, 1946. Official Record of World Health Organization 2, no. 100.

9

The Variable Value of Life and Fairness to the Already Ill

Two Promising but Tenuous Arguments for Treatment's Priority

PAUL T. MENZEL, PhD ■

If the presence or absence of life is the actual consequence of prevention or of treatment, preventing death and successfully treating life-threatening illness are equivalent in results. If, similarly, avoiding disease-caused suffering and being effectively treated to avoid suffering reach the same endpoints, prevention and treatment are again equivalent in results. But then an outstanding apparent *moral* fact stares us in the face: with treatment and prevention accomplishing the same gain in life and health, what is achieved by each would seem to have *equivalent value*. How could this *not* be true? If any of us loses our life from lack of adequate prevention, surely, it seems, we lose something *just as valuable* as we do if we lose our life from lack of effective treatment.[1]

This essential equivalence of the value of the results is robust. If for both of us it holds intrapersonally (that is, for me, and also, separately, for you), then it

---

1. If there are differences here that point away from equivalent value, they if anything lean toward prevention, not toward priority for treatment. Prevention may often have consequential advantages that affect its comparative value vis-à-vis treatment even though we are comparing prevention of exactly the same poor health state, for the same length of time, as a treatment cures. Most diseases create burdens in their emergence even when they can be fixed by a treatment, which saves as much life, or avoids as much morbidity.

also applies *interpersonally* (*between* you and me). To see this compare what *you* would lose from lack of prevention with what *I* would lose from lack of treatment, or vice versa. There is still equivalent value in the results. Moreover, things don't seem to change if we state the value of the results in positive terms rather than in the negative terms of losses: if I preserve my life by effective prevention, what I *gain* has the same value as what I gain if I survive an illness with effective treatment. In both cases, what is gained is *my life*. It seems utterly implausible to claim, other things being equal (such as the personal effort required in prevention, say, or the irretrievable burdens involved in the emergence of a disease), that the life saved by prevention is worth less than the life saved by treatment, or that *actually losing life* from lack of prevention is any less a tragedy than losing life from failure to treat. Either claim reflects a striking lack of imagination.

Given this apparent equivalence of value, the initial case against moral priority for treatment, and for a relationship of moral equivalence with prevention, is very powerful. I will refer to this as "the initial case" for moral equivalence. Can any subsequent consideration overcome this case and pull us back toward priority for treatment?

In this chapter I will claim, first, that three arguments made for treatment's priority quickly dissolve in the face of the equivalent value just described. Then I pursue the intricate matter of identifiable as compared to statistical lives, analyzing the distinction to see the respects in which it does, and does not, apply to the distinction between prevention and treatment. This analysis sets the stage for an argument that may be more promising: that actually, the very value of the lives and health at stake in cases of prevention and treatment, respectively, is frequently *not* equal after all, but variable in the direction of being lower for prevention. Finally, I explain how a second argument is also promising: in any context in which we are about to abide by a new policy of moral equivalence, it is difficult to be fair to those in the transition generation who are already ill. I will also argue, however, that neither of these "promising" arguments is compelling. The first, invoking variable values of life, is persuasive only within certain limited contexts; it thus generates only a selective priority for treatment. The second, concerning fairness to the already ill, loses its moral attraction once we realize its long-term historical consequences.

THREE DUBIOUS ARGUMENTS

Three arguments for treatment's priority are demonstrably weak, particularly in the face of the prima facie equivalence of value articulated in the initial case.

Psychological Difficulty and the Difficulty of Imagination

It is psychologically easier for people to identify with a person's needs in treatment than in prevention.[2] Thus, people are more easily motivated by a call for treatment than an appeal for prevention. One important element in this difference of ease of motivation is undoubtedly variations in imagination: since prevention's consequences are usually more distant in time and lower in probability, pulling its consequences fully into our consciousness requires more imagination than pulling the consequences of treatment vividly into our consciousness (see Faust, Chapter 7 in this volume).

But on what grounds would this be a *moral* argument? All morality and moral sensitivity require imagination—at its very foundation, arguably, the moral life starts with such imagination. Thinking and acting in moral terms require us to bring into our consciousness and caring what is often further away—present, for example, not in ourselves but in others, or not just in our friends and loved ones but in those we dislike. Regarding treatment and prevention, the moral question is whether we *should* more easily identify with someone's needs in treatment than in prevention, and whether we *should* be more easily motivated when the apparent *value* gained or lost is equivalent. The fact of variable difficulty does not make for *moral* difference.

Symbolic Value

Some (e.g., Calabresi 1965; Fried 1970, 217–8) say that by spending more effort and resources on treatment than on prevention we symbolize our belief that life has no price (or nearly none). We need to symbolize this belief, for we cannot just apply it as a policy across the board. If we did, we could not limit what we would spend on saving life and reducing risk, and we would effectively bankrupt ourselves. The best we can do is to symbolize the belief. To do that authentically, however, something superficial such as loudly proclaiming the belief will not do. We need to actually live by it in selective cases. But in what cases? This line of thought would plausibly suggest that it should be those cases that are most powerful and vivid. Those cases, arguably, are, for the most part, rescue situations, and in medical rescue circumstances it is treatment, not prevention, that is the issue. If we deny acute care then our professed belief that life

---

2. The same greater psychological difficulty of imagination is cited as a reason that people value identified lives more highly than indeterminate, statistical ones. See Small and Loewenstein (2003).

is priceless is revealed as disingenuous. By contrast, the consequences of a rejection of prevention disappear into the relative fog of the future.

Immediately, though, the equivalent value of prevention's and treatment's results intrudes. If spending almost without limit on possibly effective acute care truly represents and symbolizes what life is really worth—namely, that it is priceless—then *why isn't life also priceless when it is preserved by prevention*? To repeat the initial case: to anyone who has their health destroyed by lack of prevention, the loss in value seems to be the same as if their health was not restored through treatment. *Moreover*: if, on the other hand, life is *not* priceless—that is, it has some kind of limited worth, implying a boundary on what we should spend to preserve it—why shouldn't its worth be *as great* when saved by prevention as when restored by treatment? The conclusion is that whether or not life is priceless, prevention does not shrink in moral importance compared to treatment.

Dying and Exposure to Risk

One of Benjamin Freedman's unique arguments in his 1977 defense of treatment's priority builds on a comparison between killing people and exposing them to risk. Suppose, as a first premise, what seems plausible:

1. It is worse to kill one person who is in reasonably good health 5 years before the expected end of his or her lifespan than it is to give 10 people their first cigarettes, a "gift" that carries the statistical likelihood that one of them will die 5 years prematurely from the hazards of smoking. [A.]

Freedman then inserts his second premise:

2. If it is worse to kill one than to expose 10 to a 1-in-10 risk of the loss of a similar amount of life, then it is better to cure one dying person than it is to prevent 10 from being exposed to that risk. [If A, then B.]

He can then draw his conclusion as a matter of elementary logic:

3. It is better to cure one dying person than it is to prevent 10 from being exposed to a 1-in-10 risk of dying 5 years prematurely. [B.]

Applying this to prevention and treatment in particular, Freedman (1977) comes to his conclusion: "it is better to save lives than to preserve health."

Treatment is better than prevention even if it has no greater life-preserving effect.

In response, we might first note that the final conclusion does not follow as a translation of concluding proposition 3. If we see prevention only as "preserving *health*" and compare *that* with curing a *dying* person, of course we see a difference. We are probably not clearly holding in our consciousness the fact that the relevant health preserved is the removal of a distinct threat to life. Once we have the appropriate comparison, in which the loss from not curing is the same loss as what occurs from not preventing, the equivalent value of the results achieved regains its moral power.

To be fair to his full argument, though, we still need to consider Freedman's proposition 3 in its own right. It says that a certain kind of treatment (lifesaving) is better than a prevention that only reduces risk to life. If premises 1 and 2 are correct, 3 follows, and Freedman will have shown indeed that lifesaving treatment is better than risk-reducing prevention, even prevention that reduces risk *to life*.

The second premise, in particular, is complex and deserves to be analyzed,[3] but let me bypass that task, grant Freedman this premise, and concentrate instead on the first. People may be attracted to it because they feel uncertain that one in 10 smokers actually will die prematurely. And, indeed, for *10* people, the prediction that *one* will die is very uncertain. Preventive programs applied to larger numbers, however, involve greater statistical certainty. If we are talking about a thousand smokers, for example, we can hardly say, "well, perhaps a lot fewer than a hundred will die." We may very well know that proportionately 1 of 10 will die from exposure to cigarettes with *as much* certainty as we know that the one will die from an attempt to kill him or her specifically. But then premise 1 is no longer attractive.

In analyzing premise 1 in this way, we notice that *it is really an expression of the familiar proposition that identifiable victims carry more weight morally than*

---

3. It might be unpacked thus: (2a) If it is worse to kill one than to expose 10 to a 1-in-10 risk of losing the same amount of life, then it is worse to let one die who we could have cured than not to prevent 10 from being exposed to that risk. (2b) If it is worse to let one die who we could have cured than it is not to prevent 10 from being exposed to a 1-in-10 risk of the same loss of life, then it is better to cure one dying person than to prevent 10 from being exposed to that risk. This sequence involves comparative evaluations of six different items: killing one person and actively exposing 10 to the statistically equivalent risk of killing one; letting one person die (who we could have cured) and not preventing 10 from being exposed to the statistically equivalent risk of one person dying; and curing one dying person and preventing 10 from being exposed to the statistically equivalent risk of one person dying. Note that premise 2 unpacked into this 2a/2b sequence does not seem to involve the claim that killing is worse than letting die; it only compares killing with exposure to risk and letting die with not preventing exposure to risk.

statistical ones—when risk is concentrated in one or a very small number of people, then susceptibility is worse, even if the results are objectively similar, than when risk is spread over a larger number. If, of course, we accepts this proposition, then indeed we will be inclined to grant treatment some priority over prevention. What is revealed in this, however, is that Freedman's first premise *already* harbors the view that failing to treat is worse than failing to prevent. Constructing an argument with such a premise begs the question in favor of priority for treatment; the argument collapses.

Emerging from this analysis of Freedman's argument, the commanding questions are whether there is reason to think that the distinction between statistical and identifiable lives is morally relevant, and how closely this distinction tracks the distinction between prevention and treatment.

STATISTICAL VS. IDENTIFIABLE LIVES

In our preconception of the difference between prevention and treatment, we usually think that those who benefit from treatment do so as "identifiable," specific individuals. By contrast, those benefited by preventive services remain nameless—"statistical." Both before and after the provision of preventive measures, we do not know specifically who the beneficiaries of prevention are. Although partially accurate, this preconception that the prevention/treatment distinction reflects the statistical/identifiable distinction greatly oversimplifies their relationship.

To see this, all we need to do is distinguish *recipients* from *beneficiaries*. In regard to this distinction, the subjects of preventive services come in several combinations.

(a) *Neither the recipients nor beneficiaries are identifiable*. In typical "public health" measures, even the recipients are only a collective, anonymous group.[4] Clean water, for example, goes to anyone in a catchment area. Some recipients may be known individuals at the time a measure is instituted, but that is material to neither the measure's execution nor its perceived value. As for beneficiaries, the measure is thought to have many, but who exactly they are—who, that is, are the persons who would have suffered from less clean water had the measure not been taken, and therefore who will actually have been helped—may never be known.

---

4. At least they remain anonymous individually because we keep them that way. Halley Faust has noted to me that almost always we could, technically, enumerate and identify each member of the group. Sometimes we actually do that in a survey or census.

(b) *Recipients are identifiable but beneficiaries are not.* In "clinical" preventive services, on the other hand—vaccinations, screening tests, etc.—the recipients are individually identifiable. Here, too, however, the identity of the beneficiaries remains unknown. For one thing, the risk diminished by these measures is usually already so low that it becomes very difficult to discern who benefits. Certainly people do not know who benefits when the measure is administered, and seldom do they know even later. If a vaccinated person ends up not getting the flu, we still do not know the person has benefited; he or she may well not have contracted the flu anyhow. And even when a nonvaccinated person gets influenza, we cannot be sure that this occurred because of a lack of vaccination; he or she might have contracted the flu regardless.

(c) *Beneficiaries as well as recipients are identifiable.* Such cases are not as common a category for prevention as the previous two, but some secondary prevention efforts, particularly screenings, fall into this category. A screening may turn out quickly to have an identifiable beneficiary: an early stage cancer is found, for example, that can then be cured. If it is a very aggressive form highly likely to have been fatal had it not been caught early, the patient has almost certainly benefited from the screening: without it, the patient would have died. Some primary prevention activities may also qualify: almost all the recipients of chlorinated water in a very highly cholera-infested area are beneficiaries, for example.

The subjects of treatment also come in several combinations.

(d) *Neither recipients nor beneficiaries are identifiable.* We may think that there are no treatments with these characteristics. There are, though, if we include policy decisions about treatments (coverage for them by Medicare, say). In this case, typically a treatment's individual recipients are no more known than they are in most other policy decisions.

(e) *Recipients are identifiable but beneficiaries are not.* At the time of treatment's clinical provision, of course, the identity of recipients is known. Who will actually benefit, however, may not be known—not beforehand, and not even after the treatment has had time to play out. Spinal surgery, for example, may "result" in the patient being relatively pain free a year later, and both surgeon and patient may naturally tend to think of the patient as having benefited from that procedure. Yet appropriate rest and good physical therapy—along with medication, exercise, whatever—may have yielded the same result. Or prostate surgery may leave its recipient alive for 20 years, believing that he has benefited, when the tumor would have grown so slowly as not to be fatal.

(f) *Beneficiaries are identifiable after the treatment has had time to take effect.* With some treatments, the beneficiaries are identifiable afterward. A certain sort of relatively advanced malignant tumor, for example, may have always resulted in death when not surgically removed or radiated. If such a patient survives for years after treatment, we justifiably see this individual as having benefited.

(g) *Beneficiaries are identifiable, even at the time the treatment is provided.* There are two forms of this situation. (1) The beneficiary of treatment is identifiable beforehand because treatment has an extremely high likelihood of benefit. Certain kinds of emergency trauma surgery, for example, may have such a good track record, and be so necessary to avoid an otherwise certain death, that we are justified in already seeing the individual patient as a beneficiary at the point of action. (2) Beneficiaries are identifiable at the point of provision because a considerable enough reduction of risk is already seen as a benefit. A given individual treatment might not work when it lowers a 90% risk of death to 40%, for example, but the proportion of reduction in the high-risk situation is so great that many people see the reduction of risk itself as a benefit to the patient. If the patient does not survive, of course, it cannot be claimed, in the primary sense of medical benefit, that the treatment has benefited the patient, but it is still not implausible to say that in a sense the patient "benefited" from the treatment. After all, the patient went from having very little chance of survival (10%) to having a better than 50–50 chance! Some patients living through such a scenario will experience that increased chance as a benefit.

Thus, there is some correlation of statistical/identifiable with prevention/treatment, but the match is not complete. Prevention and treatment both have their contexts in which recipients are not identifiable, and both have contexts in which they are. Even treatment has its contexts where, *after* its provision, its beneficiaries are not identifiable, just as is the case with most prevention. Also, one category is almost exclusively the province of treatment: where we know, when the care is given, who will benefit. That is, to be sure, less frequently the case in treatment than commonly thought, but it is still more commonly the case with treatment than with prevention. If we have strong evidence that treatment is highly likely to succeed, we slide over into presuming that we can already identify an individual who benefits.

These associations are spotty, and four distinctions other than statistical/identifiable track the prevention/treatment difference better.

(1) The "baseline risks"[5] to the recipients of prevention are typically low. In treatment they are typically higher, and sometimes much higher. That is, patients receiving treatment start from a higher risk situation than recipients of preventive measures typically do. We must be careful not to overgeneralize on this score. Male prostate cancer, for example, may carry a very low risk of loss of life or worse quality of life if it is left untreated. Nonetheless, once diagnosed

---

5. The term is prominently used by Eeckhondt and Hammitt (2001) and Hammitt and Treich (2007).

with prostate cancer, the person is seen as "having a disease" and "under threat." What they can be provided is seen as "treatment," despite the fact that baseline risk may be no higher than it is in many cases of prevention.

(2) Partly due to the fact that treatment is typically applied in a context of higher baseline risk, the magnitude of the reduction in the risk that treatment accomplishes is usually greater than the magnitude of the reduction in risk that effective prevention accomplishes.[6] Note again, however, that, as with baseline risk, this difference does not always characterize treatment. Some treatments reduce baseline risks by only a very small amount.

(3) Usually the bad events that prevention can avoid lie further into the future than do the bad events that treatment helps avoid.

(4) It is a fourth characteristic, however, that most frequently characterizes the treatment/prevention difference: treatment is provided to people who are already seen to be "in trouble." They perceive themselves to be under threat, and others, too, share that perception. By contrast, prevention is provided before people are seen as being under such levels of threat. Often this fourth distinguishing characteristic is the colloquial rendition of relatively high baseline risk, the first differentiating characteristic of treatment noted previously, but it would be a mistake to think that all cases of "being in trouble" involve high baseline risk. In some cases of prostate cancer, for example (see the previous discussion of baseline risk), people are seen as having a disease and being under threat despite a low risk.

To summarize this, the recipients of prevention can be identifiable individuals just as much as the recipients of treatment usually are. Often the actual beneficiaries of treatment are no more individually identifiable than the people who benefit from prevention. Nonetheless, proportionately more patients who receive and benefit from treatment are identifiable individuals than those who receive and benefit from prevention. Although the "statistical" vs. "identifiable" lives distinction is thus bound to be associated with the difference between prevention and treatment, it does not track the difference well. Three characteristics track it more accurately, though not perfectly. Treatment, generally, is marked by higher baseline risk, greater magnitude of the reduction of that risk, and relatively immediate as distinct from distant future benefits. Conversely, prevention, generally, is marked by lower baseline risk, smaller magnitude of the net risk reduction, and more distant future as distinct from

6. By "magnitude of risk reduction" here I mean the amount of absolute risk, not relative risk, that is reduced. Take the following two risk reductions. Reduction A is from a 1:2 risk to 1:4. That is a reduction of 1:4 in the magnitude of risk and a 50% reduction in the baseline risk. Reduction B is from 1:10 (i.e., 10:100) to 1:100—a 90% reduction in the baseline risk, but only a reduction of 9:100 in the magnitude of risk. A is a greater reduction in magnitude of risk than B, but B is a greater relative risk reduction than A.

near-term benefits. A fourth characteristic even more centrally distinguishes treatment from prevention: recipients of treatment are perceived to be already "in trouble." This perception naturally results from the higher baseline risk of most treatment situations, and it even characterizes treatment when baseline risk is low.

VARIATION IN THE VALUE OF LIFE

We are now prepared to revisit the claim with which we started—that when the same sort of life and health results from prevention as results from treatment, the value of that life and health in the two cases is equivalent. Could it be that the value of a life[7] saved by treatment really is greater than the value of a life saved by prevention? There is, indeed, a sense of "the value of life" in which the values vary with the different perspectives of those doing the valuing, and some of these differences in perspective highly correlate with the difference between prevention and treatment.

Let us look at an array of possibly relevant differences in perspective first, and then concentrate on those that most affect the valuation of life. Contexts can vary by whether they involve:

1. *Identifiable or statistical recipient*: the person who receives the lifesaving/health preserving measure is either an identifiable individual or is not.
2. *Identifiable or statistical beneficiary*: the individual who actually benefits from care or prevention can either be identified or cannot.
3. *High or low baseline risk*: the risk to life without treatment or prevention can range from very high (even certain death) to very low.[8]

---

7. For the sake of manageable phrasing, I will couch the discussion in terms of the value of lives saved and not keep mentioning other aspects of health that may be repaired by treatment and preserved by prevention. Note though that patterns in the preference data about variation in the implied value of life may not always transfer over to variation in the value of morbidity improvements implied by risk preferences. Much fewer empirical data are available for health-related quality-of-life damaging risks than for risks about life itself.

8. Jenni and Loewenstein (1997) refer to a factor that is related but is not identical to baseline risk, "certainty and uncertainty." Very high baseline risk in treatment situations would constitute relative certainty that something bad would happen without treatment; low baseline risk would constitute a very uncertain prospect of harm. Included in their certainty/uncertainty factor, however, is also another element: certainty/uncertainty about what the risk is. We might face a range of risk (e.g., "from zero to 1:500"), or a more specific and definite but statistically equivalent risk (for this case, 1:250). Depending on the elements of certainty/uncertainty involved in a scenario, Jenni and Loewenstein found either a modest or no

4. *Magnitude of risk reduction*: the amount of risk reduced by treatment or prevention can vary from total elimination of certain death to very small reduction of a risk.[9]

5. *Near-term or long-term benefits*: the benefits of treatment or prevention can accrue almost immediately, or they can be far off in the future.

An additional contrast concerns when the evaluation takes place—before or after a risk materializes:

6. *Ex ante or ex post evaluation*: valuation of life can be expressed either before or after the results of decisions that reduce risk to life are known.

The contrast between *ex ante* and *ex post* perspectives intersects strongly with the second and third contrasts in the list above. Usually, *ex ante* beneficiaries remain statistical, though *ex post* beneficiaries become identifiable. Similarly, the baseline risk of a situation, seen *ex ante*, is frequently lower than it is *ex post*, when it has become much higher. For example, when people choose whether to pay a certain extra premium to add coverage insuring themselves for a certain sort of treatment (an *ex ante* perspective), they are choosing from a position of relatively low baseline risk. But later, if and when the risk materializes and they find themselves candidates for the care in question (an *ex post* perspective, in relation to the insurance coverage decision), they face a much higher baseline risk. Because of these associations of *ex ante* with low baseline risk and *ex post* with higher baseline risk, the difference in *ex ante* and *ex post* perspectives is already largely accounted for by attending to variations in baseline risk. I will therefore not deal with *ex ante* vs. *ex post* as a separate contrast in perspective.[10]

Other sensible simplifications of our discussion can be made. The previous section revealed that the first two contrasts in the list above—identifiable vs.

increase in concern about fatalities as a wide variance (uncertainty) moved to a narrow variance or specific risk (certainty).

9. Jenni and Loewenstein (1997) refer to a related but not identical factor, "proportion of the reference group that can be saved." To have a relatively high proportion of a reference group capable of being saved, the baseline risk itself must be high, and the magnitude of reduction in that risk must be great (e.g., reducing a 3:4 risk to 1:4). Daniels (in Chapter 8 of this volume) is among those who have referred to this as "concentration of risk."

10. Jenni and Loewenstein (1997, 248) found that the role of the *ex ante/ex post* difference in the identifiable victim effect (the greater importance of identifiable than statistical victims) was either insignificant or the reverse of the usually expected greater value of developments seen *ex post* compared to those seen *ex ante*.

statistical recipients and beneficiaries—fail to track the prevention/treatment difference as well as the third, fourth, and fifth contrasts. Thus we can bypass the discussion of the identifiable vs. statistical distinction to concentrate on the contrasts of baseline risk, magnitude of risk reduction, and temporal distance of results.[11] Because temporal distance of results will be pursued in Chapter 11 in the assessment of the practice of discounting the value of future health benefits back to present value, in this chapter I will confine the discussion to differences in perspective created by varying *baseline risk* and *magnitude of risk reduction*.

What might these two variables mean for the value of life? What constitutes the value of life is, of course, a highly contested matter. Without trying to justify a particular substantive view, one sort of value has to be acknowledged as prominent in the last century, especially in economics and social science, but also in selected philosophical circles: this is what I will call "subjectively assigned value" (SAV), value constructed by human beings in the very act of expressing various preferences. Although SAV may be undergirded by many objective aspects of human nature (we *are* mortal, for example), when expressions of preference constitute such a value, they effectively *assign* a value to life. In a democratic and consumer-oriented society, it is not surprising that this sort of value plays a prominent role.

One way to discern such value in the case of life is to observe what sacrifices people are willing to make to preserve life. The sacrifice most frequently used by economists and psychologists is how much money people are willing to pay to reduce or eliminate a risk to life (or, concomitantly, how much money they demand and will take to endure an increase in risk). To be sure, a host of issues surround such "willingness to pay" (WTP) models of valuing life, including the need to neutralize differences in income and the potential for inconsistent and irrational preferences.[12] The point of using the model here is not to claim that tradeoffs between money and preserving life constitute a preferred method of discerning a value of life, but only to illustrate how subjectively assigned value operates, especially how differences in perspective can generate different preferences and thus different values.

11. Admittedly, there may be some residual element in the matter of being an identifiable victim that is not a function of baseline risk or perceived magnitude of risk reduction. Small and Loewenstein (2003) find a modestly lower willingness to contribute to what respondents are told is saving *a* victim who has not yet been selected, compared to saving *the* one victim who has already been selected (both remain unnamed and undescribed). We might view this as the "pure" effect of identifiability per se.

12. On these and a variety of other issues concerning the value of life as inferred from tradeoff preferences, including WTP, see Menzel (1990, Chapter 3) "Consent and the Pricing of Life."

For instance, suppose that in a WTP valuation people are willing to pay $50 to definitively eliminate a 1:10,000 risk to their lives. The implied value of life they thus express is $500,000 (50 × 10,000). Immediately we begin to suspect that different values will be implied by the different preferences that people typically register in different situations. Facing a very high risk such as nearly 1:1 (a "death sentence," as we say), people who want to live will pay almost everything they can get their hands on to survive. Even a 1:2 risk, although greatly lower than 1:1, will elicit almost unlimited efforts to survive. That is easy to see if we reverse the trade into asking what money people are willing to *take* to incur a 1:2 risk. The economist Ezra Mishan quipped that he had yet to meet a colleague "who would honestly agree to accept any sum of money to enter a gamble in which, if at the first [and only] toss of a coin it came down heads, he would be summarily executed" (Mishan 1985, 159–60). We can thus say that when expressed from a 1:2 risk situation, the implied value of life is millions of dollars, if not effectively infinite, whereas in facing a 1:10,000 risk the value of life is only $500,000.

One of the factors on which the value of life implied by consent to risk and willingness to sacrifice depends is thus baseline risk. The wider trajectory of variations we suspect on the basis of the simple two-risk comparison just used is born out by many empirical studies (Jenni and Loewenstein 1997; Eeckhondt and Hammitt 2001, 261; Pratt and Zeckhauser 1996; Horowitz and Carson 1993; Viscusi and Evans 1990; Weinstein, Shepard, and Pliskin, 1980; Jones-Lee 1974).[13] My willingness to pay drops off *more than proportionately* as the risk drops from 1:2 to 1:10 to 1:100 to 1:1000. By the time the risk reaches 1:100,000, I probably dismiss it and refuse to pay anything to reduce or even eliminate it. Suppose, in this series, that the sum I am willing to pay drops from $1,000,000 to $100,000 to $5000 to $100 before it tails off to nothing. The values of life implied by these declining values of risk reduction decrease from $2,000,000 to $1,000,000 to $500,000 to $100,000 to $0. See Table 9.1, which though constructed hypothetically, represents the pattern of the values found in the empirical studies just cited.

There is a second significant factor. Often a certain *magnitude of risk reduction* is seen as the direct health gain from a preventive service, as it is for some treatments, too. Although such magnitude does not have as much of an effect on the implied value of life as baseline risk does, it, too, can be

---

13. For one set of complications, though largely focused only on variations in small probabilities, see Hammitt and Graham (1999).

Table 9.1. VARIATION OF VALUE OF LIFE WITH BASELINE RISK

Baseline Risk	Willingness to Pay (WTP)	Implied Value of Life
1:2	$1,000,000	$2,000,000
1: 10	$100,000	$1,000,000
1:100	$5,000	$500,000
1:1000	$100	$100,000
1:10,000	$0	$0

a significant variable.[14] If a treatment can cut an 8:10 risk of dying in half to 4:10, for example, it will be seen as a "life saver," though half its recipients do not survive. Although high baseline risk probably remains the main driver, the magnitude of the reduction in risk has a role, too. To see this, imagine variations in the magnitude of the reduction of the 8:10 risk, with that baseline risk kept constant. Suppose the risk can be reduced from 8:10 to 7:10, from 80:100 to 79:100, from 800:1000 to 799:1000, or from 8000:10,000 to 7999:10,000. If I am willing to invest $50,000 in the first of these reductions, I might plausibly invest only $2000 in the second, and only $100 in the third and nothing in the last, which I really do see as just futile. The values of life implied in such a series are, respectively, $500,000, $200,000, $100,000, and $0 (see Table 9.2).[15]

To summarize, typical preferences about investment in safety and lifesaving imply higher valuations of life in situations in which the payoff is a relatively large reduction of a high baseline risk.[16] This situation of a considerable

14. Studies of the effect of such magnitudes of *change* in risk, as distinct from studies of the effect of the size of risk itself (baseline risk), are few, and they have focused on changes in small risks (e.g., Etchart-Vincent 2004). These studies do not pursue the situations most relevant to the treatment/prevention difference, in which treatment situations typically involve higher risks.

15. The table is hypothetical. See the previous note about the data on which it is patterned. Because we have few good data on this aspect of variation in implied value, perhaps it can only be said that a high magnitude of risk reduction gets *seen* as "life saving," analogous to how not being able to get treatment in high baseline risk situations gets experienced as a "death sentence." Not only when baseline risk is high, but especially when there is a great reduction in a high baseline, the implied values of life are high.

16. One study by Corso et al. (2002) has looked at WTP for treatment as opposed to prevention directly. To do so the authors kept the baseline risk and magnitude of risk reduction the same in a treatment scenario as in the comparison prevention scenario—both risks were low (a 1:25,000 risk dropped to 1:50,000). We could hardly say that treatment given in such a situation would be to a person "already in trouble." Because of that I would argue that this study's findings do not accurately speak to the real life treatment/prevention difference. Obviously, there is need for additional research here.

Table 9.2. Variation of Value of Life with Magnitude of Risk Reduction

Initial Risk	Resulting Risk	Magnitude of Risk Reduction	Willingness to Pay (WTP)	Implied Value of Life
8:10	7:10	1:10	$50,000	$500,000
80:100	79:100	1:100	$2,000	$200,000
800:1000	799:1000	1:1000	$100	$100,000
8000:10,000	7,999:10,000	1:10,000	$0	$0

reduction of a relatively high risk often—though certainly not always—characterizes treatment. It rarely characterizes prevention.

THE MORAL RELEVANCE OF PREFERENCE VARIATION

What does this description and analysis of SAV preference data mean for the normative debate about the relative priority of treatment and prevention? Should we claim that as a matter of fact (the fact of people's typical preference variations), the value of lives saved by treatment is often greater than the value of lives saved by prevention? The claim is literally true, but the problem with the claim is that the real life actually lost from lack of prevention is still the same life qualitatively and quantitatively as the life lost from failure to treat, no matter how much lower the baseline risk and amount of reduction in it is in foregoing prevention. It is easy to agree that the preferences previously noted, with their nonproportionate variation, indicate how much people value various reductions in different risks. How, though, should we interpret the values thus expressed: only as the values they *literally* are—the value of *safety* and *risk reduction*—or also as indicators of the value of *life*?

Answers to this question are difficult (see, for example, Menzel 1990, Chap. 3). On the one hand, when life is lost, what is lost seems to be much more than safety. Moreover, the preferences that imply an apparent value of life can seem superficial. Are they deeply grounded? Think carefully about their variation—as risk and risk reduction decrease we see a disproportionately lower willingness to invest. To be sure, I have a more difficult time imagining myself losing my life if I'm one of 25,000, one of whom will lose his or her life, than I do if I'm part of a much higher risk subgroup of 10, say, within the 25,000. But why should that lead us to say that my life preserved by prevention in the 1:25,000 risk situation is less valuable than my life saved by treatment when I'm one of 10? The value of *real life* cannot be determined simply by values of risk reduction.

On the other hand, *it is hard to know where to look to find the value of life if we do not find it in some desire or preference for life.* And in turn, how can such desire and preference be discerned except by observing it in the willingness to trade and sacrifice something for life? We cannot (at least not normally) just start trading lives and deaths themselves. Risk to life is the thing closest to life and death that can be traded. Valuations of life that emerge from decisions about risk reduction would appear to involve the most conceivably appropriate process for valuing life.

There is an additional, more positive reason for taking values of risk reduction as indicative of something substantive about the value of life: consent. Even if we are clear that the values of life that emerge from preferences about risk reduction are values of life only of a specific, restricted sort, they nonetheless gain some moral force from consent. When life and health are at stake, we have to make decisions before we know everything. In some cases we make decisions when we are looking at high risk ("death in the face," so to speak). In others we are looking at relatively low risk. At either end of this variation, we are expected to abide by our choices and not complain afterward. We would not put much stock in the complaint of someone on her death bed who complains that her life was not taken seriously if she knowingly had decided to forego prevention modalities that would have caused her to avoid her now in-the-face-of-death situation.

If preferences really do represent how people choose in these different situations, and if they are expected to abide by their choices, their choices would seem to have gained some of the moral force of consent. Then in a society in which noncoerced choices are taken seriously why shouldn't society's action be based on the values of life signaled by those preferences? If social institutions justify giving some priority to treatment over prevention by citing the varying values of life expressed in low-risk and high-risk situations, society is, at bottom, just respecting people's choices.

That is hardly, however, the end of the story of considering consent in assessing whether varying values of life should matter in health care policy. A more prior consent can put in question the argument for qualified priority for treatment just articulated. Take Norman Daniels' case (Chapter 8 of this volume) comparing Alice, who will die unless she gets five doses of a rare vaccine, with Betty, Cathy, Dolly, Ellie, and Fannie, each of whom needs only one dose to be protected from the 20% chance of contracting the fatal disease they each face. Suppose that the concentration of risk in Alice leads us to think we have a stronger obligation to treat Alice than to vaccinate Betty, Cathy, Dolly, Ellie, and Fannie. The situation may look very different if we put Alice herself in a position in which she does not know whether she will be the one in whom all the risk is concentrated, or one of those exposed to a 1:5 risk. Arguably, from such a perspective of ignorance about her eventual situation, she herself will not consent to priority for the person needing all five doses. The primary reason is that she can easily imagine herself being one of the other five. She will also be able to imagine this very ease of imagination about herself: namely, that *were* she to become one of the people in the 1:5 situation, she could readily imagine herself being the one who would die. She might cast her lot with a policy of allowing the concentration of risk in one individual to break ties (i.e., to win in a case in which only *one in five* could be saved with smaller doses), but why would she consent to a policy of favoring the one person facing the concentrated risk if statistically *more* than one in five (one in four, say) could be saved by a wider distribution of the doses that the one would have to have? After all, her self-interest, from her current early-unbiased perspective, would be best served by devoting the doses to save more than one in five.

Thus, Alice hardly comes out of this exercise as a proponent of any strong priority for treatment. She can see her self-interest at stake in people who will be exposed to the 1:5 risk. If she comes out defending anything other than strict equivalence, it will be only a very weak priority for treatment to break ties when prevention and treatment are equally lifesaving.[17]

Does our hypothetical posing of such a question to Alice about what policy she would choose *before* she turns out to be the particular person in whom all the risk is concentrated—strict equivalence, weak priority for treatment, or strong priority—have any real life application?[18] Perhaps. In (a) buying into a health plan, or in (b) voting on policy decisions in a cooperative in which members actually have an explicit say in allocation policy, people who may eventually end up being either the Alices of this world, or the Bettys and Cathys, may have the opportunity to make a policy decision about priority vs. equivalence. In the first type of circumstance, for example, a plan may proudly advertise itself as emphasizing prevention, and it may already have made decisions that clearly manifest an attitude of equivalence for prevention, perhaps even priority. Accordingly, decisions to subscribe may plausibly be taken to imply consent to those policy decisions.

We are thus left with a somewhat messy conclusion.

(1) While what is lost when life is lost, whether from lack of prevention or from lack of treatment, is much more than safety, *one* perfectly

---

17. I shall refer to the view that treatment should have priority over prevention only in "tie" situations as "weak priority" for treatment.

18. One tradition in contemporary moral and social philosophy works out moral principles from a perspective of hypothetical, veil-of-ignorance consent. That tradition, one of whose founding writers is John Rawls (1971), is not remotely unified on two matters affecting whether a hypothetical, as distinct from actual, consent argument in the current discussion would apply. For an attempt to apply Rawls' approach to justice to health care in particular, see Daniels (1985), though he does not work out any implications for the prevention–treatment relationship.

plausible sense of the value of life is expressed by the willingness to purchase risk reduction.

(2) People's preferences about investing in risk reduction can be variable, but typically people express a proportionately greater willingness to invest in reducing the high baseline risk that tends to characterize treatment and almost never characterizes prevention. This generates a justified priority for treatment.

(3) The extent of the priority thus generated is greatly moderated, however, by the fact that for many treatments, the amount of risk reduction to be achieved is small. Even if there is a perfectly good sense of the "value of life" generated by investment preferences about risk reduction, and even if the value of life saved by treatment is thus typically greater than it is for prevention, not all treatment—and perhaps not even much—should gain priority over prevention. Treatments that either operate from low baseline risk or will accomplish only a very small reduction in risk warrant no priority based on the variable value of life argument.

(4) Before people know whether they will land in situations with the potential for a large reduction of high risk, it is contrary to their self-interest to prefer disproportionately greater investments in treatment than in prevention. Thus, at the level of policy decision making, equivalence between prevention and treatment—or only a weak priority for treatment at most, one that only breaks ties—gains greater natural support than it can typically gain in a "bedside" or clinical context.

Based on these conclusions, variations in the subjectively expressed value of life generate priority for treatment, but not for treatment in which patients are faced with only low baseline risk or in which they will prospectively gain only very small reductions in risk. The priority generated is a highly qualified and generally weak form of priority, and it can be overridden either by prior consent in subscribing to a revealing health plan or through a plan's decision-making processes designed to represent all members in major allocation decisions.

FAIRNESS TO THE ALREADY ILL[19]

We move to a second main argument. Forego for the moment any understanding from the previous section that treatment should have limited and

19. Substantial parts of this section replicate the substance of Menzel (1983, 174–78).

selective priority. Suppose we are at square one, not having concluded anything about whether treatment should have priority. Then imagine that when we are well, we all have the opportunity to choose between general policies of either equivalence for prevention and treatment or priority for treatment. And suppose that then, like Alice, who we earlier imagined had to express a choice *before* she becomes the person in the concentrated 1:1 risk situation, we all choose to maximize our chances of survival by choosing a policy of equivalence to govern our society.[20] None of us can complain if we are then disadvantaged when some marginal treatment from which we might benefit turns out to have been squeezed out by more cost-effective prevention. We not only made a choice for equivalence, but we had our opportunity to gain from the increase in preventive services that occurred with the implementation of our choice.

Notice, though, how very different from this the moral situation is if those who find themselves disadvantaged by prevention's newfound equivalence have *not* had the opportunity to benefit from such a policy. They lived with less prevention up to this point, and they had little occasion before now to gain from any priority for treatment since they needed little treatment. But now they are ill, or threatened with imminent illness. Whatever the precise nature of their condition, they could potentially benefit from some treatments that are not covered or available if a policy of equivalence now rules.

This circumstance—being caught disadvantaged by a policy of equivalence, without having had the opportunity to gain its benefits—is generally the situation of two segments of the population: older people at the time a shift is made from a policy of priority for treatment to a policy of equivalence, and those of any age whose dominant health characteristic is a congenital or early-onset illness for whom preventive measures are much less relevant. The more generic problem, covering both groups, is the problem of fairness to the already ill. For the former population, the difficulty is only a "transition problem" that will disappear within two generations or so after the adoption of a policy of equivalence. We might call that portion of people the "transition population."[21]

Conceptually, the easiest solution of the transition problem is to disaggregate populations: until they die off, those already ill will be governed by the degree of priority for treatment that held sway previously. Treat them as if their treatment had priority over other people's equally beneficial prevention, but apply a policy of equivalence to all others. Perhaps a successful transition strategy could

20. I choose to make the context here one of the whole society, not the more limited circle of a health plan. The arguments developed will usually apply to the context of a plan as well.

21. The relevant "transition population" includes not only those with significant illness at the time of transition, but also those who, though not yet ill, have too little time left to benefit from equivalence of prevention before their greater need for treatment sets in.

be similar to what insurance plans do when coverages change. If Medicare coverage were fundamentally to change, for example, the changes might be applied to all enrollees immediately, but we might also carry current enrollees for (say) up to 20 years on the previous coverage. In might be possible to implement such a "separation" transition strategy, but in practical terms it would appear to be difficult and in any case relatively crude. We would have to regard those over 50, say, as the "transition population," with those under 50 subject to the allocation decisions flowing from equivalence, even though a good number of people under 50, too, have major illness and are past the point of being able to obtain the largest benefits from prevention.

Suppose that the barriers to such a transition solution cannot be resolved and the only manner of implementation is universally for all. Should unfairness to the already ill then lead us simply to reject equivalence? If we cannot feasibly or very accurately disaggregate the already ill from the general population that has a long-term interest in prevention and will consent to a policy of equivalence, must the society stay locked in to priority for treatment simply because of a transition problem, though otherwise equivalence is right? This would make the decision a stark tradeoff between (1) the benefits of implementing equivalence—both lives saved and health preserved, and respect for the choice of the bulk of the population to put prevention morally on a par with treatment—and (2) fairness to those already ill.

If that is the trade-off we ultimately face, the implications are immense. If no transition strategy is acceptable and we reject moving to a policy of equivalence, we will not be putting its benefits off for just one or two generations; the transition problem will be no less significant for the next generation, and the next yet; the delay will be perpetuated ad infinitum. The comparative benefits of implementing equivalence need to be seen in light of that alternative of forgoing the huge benefits of equivalence for the long term of history. By contrast, the unfairness to the already ill lasts only through the transition generation. Defenders of justice and fairness, to be sure, often say that justice and fairness should trump even large amounts of competing well-being, but we must ask, "*This* many lives saved, *this* much health preserved, for generation after generation in perpetuity, when the loss of life and health involved in the alternative is itself a kind of unfairness to each of its victims?" Put this way, the fairness objection recedes.

I thus come to this intermediate conclusion: fairness to the already ill, within the confines of one or two generations, initially constitutes a sound moral argument against implementing a new policy of equivalence. Considering the long run of history, however, the argument ceases to be persuasive. Alternatively, we should try to ameliorate the effects of a new policy on those who have had little opportunity to benefit from it. The fairness argument should not block the change.

So far the discussion in this section has proceeded in isolation from the conclusion found in the previous section. In that section we decided that treatment did deserve priority, though only selective and relatively weak. If the variable value of life argument for such a modest degree of priority is persuasive, then the conflict created for moving closer to equivalence by considerations of fairness to the already ill diminishes. Those already ill will still get the marginal treatments justified by this limited priority, and the gap between that and what they would have gotten in the old days of stronger priority will then not be as significant as it would be if the new policy was one of total equivalence. Moreover, if the morally justified policy is one of selective and limited priority for treatment, those who are already ill have no claim anyhow on treatment beyond what is justified by that limited priority. For example, treatments for certain prostate cancers, because of the low baseline risk, do not gain the priority generated by the higher value of life saved in high baseline risk situations; those who have already contracted prostate cancer have no claim to less productive treatments for their condition than is used as the threshold of productivity for prevention. A good share of the fairness problem thus gets blunted.

In another respect—for the congenitally ill—the fairness problem's influence also gets limited. At first the problem is the most serious in their case: the congenitally ill have never been situated so as to find it in their rational self-interest to vote for something closer to a policy of equivalence. They have always been among the "already ill." Yet though the fairness argument against equivalence is even more persuasive in their case than it is for others, *it would be especially tragic to keep prevention of their own types of illness at a lower level of investment than treatment.* By spending at a lower health productivity rate for that prevention than we do for treatment, we would fail to decrease the incidence of these very diseases in future generations, condemning more people than necessary to never being situated where they can find it in their rational self-interest to vote for a more limited priority for treatment, with all the benefits of such a policy. It would be ironic, to say the least, to allow a fairness objection to lead us to act in such a way that we condemn more people in the future to be in a situation in which they can lodge the fairness objection throughout their whole lives.

CONCLUSIONS

By concentrating our question about whether treatment should have priority on the kinds of treatment for which we can make the strongest case, the question becomes more precise: *Should we provide relatively inefficient treatment to identifiable individuals at relatively high risk for relatively immediate harms, rather than more efficient preventive care to equally identifiable individuals at lower risk for more distant harms?*

Three arguments for priority for treatment are weak and unpersuasive: the argument that equal commitment to treatment is difficult psychologically, the argument that priority for treatment is justified because it symbolizes the belief that life has no price, and Benjamin Freedman's argument comparing exposing of people to risk with killing them.

Although the distinction between identifiable and statistical lives, regarded by many as the basis of priority for treatment, is legitimately associated with the treatment/prevention difference, it does not track the treatment/prevention difference well. Factors that track it better are high vs. low baseline risk, large vs. small magnitude of the reduction in risk, and relatively immediate vs. temporally distant future benefits. Even these differential factors, however, do not always mark treatment distinct from prevention. A fourth more subjective characteristic marks the difference most accurately: recipients of treatment are perceived to be already "in trouble," whereas recipients of prevention are not.

The value of life expressed by people's willingness to sacrifice to preserve life when it is threatened rises as the risk to life increases. Variations in such subjectively expressed values of life generate priority for much treatment, but not for treatment when patients are faced with only low baseline risks or when the anticipated reduction in risk is very small. The priority for treatment generated by variations in the expressed value of life is thus quite selective. Moreover, even that priority can be overridden either by the prior consent of members in subscribing to a revealing plan that emphasizes equivalence of prevention, or through the decision-making processes of a health plan designed to represent the membership in major allocation decisions.

Fairness to the already ill at a time of transition to any new policy of equivalence may appear to constitute a sound moral objection to implementing such a policy, but considering the role such an objection would play in the long run renders the objection unpersuasive. The unfair-to-the-already-ill objection should not be allowed to stop an otherwise justified move toward equivalence.

A move to full equivalence, however, is not justified. All things considered, treatment should have selective priority over prevention. It is a priority, though, that can be overridden by people's knowledgeable endorsement of a policy of equivalence that they are willing to impose on themselves in advance.

CODA: OBSERVATIONS ON A PHYSICIAN'S HYPOTHETICAL CHOICE

What implications does my analysis and position on the moral relationship between prevention and treatment have for the physician's choice in the thought experiment described in the introduction to this volume (Chapter 1)—seeing Bill to diagnose and treat his heart attack symptoms, seeing John to prevent a similar heart attack in his future, or lending an essential hand to an equally cost-effective community effort to reduce cardiovascular disease?

In the stipulated situation, Bill's and John's baseline risks appear to be equal, as are the magnitudes of the reduction in their respective risks that would be accomplished by a physician's attention. Both baseline risk and magnitude of individual risk reduction, however, are higher for John and Bill than for any recipients of the health department's prospective community heart disease prevention program. Therefore, because the community prevention program is not likely to be more cost-effective than attending to Bill or John, the physician should see one of them rather than participate in the health department's critical conference call. (To be sure, the benefit for the one person who would eventually be helped by the health department program would be as great. Yet either that person is not situated to know what their baseline risk and prospective magnitude of risk reduction are, or, if they recognize themselves as a recipient at risk, their perceived baseline risk is very low, just as it is for the thousands of other like recipients around them.)

But which—Bill or John—should the physician see? Both have appointments and are the doctor's established patients. Though what John would receive from the physician is clinical prevention, not treatment, he already perceives himself to "be in trouble," or at least in likely enough trouble to create his anxiety. Thus there is no morally relevant characteristic on the basis of which to give preference to one over the other.

There is still one remaining difference that will lead some toward seeing Bill instead of John. Without treatment, Bill's consequent loss of health and life will occur 12 years earlier than John's identical loss from lack of prevention. *If* a life saved in the future is not as valuable as a life saved now—that is, the correct moral equation about temporal location of a good is one that reflects economists' practice of "discounting back to present value"—then the physician should provide Bill with treatment before providing John with clinical prevention. Such time discounting of future nonmonetary benefits, however, is morally highly questionable, and especially so for situations such as Bill vs. John in which the trade-off is between early-result treatment for one person and later-result prevention for another (see Chapter 11 of this volume).

Nonetheless, it may be too much to expect any physician—and any human observer making a moral recommendation—not to gravitate strongly toward treating Bill. To be sure, the hypothetical situation is meticulously described to exclude the possibility that the physician can see John later while still being able to do it soon enough (now) for preventive care to be effective, but every provider has experienced people such as John whose medical future is not closed when they do not receive immediate preventive care. They have undoubtedly also experienced many of the Bills of this world for whom treatment cannot wait. It is almost inevitable that they will think that there is at least some chance that John's preventive care can wait. Understandably, they thus will not truly respond to the *exact* question posed by the thought experiment.

ACKNOWLEDGMENTS

Halley Faust (co-editor of this volume) has been immensely helpful in repeatedly perceiving weaknesses and suggesting repairs. Benjamin Sachs (New York University, Center for Bioethics) has also offered helpful observations.

REFERENCES

Calabresi, G. 1965. The Decision for Accidents: An Approach to Nonfault Allocation of Costs. *Harvard Law Review* 78:713–52.

Corso, P.S., Hammitt, J.K., Graham, J.K., Dicker, R.C., and Goldie, S.J. 2002. Assessing Preferences for Prevention versus Treatment Using Willingness to Pay. *Medical Decision Making* 22 (Suppl):S92-S101.

Daniels, N. 1985. *Just Health Care*. Cambridge, UK: Cambridge University Press.

Eeckhondt, L.R., and Hammitt, J.K. 2001. Background Risks and the Value of a Statistical Life. *Journal of Risk and Uncertainty* 23 (3):261–79.

Etchart-Vincent, N. 2004. Is Probability Weighting Sensitive to the Magnitude of Consequences? As Experimental Investigation on Losses. *Journal of Risk and Uncertainty* 28 (3):217–35.

Freedman, B. 1977. The Case for Medical Care, Inefficient or Not. *Hastings Center Report* 7 2(Apr):31–9.

Fried, C. 1970. *An Anatomy of Values*. Cambridge, UK: Cambridge University Press.

Hammitt, J.K., and Graham, J.D. 1999. Willingness to Pay for Health Protection: Inadequate Sensitivity to Probability? *Journal of Risk and Uncertainty* 8:33–62.

Hammitt, J.K., and Treich, N. 2007. Statistical vs. Identified Lives in Benefit-Cost Analysis. *Journal of Risk and Uncertainty* 35:45–66.

Horowitz, J.K., and Carson, R.T. 1993. Baseline Risk and Preference for Reductions in Risk to Life. *Risk Analysis* 13 (2):457–62.

Jenni, K.E., and Loewenstein, G. 1997. Explaining the "Identifiable Victim Effect." *Journal of Risk and Uncertainty* 14:235–57.

Jones-Lee, M.W. 1974. The Value of Changes in the Probability of Death or Injury. *Journal of Political Economy* 82:835–49.

Menzel, P.T. 1983. *Medical Costs, Moral Choices: A Philosophy of Health Care Economics in America*. New Haven, CT: Yale University Press.

———. 1990. *Strong Medicine: The Ethical Rationing of Health Care*. New York: Oxford University Press.

Mishan, E.J. 1985. Evaluation of Life and Limb: A Theoretical Approach. *Journal of Political Economy* 79 (Jul):687–706.

Pratt, J.W., and Zeckhauser, R.J. 1996. Willingness to Pay and the Distribution of Risk and Wealth. *Journal of Political Economy* 104:747–63.

Rawls, J. 1971. *A Theory of Justice*. Cambridge, MA: Harvard University Press.

Small, D.A., and Loewenstein, G. 2003. Helping *a* Victim or Helping *the* Victim: Altruism and Identifiability. *Journal of Risk and Uncertainty* 26 (1):5–16.

Viscusi, W.K., and Evans, W.N. 1990. Utility Functions That Depend on Health Status: Estimates and Economic Implications. *The American Economic Review* 80 (3): 353–74.

Weinstein, M.C., Shepard, D.S., and Pliskin, J.S. 1980. The Economic Value of Changing Mortality Probabilities. *Quarterly Journal of Economics* 94:373–96.

10

The Slow Transition of U.S. Law toward a Greater Emphasis on Prevention

THADDEUS MASON POPE, JD, PhD ■

United States law has long emphasized treatment over prevention. Only over the past decade have legal measures begun to materially target many of the root causes of morbidity and mortality. This revitalization of public health law is long overdue. But it presents difficult (and, as yet, largely unanswered) ethical and policy questions.

This chapter has four primary aims. First, it describes the traditional neglect of public health law. Second, it describes a built-in bias of the common law toward treatment over prevention. Third, this chapter describes many of the most notable recent legal developments that increasingly emphasize the prevention, rather than the medical treatment, of health problems. Finally, this chapter examines normative problems raised both by these new, arguably more paternalistic, public health laws and by others that are likely to follow.

The law has been very slow to address the greatest public health epidemics of the past several decades: smoking, obesity, alcohol abuse, diabetes, and sexually transmitted disease. Certainly food and alcohol labeling laws require the disclosure of some risk information. Smoking has been taxed, banned in many public indoor spaces, and restricted in marketing and advertising. But because these public health problems result from individual lifestyle choices, because they correlate to powerful corporate market interests, and because they affect only statistical future lives; state and federal governments have been loath to intervene to the extent necessary to prevent significant morbidity and mortality.

Furthermore, the paucity of legislative and regulatory public health measures may not be the only legal problem. In the absence of such measures, public health is regulated by tort law. But tort law is itself biased toward treatment rather than prevention. For example, compensation is provided only after an injury has already occurred. In the Thought Experiment in this book's introduction, the doctor can treat only Bill or John. Either Bill must be turned away and not receive treatment for his condition that is already starkly revealing itself, or John must be refused individual preventive care. In neither case does the doctor likely face liability (probably under a theory of abandonment) for that decision unless or until the neglected patient is actually later injured. Moreover, even at that point, the patient-plaintiff has a formidable challenge to establish "but for" causation: that had he received the prevention services (arguably promised by the doctor's secretary), then he would probably not have been injured. And that is likely to be even harder for John to prove in his situation, if his individual prevention has been foregone, than it is in Bill's situation in which treatment has been foregone.

Society is fully prepared to come to the rescue of the injured or sick individual, but is far less prepared to provide the resources and legal incentives to prevent those injuries and illnesses from occurring in the first place. Admittedly, because prudent individuals and entities (or at least their insurers) do not want to pay money damages, tort law arguably motivates them to make products and activities safer or abandon them altogether. But any deterrent (or preventive) effect of tort law is significantly diluted.

Still, the enormous (and growing) economic consequences of today's tobacco and obesity epidemics have forced some governments to take action. Over the past decade, there has been a substantial growth in legislation and regulation concerning health-harming behaviors. These laws and regulations target conduct from tanning beds to texting. Although there is hardly space to provide a complete taxonomy of such laws, this chapter reviews the most notable examples such as soda sin taxes and recent bans on outdoor smoking and trans-fats.

Although public health legal measures date to the earliest days of colonial America, for most of U.S. history those laws were aimed at preventing discrete harm to others. For example, mandatory vaccinations, isolation, and quarantine all restricted individual liberty in order to prevent the spread of contagious diseases. The individual whose freedom was overridden posed a direct threat to other people.

Today, in contrast, the greatest threats to public health come from substantially self-regarding behaviors. For example, within the constraints of existing laws, individuals who smoke (at least while alone) or become obese rarely pose any *direct* health threat to others. And they often engage in such conduct with substantial voluntariness. Therefore, interfering with the liberty of such individuals is permissible only by appeal either to a theory of justified paternalism or to a theory that prioritizes overall societal welfare (utilitarianism or most theories of communitarianism). But both potential justifications are in tension with liberal individualism, the prevailing political philosophy in the United States.

Rather than abandon long-espoused normative axioms, the best justificatory approach is to work within the liberal framework. Specifically, we should develop a new "harm to community" liberty-limiting (or coercion legitimizing) principle, a rule or test for when the state can justifiably restrict autonomy for the sake of public health. Admittedly, John Stuart Mill's familiar harm principle does not comfortably address aggregate, collective harm. But still working within a classical liberal framework, this new "harm to community" liberty-limiting principle would state relevant community-protecting reasons that can outweigh the presumption in favor of liberty.

PUBLIC HEALTH LAW: A HISTORY OF NEGLECT

Other chapters (1-6) in this volume address an alleged overemphasis on treatment at the expense of prevention. Although not a perfect fit, I want to recast this imbalance as one between the fields of medicine and public health. Admittedly, health care providers do practice clinical preventive medicine, and this may be growing in response to certain pay-for-performance incentives (Wallace 2008; Gavagan et al. 2010). Still, the primary focus of medicine is on treatment. In contrast, the primary emphasis of public health is on prevention. Medicine explains morbidity and mortality in terms of things such as cancer, heart disease, and stroke. Public health, on the other hand, looks at the root causes, such as smoking, alcohol, and diet.

But the differences between medicine and public health do not stop there. Public health concerns "what we, as a society, do collectively to assure the conditions in which people can be healthy" (IOM 1988). Public health focuses on community-level interventions. It concentrates on measures aimed at the entire population, at the broad distribution of diseases and health determinants. Medicine, in contrast, focuses on measures aimed at the individual. In addition, public health usually entails government action. Unlike medicine, public health measures are often coercive and backed by the force of law (IOM 2011).

Treatment did not always receive greater priority than prevention. During the end of the nineteenth century and the beginning of the twentieth century, public health and prevention were center stage. The nation was scourged with smallpox, cholera, polio, and measles. But through vaccination, antibiotics, better hygiene, and the control of infectious diseases, these illnesses were either eradicated or substantially reduced. Indeed, such public health achievements contributed 25 of the 30 years of life added to the average lifespan during the twentieth century (CDC 1999).

Public health was a victim of its own success. By the 1960s, communicable diseases were thought to be under control. So complacent lawmakers began to lose interest in public health (Burris et al. 2010). For the subsequent half-century, public health has been consistently neglected by policymakers. Indeed, the status of public health law at the end of the twentieth century has been described as "withering" (Gostin 2005), "anachronistic" (Meier 2007, 2009), and "deficient" (Gostin 2002). In its 1988 report, *The Future of Public Health*, the Institute of Medicine criticized the states for failing to modernize their public health laws (IOM 1988). Fourteen years later, in a follow-up report, *The Future of the Public's Health in the 20th Century*, the Institute of Medicine found that "the public health system that was in disarray in 1988 remains in disarray today" (IOM 2002; DHHS 2000).

TORT LAW: EMPHASIS ON TREATMENT, NOT PREVENTION

Fortunately, a withering, deficient public health system does not happen in a legal vacuum. When government refuses or fails to act to protect health and safety, tort law becomes more important. This is because the tort system is the default legal response to physical harm. In contrast to Europe, the United States has traditionally more heavily relied on tort than on regulation (Owen 2005, 49–50; Weiner and Rogers 2002). But tort (and its focus on compensating injuries) is not a perfect substitute for regulation (which usually focuses on preventing injuries).

The tort system is paradigmatically about retroactive compensation. When someone suffers harm due to someone else's action, tort often provides a remedy. Under negligence, the major theory of tort liability, a plaintiff must establish five elements: (1) the defendant's duty of care, (2) breach of that duty, (3) factual causation, (4) proximate causation, and (5) damages (Dobbs 2000). Lives, health, and suffering usually cannot be restored. But an injured person may get money damages by bringing a lawsuit and receiving a favorable verdict or settlement.

Nevertheless, the scope of liability is limited. Injured individuals typically can get compensation only from those who affirmatively cause harm. Generally, there is no obligation to prevent harm or protect others from harm. Tort law treats actions differently from omissions. It protects negative rather than positive rights. This is tort law's "no-duty-to-rescue rule" (Parmet 2009, 225).

For example, in the Thought Experiment (Chapter 1) the doctor must choose just one of three mutually exclusive options: (1) treat Bill, (2) treat John with individual prevention, or (3) help secure a health promotion grant. Although not voting on the grant will result in preventable harm, the doctor faces no liability for failing to act. In contrast, the doctor may owe duties to Bill and John, but only because each had already been scheduled for an appointment. This creates a treatment relationship and a duty to treat that would not otherwise exist [*Lyons v. Grether*, 239 S.E.2d 103 (Va. 1977)].

There are exceptions to the no-duty-to-rescue rule. Notably, those who are in special relationships assume protective duties. For example, in *Truman v. Thomas*, the California Supreme Court held that a physician had a duty to inform the patient of the importance of Pap smears [611 P.2d 902 (Cal. 1980)]. The court found that the Pap smear test is an accurate detector of cervical cancer, that the potential harm of failing to detect the disease at an early stage was death, and that the test itself posed relatively minor risks. Consequently, the physician had an informed consent duty to ensure that the patient appreciated the serious danger entailed in not undergoing the test.

A second famous case, also from the California Supreme Court, illustrates another exception to the no-duty-to-rescue rule. In *Tarasoff v. Regents of the University of California*, the court held that mental health professionals have an affirmative duty to warn potential identifiable victims of intended harm by their clients [17 Cal.3d 425 (1976)]. In the court's language: "When a therapist determines, or pursuant to the standards of his profession should determine, that his patient presents a serious danger of violence to another, he incurs an obligation to use reasonable care to protect the intended victim against such danger." The therapist can discharge this duty by warning the intended victim, notifying the police, or taking other steps reasonably necessary under the circumstances.

The sorts of tort duties articulated in *Truman* and *Tarasoff* are focused not only on compensating but also on preventing harm. Indeed, in *Tarasoff*, the provider's prevention duty extends not only to the patient (with whom the provider is joined in a treatment relationship) but also to third parties whose health is imminently threatened by that patient. Health care providers must not only treat the injury and illness of their patients but must also undertake to prevent illness and injury. Still, in order to bring a claim for breach of such tort duties, the individual must have actually suffered injuries caused by the breach of duty. Even here, tort law is still primarily retrospective.

But there are yet other mechanisms by which tort law serves a more prospective role, other mechanisms by which tort law serves not only to compensate but also to deter (Schwartz 1997; Leonard 2010). Tort law can be forward-looking and promote safety and reduce future harm. Sometimes it does this by catalyzing regulatory action through uncovering, exposing, and publicizing health risks. For example, tort litigation against asbestos and pharmaceutical companies triggered greater regulatory oversight over those industries and products (Wagner 2007).

Tort law can even promote safety and prevention more directly. Perhaps the most notable example is the 1998 Tobacco Master Settlement Agreement (MSA). During the 1990s, all 50 states sued the major tobacco manufacturers seeking recovery for Medicaid and other expenses incurred in the treatment of smoking-related illnesses. Florida, Minnesota, Mississippi, and Texas settled individually. The other 46 states entered into an MSA with the manufacturers. The MSA provided the states $206 billion and required the manufacturers to restrict advertising and to fund health education programs (NAAG 1998).

But the tobacco MSA remains the exception rather than the rule. The tort system is still almost entirely retrospective. It compensates harm that has *already* occurred. Tort law focuses on prevention and promotes safety only *indirectly*: by threatening that future tortfeasors will be taxed with the harm that they cause. In other words, people are deterred from acting carelessly or negligently because they want to avoid the potential costs of liability (Calabresi 1970, 244–65). In serving this deterrence function, tort law resembles a "police presence." Just as people drive more slowly when they see a police car, people behave more safely when tort is around (Bell and O'Connell 1997, 69).

Tort law deters unsafe conduct in at least three ways (Bell and O'Connell 1997, 68–77). First, it forces people to factor into their cost–benefit analysis the full expense of the injuries their conduct will cause. Cheaper though riskier conduct may, after taking into account the costs of liability, not be cheaper (and more attractive) after all. Second, to the extent that comparatively riskier activities and goods are available, tort makes them more expensive than safer alternatives, reducing their consumption. Third, tort may encourage safety advances due to the market demand for safer products.

Unfortunately, this deterrent (or regulatory) effect of tort law is not terribly effective (Schuck 1988, 290). Studies on tort law's deterrent effect have reached mixed conclusions (Parmet 2009, 236–37). After all, tort law does not fulfill even its compensation role in a consistent way. The probability of sanction is low, unpredictable, or both (Corbett 2006). Penalties are triggered only when someone is injured (Shavell 1987, 278). A majority of those who are injured do not sue. Often, the expected monetary recovery is too small to warrant the expense of litigation. Consequently, any deterrence message is often only faintly heard and imperfectly obeyed (Schroeder 2002; Parmet and Daynard 2000).

Furthermore, because the burden of proof in litigation is higher than in regulation, many of those who sue have trouble proving that their injuries were caused by the defendant's negligent conduct (Hyman and Silver 2005). For example, consumers lost every single one of over 800 lawsuits against tobacco manufacturers between 1954 and 1994 (LaFrance 2000). Obesity-related tort litigation faces similar substantial hurdles (Mello et al. 2006). Even if a manufacturer raises the risk of morbidity or mortality from 5 in 1000 to 9 in 1000,

that evidence is not sufficient for tort recovery. Tort law's individualized causation requirement demands that the defendant's conduct be more likely than not
the cause of the plaintiff's injuries (Parmet 2009, 227–31). Where the defendant
raises the risk from 5 in 1000 to 9 in 1000, the baseline risk (5 in 1000) is more
probably the cause than the defendant's conduct (4 in 1000).

Tort law remains a fine stop-gap.[1] But it cannot replace regulation (Jacobson
and Warner 1999). First, because lawsuits are anchored in the facts and circumstances of individual litigants, tort law cannot be as circumspect and comprehensive as regulation. Second, tort law is of little use where the harm is diffuse.
Where many people are harmed in a small way, the potential monetary damages of no single individual can justify (to a rational plaintiff's attorney) the
high transaction costs of litigation. Third, tort law is comparatively less useful
when the harm cannot be traced to an identifiable source (Rose-Ackerman
1994, 152). Fourth, tort law is limited when individuals contribute to their ill
health through their own voluntary behavior (Gostin 2000, 289–90). In sum, in
the absence of affirmative action by legislatures and administrative agencies,
the focus of the law remains principally on treatment, not prevention.

GROWTH OF PUBLIC HEALTH LAW: INCREASING EMPHASIS ON PREVENTION

Encouragingly, it now looks like the United States is getting beyond a withering
public health system and an overreliance on tort law. The beginning of the
twenty-first century marks a significant increase in attention to public health
law (Gostin and Taylor 2008). Indeed, public health law over the past decade
has been variously described as undergoing a "renaissance" (Gostin 2002), a
"modernization" (Meier 2009), a "reemergence" (Parmet 2009, 271), a "revitalization" (Gostin 2005), and a "renewal" (Magnusson 2009).

This revitalization (or resurrection) was prompted by at least three separate
developments. First, new infectious diseases such as SARS and West Nile virus
emerged and old ones such as tuberculosis reemerged (NIAID 2008). Second,
with the 9/11 and anthrax attacks of 2001, the threat of bioterrorism became all
too real (IOM 2002, 106). Third, in an era of health coverage reform, the financial cost of treating disease and injury that could have been prevented has been

---

1. The tort system is one of seven basic legal tools to promote public health. The other six
are (1) taxation and spending, (2) altering the information environment (e.g., labeling,
advertising), (3) altering the built environment (e.g., zoning to encourage physical activity), (4) altering the socioeconomic environment, (5) direct regulation, and (6) deregulation
(Gostin 2000 IOM 2011).

increasingly recognized to be imprudent and unsustainable [H.R. 3590, 111th Cong., 1st Sess. (2009) (Rangel, D-NY), enacted as Pub. L. No. 111-148 (2010)].[2]

Federal Public Health Laws

Public health law remains primarily a matter for state and local governments (IOM 2002, 102–4). But the federal Congress has recently enacted major new legislation and various federal agencies are busy promulgating rules and regulations. Notable among these laws are (1) the Patient Protection and Affordable Care Act, (2) the Family Smoking Prevention and Tobacco Control Act, (3) First Lady Michelle Obama's "Let's Move" initiative, and (4) the Food and Drug Administration's (FDA's) regulation of salt.

PATIENT PROTECTION AND AFFORDABLE CARE ACT
Perhaps most notable among recent federal laws, on March 23, 2010, President Obama signed the Patient Protection and Affordable Care Act (PPACA 2010). Although the legislation has attracted public attention primarily for its expansion of affordable health care coverage, it devoted one of five main titles to public health. Title IV, captioned "Prevention of Chronic Disease and Improving Public Health," spans 50 pages and creates at least four important new public health laws (Koh and Sebelius 2010). Although leading experts have rightly criticized PPACA for not doing enough to advance public health, it is still a major achievement in improving prevention and wellness (Gostin et al. 2011). The key prevention provisions are enumerated in Chapter 1 of this volume, by Faust and Menzel. I will note some additional items of importance.

Regarding the PPACA's National Prevention, Health Promotion, and Public Health Council (Section 4001), it might be suspected that the Council will end

---

2. In Chapter 3, Louise B. Russell finds that prevention often costs *more* than treatment. This seems inconsistent with an assumption driving the public health portion of federal health care reform. In fact, there is no contradiction. Russell and I are focusing on different targets. Russell focuses on "tertiary" prevention which operates at the individual level. In contrast, I focus on "primary" and "secondary" prevention which operate at the population level. In other words, Russell focuses on preventive clinical "interventions." For example, 1000 individuals may need to take medication over some period of time, so that 50 can avoid surgery. Russell's point is that although the medicine is cheaper than the surgery, the cumulative cost of the medicine, across both the population of individuals and across time, is greater. In contrast, my focus is not on preventive clinical interventions, but on public health laws. Law often works to change behavior without incurring the costs of enforcement against the protected population. It is, for example, unclear that costs outweigh savings when soda or tobacco consumption is limited.

up as yet another obscure and impotent government entity. But its role is not to replace or supplement, but rather to increase the efficiency and effectiveness of existing regulatory bodies.

The PPACA (Section 4003) materially expands research and education mechanisms. It amends the current law authorizing the U.S. Preventive Services Task Force [supported by the Agency for Healthcare Research and Quality (AHRQ)] to more clearly articulate both its purpose and expectations for development and ongoing review of evidence-based clinical preventive services. In the same section, PPACA authorizes the creation of a new "Community Preventive Services Task Force" [supported by the Centers for Disease Control and Prevention (CDC)] to focus on the development and evaluation of population-based prevention programs. In section 4004 PPACA mandates several health promotion outreach and education campaigns. It provides grants for school-based health centers (Section 4101), community transformation (Section 4201), and testing approaches that encourage Medicaid beneficiaries to modify their behavior to prevent chronic diseases (Section 4108).

Finally, the PPACA goes beyond just funding and education. For example, it authorizes an excise tax on indoor tanning services (PPACA 2010, Section 10907). Such so-called "sin taxes" are designed to deter harmful conduct by raising its price (Haile 2009). In June 2010, the IRS issued proposed regulations outlining a 10% tax on tanning (IRS 2010). But PPACA uses carrots as well as sticks. For example, it authorizes employers to reduce, by up to 50%, the cost of health insurance premiums for employees practicing healthy behaviors (PPACA 2010, Section 2705).

Family Smoking Prevention and Tobacco Control Act

While tobacco has long been the target of taxation and indoor air quality laws, it is still responsible for 400,000 deaths and 8.5 million chronic illnesses annually (CDC 2008). Accordingly, the FDA tried to regulate the tobacco industry during the Clinton Administration. But the Supreme Court struck down the regulations, ruling that Congress had not given the agency sufficient authority for such action under its authorizing statute, the Food, Drug, and Cosmetic Act of 1938 [*FDA v. Brown and Williamson Tobacco Corp.*, 529 U.S. 120 (2000)].

Nearly a decade later, Congress finally responded. In June 2009, President Obama signed the Family Smoking Prevention and Tobacco Control Act (Pub. L. No. 111-031). The Act specifically gives the FDA the power to regulate the tobacco industry. It also limits advertising and requires cigarette warning labels to cover 50% of the front and rear of each pack. In March 2010, the FDA issued regulations designed to curb both access to and the appeal of tobacco to children (FDA 2010a). Because many of the provisions became effective only in the summer of 2010, it is too soon to evaluate their impact. But the FDA is continuing (1) to build a science base for further regulation, (2) to issue industry guidance, and (3) to award state contracts to enforce the Tobacco Control Act.

MICHELLE OBAMA'S "LET'S MOVE" INITIATIVE

In February 2010, First Lady Michelle Obama announced her "Let's Move" initiative, an ambitious program to end childhood obesity (Let's Move 2011). The program calls for numerous measures that target what Obama calls the four key pillars: (1) getting parents more informed about nutrition and exercise, (2) improving the quality of food in schools, (3) making healthy foods more affordable and accessible for families, and (4) focusing more on physical education. These initiatives are mirrored in the Healthy, Hunger-Free Kids Act, enacted in December 2010 (Pub. L. No. 111-296). This legislation establishes nutrition standards both for school meals and for other food sold on school campuses.

FDA REGULATION OF SALT

Today's average sodium intake is several times what the body requires. Too much sodium in the daily diet is a major contributor to high blood pressure. High blood pressure, in turn, increases the risk for heart attacks, strokes, heart failure, and kidney failure. Responding to this threat, in April 2010, the Institute of Medicine released a report stressing the urgent need to reduce sodium intake in the United States (IOM 2010). At the same time, the Department of Health and Human Services announced that it is establishing an interagency working group to support the reduction of sodium levels in the U.S. food supply (FDA 2010b). The FDA, which already has the regulatory authority to limit the amount of salt added to processed foods, is carefully reviewing the IOM recommendations.

State and Local Public Health Laws

Although the federal government has been unusually active in recent years, most public health regulation still occurs at the state and local level. Jurisdictions across the United States have recently implemented various new measures addressed at preventing disease and injury from varied activities. These include (1) motor vehicle safety measures, (2) tobacco smoking bans, (3) tanning restrictions, (4) school nutrition and exercise mandates, (5) menu-labeling mandates, (6) soda taxes, and (7) trans-fat-labeling mandates and bans.

MOTOR VEHICLE SAFETY MEASURES

A total of 40,000 people die and nearly 2.5 million people are injured each year in U.S. motor vehicle traffic crashes (NHTSA 2009). To address this, every state except New Hampshire requires the use of safety belts. Forty-seven states require motorcycle riders to wear helmets (though most apply only to minors). Recently, the states have been strengthening both DUI/DWI laws and licensing renewal procedures for older drivers. Even more recently, a majority of state and local jurisdictions have enacted bans on the use of handheld cell phones and/or text messaging while driving (GHSA 2010; IIHS 2011).

Tobacco Smoking Bans

Smoking is banned in airplanes, restaurants, and other indoor spaces in a majority of U.S. jurisdictions, and this number has been expanding every year (ANR 2011). Moreover, over the past few years, an ever-growing number of jurisdictions has banned smoking in outdoor spaces such as bus stops, beaches, sidewalks, parks, golf courses, and patios (Broder 2006; Francisco 2006). This is notable because the concentration of environmental tobacco smoke outdoors is insufficient to be harmful to others. Many of these laws are aimed at the protection of harm to the smoker (Pope 2000). States have also been increasing tobacco excise taxes and expanding programs to help smokers quit (NCSL 2010a; American Lung Association 2010).

Tanning Restrictions

As with tobacco smoking bans, children are a primary target of much public health regulation. Indeed, sometimes children are the near-exclusive focus. Such is the case for tanning restrictions. Not only is high-risk exposure to ultraviolet light common among teens, but also blistering sunburns and overexposure during childhood greatly increase the chances of developing skin cancer later in life. Accordingly, policymakers in many states have begun regulating minors' use of tanning devices such as tanning beds (NCSL 2010b). Although some states only require parental permission, others categorically prohibit the use of tanning devices by minors under a certain age. More than 20 states introduced new legislation in 2010.

School Nutrition and Exercise Mandates

Although tanning can be dangerous, the major threat to child health is obesity. Nearly 20% of U.S. children are obese, placing them at risk for health problems both during their youth and as adults (Ogden et al. 2010). Consequently, children have been a special target of antiobesity laws. At least within the school environment, jurisdictions across the country have banned candy and sweetened beverages, imposed nutrition standards, and mandated expanded physical education (Winterfield, Morandi, and Shinkle 2010). Nevertheless, these laws vary significantly in effectiveness, and many jurisdictions still have no school nutrition regulations whatsoever.

Menu Labeling Mandates

Obesity is hardly a problem limited to children. Nearly 65% of U.S. adults are overweight and 31% are obese (Flegal et al. 2010). One contributing factor is the dearth of restaurants that provide nutrition information. Without such information, people get more calories, fat, and salt than they realize. In response, in 2006, New York City enacted a measure requiring restaurants to disclose calorie and nutrition information on menus and menu boards (N.Y.C. Public Health Code, section 81.50). California enacted a statewide requirement in 2008 (Farley 2009). Maine, Massachusetts, New Jersey, and Oregon followed in 2009 and 2010, along with a significant number of cities and counties (NCSL 2011).

Data on the effectiveness of menu labeling are mixed. On the one hand, people ordering from a calorie-labeled menu do order fewer calories, especially if the information is presented along with recommended daily caloric intake (Roberto et al. 2010; Pulos and Leng 2010). Similarly, parents order fewer calories for their children when ordering from a labeled menu (Tandon et al. 2010). On the other hand, some studies have found that labeling did not change the number of calories purchased by more price-sensitive lower-income individuals (Elbel et al. 2009).

Soda Taxes

Sweetened soft drinks are an increasingly popular target of food-focused public health laws. All 50 states, the federal government, and many municipalities impose excise taxes on cigarettes. Numerous studies have confirmed that the cumulative effect of these taxes has decreased consumption (CDC 2009; Chaloupka and Davidson 2010). Looking to duplicate this success, many jurisdictions have been imposing taxes on sweetened beverages. Although the size of these taxes is typically still too small to affect consumption, many state and local governments are exploring more substantial taxes (Rudd Center 2011).

Trans-Fat Labeling Mandates and Bans

Like soda, trans-fats have been a special focus of healthy food laws. Consuming trans-fats can cause arteries to become clogged, increasing the risk of heart attack and stroke. Although the FDA had mandated nutrition labels on packaged food since 1994, those regulations did not address trans-fat content [Nutrition Labeling and Education Act, 21 U.S.C. sec. 343(q)–(r)]. Then, in 2003, the FDA mandated the disclosure of trans-fats in packaged foods (FDA 2003). Nevertheless, over the next several years, many jurisdictions determined that disclosure was insufficient. So, they just banned trans-fats outright. In 2008, California enacted a law that banned trans-fats in some food by 2010 and in all food by 2011 [Cal. A.B. 97 (Mendoza), enacted as Ch. 207, codified at Cal. Health and Safety Code, sec. 113377]. More than 10 local governments have imposed similar bans. And many other states and cities have considered, or are still considering, such measures (NCSL 2011).

Summary

Given both the broad scope of public health and the huge number of relevant jurisdictions, this review of recent public health law measures is necessarily less than comprehensive. But it should be sufficient to illustrate two general trends. First, governments are increasingly prepared to legislate and regulate for the protection of public health. Second, the increasingly frequent target of these laws is lifestyle and personal behavior. But bringing the coercive power of the law to bear on the realm of private conduct presents special and difficult ethical challenges.

NORMATIVE PROBLEMS RAISED BY NEW PUBLIC HEALTH LAWS

One of the primary explanations for the traditional relative neglect of public health law has been the emphasis in the latter half of the twentieth century on autonomy and individualism (Gostin 2003). Public health at the beginning of the twentieth century focused on microbial and environmental factors. Public health laws were aimed at preventing discrete harm to others––for example, mandatory vaccinations, isolation, and quarantine to prevent the spread of contagious diseases. The individual whose freedom was overridden posed a direct threat to society.

Today, in contrast, the greatest threats to public health come from primarily self-regarding behaviors such as diet and exercise. For example, within the constraints of existing laws, individuals who smoke (at least while alone) or become obese rarely pose any direct health threat to others. But they can adversely affect the "public" health in two indirect ways. First, these individuals are part of the community. At some point, the cumulative effect of their health-harming behavior rises to public concern. Second, as these individuals may need extra (often government) support due to their health-harming behavior, they impose negative externalities on society. They effectively force other community members to subsidize their unhealthy ways.

Laws addressing contemporary public health threats often require significant interference with individual liberty.[3] They tell people whether and where they

---

3. As indicated in note 1, not all public health laws require limiting liberty. Education, such as menu labeling, is empowering not coercive. Unfortunately, merely supplying information

can drink, smoke, or tan. The PPACA, for example, focuses specifically on "life-style behavior modification" such as smoking cessation, proper nutrition, and appropriate exercise (PPACA 2010, Section 4001). The "new" public health laws, in short, are restricting personal conduct that has long been considered to lie squarely within a private sphere of individual liberty.

Of course, if individuals engage in health-harming behaviors without suffi-cient information or without sufficient voluntariness, then their liberty may be restricted on soft/weak paternalistic grounds. Public health laws with such a rationale (e.g., those aimed at children, menu labeling) have a firm ethical and legal basis. Such liberty limitation has been supported by liberal political philosophical thinkers from Mill to Feinberg (Pope 2000; Thomas and Buckmaster 2010). Even today, soft paternalism is being rejuvenated in the form of "libertarian paternalism," as behavioral economics shows just what poor decisions we make (Thaler and Sunstein 2009).

But putting soft paternalism aside, individuals engage in many health-harm-ing behaviors with no significant cognitive or volitional defects. Therefore, interfering with this liberty demands a fundamentally different moral justifica-tion: either a theory of justified paternalism or a theory of the power of overall societal welfare to justify coercion of the individual.

These moral justifications are the products of two main competing frame-works for balancing public health and individual liberty: the classical liberal framework and the communitarian framework. There is a recently revitalized and growing debate over whether trade-offs between individual liberty and public health ought to be assessed (1) in an autonomy-focused bioethics framework (classical liberalism) or (2) in a different ethical framework (arguably) more amenable to strong arguments for public health measures (communitarianism).

Classical Liberalism

When determining the justifiability of limiting liberty, a fundamental way to structure the normative inquiry is by asking *for whom* has the conduct been

is usually insufficient to change behavior. But even more direct regulation can be effective without limiting freedom of choice. Behavioral economists have proposed measures to exploit human biases such as the tendency to stick with the *status quo* or default options. For example, an intervention to arrange the food in a cafeteria line so that the healthy foods appear first increases the amount of healthy food chosen without limiting an individual's lib-erty and without limiting the individual's ability to choose unhealthy options (Loewenstein et al. 2007). Similarly, making salad rather than French fries the default "side" option results in the consumption of more healthy food without restricting choice.

restricted? There are three principal categories of potential beneficiaries: (1) the individual, (2) identifiable third parties, and (3) the community. These categories often overlap. But we can often reasonably discern that a law or regulation is intended primarily or predominantly to benefit just one type of beneficiary.

The liberal framework starts with a presumption in favor of liberty. But it is a presumption that can be rebutted. The reasons for which the presumption can be rebutted are often referred to as "liberty-limiting principles" (Feinberg 1984, 1986, 1988). Individuals who pose significant harm to others may have their conduct restricted on the basis of the "harm principle." If they pose harm to themselves without substantial voluntariness, then their conduct may be restricted on the basis of "soft (or weak) paternalism." And if they pose harm to themselves with substantial voluntariness, then their conduct may be restricted on the basis of "hard (or strong) paternalism" (Pope 2000).

But liberalism lacks a population-level liberty-limiting principle that addresses the aggregate harm of many individuals against the community itself (Nuffield Council 2007).[4] Scott Burris observes that "to accept the rhetorical structure of market individualism is to accept a political language that has no words for public health" (Burris 1997, 1608). Bruce Jennings similarly argues that "public health ethics must go beyond the Millian paradigm and its individualism" because it is "incapable of sustaining the normative justification for public health practice outside a very narrow range" (Jennings 2009, 130–31).

Admittedly, the "moralism" liberty-limiting principle concerns community-wide, collective impact. But moralism permits liberty limitation only to prevent drastic social change, a coarsening effect, or degraded taste (Feinberg 1988). Its focus is on public morals, not public health. Although public health and public morals have long been somewhat connected, it is not clear that moralism can do the job here, without changing its distinctive focus on nonphysical harm.

---

4. Feinberg suggests that when just 100 or even 10,000 persons devote their lives to heroin shooting or opium smoking, the harm is self-regarding and not the business of the state. But Feinberg maintains that when some significant percentage of the whole population chooses to live that way, "they become parasitical and the situation approaches the threshold of serious public harm . . . and can be emphatically prohibited by the harm principle" (Feinberg 1986, 23). But this is an awkward use of the harm principle, and Feinberg does not develop the point. Appeal to the interest of the community itself is a different type of consideration than that represented by the harm principle (Feinberg 1984, 221–32). Notably, the world's leading public health law theorist describes the public health approach as following not the harm principle itself, but rather "a version" of the harm principle (Gostin 2010). The "public" interest should be protected by a separate liberty-limiting principle that states reasons and has specifications relevant to its unique context.

Communitarianism

Liberalism remains the default framework in public health ethics (Gostin and Gostin 2009). "American political culture values liberty over . . . social solidarity" (Oberlander 2006, 252). In contrast, the communitarian framework is much newer (Beauchamp 1980, 1985, 1989; Beauchamp and Steinbock 1999; Lappe 1986). But it has obtained significant attention in just the past few years, with the revitalization of theoretical legal and philosophical interest in public health (Gostin 2000).

To the extent that liberalism attends to the public interest, it is stingily skeptical. Liberalism demands that liberty limitation be carefully, narrowly, and thoroughly justified. Communitarianism, in contrast, holds that individual rights and social responsibilities are equivalent, and that liberty and the common good have equal standing (Etzioni 2002). Communitarians maintain that liberalism does not sufficiently recognize the value of community (Gostin 2010). In balancing public health against individual liberty, whenever there is a close call, liberalism resolves the close balance in favor of liberty. In contrast, communitarianism gives the state a bit more latitude. Without a presumption in favor of liberty, communitarianism makes it easier for public health officials to restrict liberty (Parmet 2009, 3, 10, 273).

For example, communitarians may demand less evidence of less harm before moving to take coercive liberty-limiting government action. Certainly, a "precautionary principle" can be espoused and applied by liberal states too (Cranor 2004). Where there are threats of serious or substantial damage, lack of full scientific certainty is not necessarily an ethical or legal obstacle to implementing effective preventive measures (Cameron 2006). But liberalism supports only less restrictive "weak precaution," whereas communitarianism also supports "strong precaution."

Liberalism vs. Communitarianism

Communitarian proponents have identified a flaw in the liberal framework. Although that framework has worked for many issues in bioethics (from clinical trials to end-of-life decisions), it is not, as currently formulated, capable of adequately dealing with ethical issues in contemporary public health (Jennings 2009; Etzioni 2011). But this does not mean that we should, as some have proposed, just switch the whole framework and throw out the liberal presumption in favor of autonomy.

Assuredly, the liberal framework needs a tune-up in order to provide a useful framework for analyzing ethical issues in public health. Liberalism needs a new "collective good" liberty-limiting principle. Indeed, historically, liberalism has developed a range of "collective good" "rules." Jeremy Bentham, for example, had separate principles for offenses to others, for offenses to self, and for public offenses. Bentham defined "public offense" as "mischief upon an unassignable indefinite multitude" (Bentham 1780).

The problem is that no such principle ever established any traction or currency. Perhaps liberal theorists failed to carve out a separate liberty-limiting principle along the lines that Bentham anticipated because it never appeared necessary. Until recently, when public health ethics started receiving significant scholarly attention, there was no recognized need for a "collective harm" principle.

Certainly, communitarianism may be able to explain things that liberalism cannot—our duty to future generations and our duty to the community. But the scope of rightful state power has always been outlined in liberal terms. This is our social, legal, and Constitutional tradition. Liberalism "fits" better with our post-1960s individualistic tradition. Coherence, sometimes referred to as "external validity" or Rawlsian "reflective equilibrium," is one of the most important criteria used to evaluate normative theories.[5] We want a theory that is consistent with our generally accepted judgments about when intrusions on individual liberty for the sake of public health are justified. Liberalism is under attack by feminist theory, care theory, and critical race theory. But liberalism is still the prevailing regime. It is, as Larry Gostin notes, the *de facto* political philosophy of contemporary America (Gostin 2003).

An ethical theory does not need to match a society's considered judgments completely. One of the virtues of ethical theories is that they suggest new ideas. But, on the other hand, we do not want a theory that would require radical changes in our practices and traditions (Daniels 1979). By throwing out the presumption in favor of autonomy, communitarianism requires just this sort of radical change and it rings familiar to the dangers warned of in classic dystopian literature such as *1984*, *Fahrenheit 451*, and *Brave New World*. Indeed, an unrestricted focus on the good of the community at the expense of individual liberty rings familiar to core Nazi tenets (Binding and Hoche 1920).

Still, coherence is not enough. We also need our ethical theory to be clear and to have explanatory power. Although liberalism may not be able to explain public health ethics adequately, it can evolve to do so. We need to specify a new, separate "collective harm" liberty-limiting principle distinct from the harm principle. The new principle will need qualification and specification. But that is a project both more manageable and more appropriate than constructing a whole new communitarian framework. Liberalism is the predominant framework for all sorts of policy issues in our culture. With a few adjustments, liberalism can also handle the population-focused nature of public health.

---

5. Other criteria for evaluating theories are clarity, consistency, simplicity, elegance, explanatory power, depth, constructivity, fertility, and falsifiability (Caldwell 1994, 231–33).

Communitarianism Masks Hard Paternalism

At the heart of the argument for the appropriateness of a communitarian frame-work is the point that public health is societally organized. Public health measures are aimed at the population, so everyone gains what each could not achieve alone. Certainly, many public health objectives are only collectively obtained. People cannot, by themselves, secure (1) clean air and water, (2) safe roads, (3) control of epidemic diseases, (4) well-planned cities, or (5) security from bioterrorism. Health is significantly influenced by social and environmental factors (IOM 2011).

But not all public health issues are collective issues. Many public health threats (diet, extreme sports, unprotected sex, safe driving, tobacco, helmets, seatbelts, illicit drugs) are typically considered to be under individual control. This is demonstrated, for example, by the frequent inability of those injured from engaging in such activities to recover damages in tort lawsuits. Admittedly, plaintiffs sometimes recover because defendants failed to disclose the true risks or because the plaintiff acted under coercion or duress (Gostin 2000, 290; *American Law of Products Liability* 2010, Section 41:1-38). But, often, plaintiffs cannot recover because they consented or "assumed the risk." *Volenti non fit injuria* (to a willing person, no injury is done) remains an influential and consequential legal doctrine.

With notable exceptions, we decide for ourselves whether to use illicit drugs, engage in unprotected sex, eat unhealthy foods, smoke cigarettes, or wear seatbelts. The communitarian model could, consistent with its proponents' arguments, work well for population-focused collective goods such as clean air and water. In contrast, although activities under individual control are appropriate subjects of public health, they do not comfortably fit within a communitarian ethical framework for public health ethics.

With regard to substantially voluntarily assumed risks, it is unclear that any collective good is promoted. Because only some subgroups confront the risks, public health interventions help only those same specific individuals or groups. Furthermore, the very population of persons engaging the risks values the conduct more highly than the rest of the population. Restricting the liberty of a particular individual or group for the good of just that same individual or group is paternalism, not protection of the community (Siegel 2001). That fact ought not be masked or hidden.

Certainly, at some point in the aggregate, even self-regarding harmful conduct can impose negative externalities on society. But, as discussed below, that point must be specified and defended. Otherwise, communitarianism obliterates the longstanding distinction between self-regarding and other-regarding conduct.

Admittedly, all self-regarding conduct suffers from some cognitive and volitional defects. But not all of these are material. The division between substantial voluntariness and nonsubstantial voluntariness is not always clear. Which actions are confronted with substantial voluntariness? Do individuals understand the risks? Do they freely confront them? The boundary may be more of a gray zone than a line, because voluntariness runs along a continuum. But as with many familiar concepts such as "night and day," "bald and not bald," and "tall and not tall," the distinction is sufficiently clear in many cases. Unless we are prepared to abandon all sorts of contractual and other self-responsibility, we must recognize some conduct as sufficiently voluntary to be free from soft paternalistic liberty limitation.

Counterarguments for Communitarianism

Communitarians have two classic responses to the "charge" of masking hard paternalism. First, they might deny that the health-harming behavior really is self-regarding. Second, communitarians might deny that the health-harming behavior really is substantially voluntary.

First communitarians may claim that the aggregate effect of many separate, individual choices affects public health. They may attempt to show that what appears to be primarily self-regarding harmful conduct affects, in the aggregate, not just the subgroup but also adversely affects public health community-wide. For example, a Johns Hopkins study showed that increased obesity means that there will be fewer young adult males qualified to serve in the military (Nolte et al. 2002). So, obesity could impact the national defense. The cumulative effect of externalities, which on their own are insufficient to trigger the harm principle, may warrant liberty limitation to avert population-wide harm.

Motorcycle helmet laws may be the classic example of looking to public harm as the justificatory basis for liberty limitation. Although courts struck down early helmet laws as paternalistic, judges began upholding these laws on the basis that the risks riders posed to themselves translated into a drain on medical resources (Pope 2000). Mary Ann Glendon observes: "the cost of his medical treatment, or rehabilitation, or long-term care will be spread among many others. The independent individualist, helmet less and free on the open road, becomes the most dependent of individuals in the spinal injury ward" (Glendon 1991, 45–6). The U.S. Surgeon General similarly concluded that "the demands on medical care resources are borne by society as a whole" (DHEW 1979, 112).

But although there may be cases in which aggregate *de minimus* self-regarding harm becomes collective harm, more justification is needed before the mere invocation of "the community" justifies limiting liberty. Otherwise, the line between self-regarding and other-regarding harm can be too easily blurred or erased. Not just *any* externality under the harm principle justifies liberty limitation (Jones and Bayer 2007). Neither ought just any aggregate harm justify liberty limitation. Any collective harm liberty-limiting principle needs specification and mediating maxims. For example, at what point does the *individual* health of larger and larger groups become a matter of *public* health? How much harm to how great a portion of the population makes what would otherwise be only self-regarding into population-regarding conduct?

Furthermore, even if an appropriate threshold were defined and satisfied, the externalities may be merely economic. In that case, liberalism's least restrictive alternative principle would demand an attempt to force the internalization of the activity's costs before moving to ban the activity altogether. In other words, a state might be justified in mandating that helmetless riders pay a certain tax or purchase certain insurance, so that they would self-fund the costs of their behavior. If such a scheme were feasible, then limiting a broader range of liberty by categorically outlawing helmetless riding would be unjustified on the basis of either harm to others or harm to community.

A second argument that communitarians might make in response to the "charge" of hard paternalism is that the risks are not substantially voluntarily assumed. Indeed, individuals are often not so free and responsible as liberalism presumes. Therefore, restriction of such conduct does not really trump any values. Deeper causes and explanations of behavior come from the environment: the marketing of food, the built environment. For instance, drug abusers do not freely reuse syringes. Sterile drug injection equipment may be unavailable or there may be peer pressure to share.

But all individuals are presumed to have decision-making capacity. The regulator bears the burden of rebutting the presumption. Whether we can show that any of these voluntariness-reducing conditions actually obtains requires empirical work. It requires scientific research to determine, for example, a food's addictive properties. It requires behavioral research to determine, for example, the impact of advertising on decision making. And it requires environmental research to determine whether healthier food options are available. But all this evidence is still being developed. And even if voluntariness is affected to *some* degree, that does not mean that action is not substantially voluntary. We engage in little conduct with *full* information and *exhaustive* deliberation but we are still charged with responsibility (Pope 2005).

Hard paternalism is widely considered to be an illegitimate rationale for state regulation. But many of the current and forthcoming measures targeting tobacco use, sedentary behavior, and poor nutrition appear to be hard paternalistic. They restrict behavior that is (seemingly) both substantially voluntary and substantially self-regarding. Communitarians argue that these laws are justified on the ground that they protect "the community." But how many self-harming individuals does it take before the aggregate of that harm matures into harm to community? Without a satisfactory distinction between self-regarding and community-regarding conduct, communitarianism cannot demonstrate how any plausible range of individual liberty is preserved.

Of course, these are questions that must be answered not only by communitarianism but also by liberalism. The answers to these questions will help define the contours and mediating maxims of a new "collective harm" liberty-limiting principle. Prevention often entails restricting liberty. Attempts to justify such restriction on the basis of "harm to others" are often strained. But some liberty limitation may very well be justified on the basis of "harm to community."

CONCLUSIONS

Finally, after a nearly 50-year slumber, public health law is being revitalized. Significant regulatory attention is being directed at preventing, instead of only at treating, illness and injury. And tort law, while not abandoning its traditional focus on treatment and ex post facto compensation, is also increasingly and aggressively taking up the challenges of prevention.

Still, unlike the pre-1960s laws that primarily targeted infectious disease, the public health laws of the twenty-first century target lifestyle behavior. Consequently, today's public health laws demand a fundamentally different justification for limiting individual liberty. Classical liberalism can supply the framework for this justification. But the requisite liberty-limiting principles need further specification and modulation.

REFERENCES

American Law of Products Liability. 2010. St. Paul, MN: Thomson/West Publishing.

American Lung Association. 2010. *State of Tobacco Control 2009*. Washington, DC: American Lung Association.

ANR (Americans for Nonsmokers' Rights). 2011. Smokefree Lists, Maps, and Data. Americans for Nonsmokers' Rights. Available at http://www.no-smoke.org/goingsmokefree.php?id=519, accessed June 13, 2011.

Beauchamp, D.E. 1980. Public Health and Individual Liberty. *Annual Review of Public Health* 1:121–36.

———. 1985. Community: The Neglected Tradition of Public Health. *Hastings Center Report* 15 (6):28–36.

———. 1989. Injury, Community, and the Republic. *Law, Medicine and Health Care* 17 (1):42–49.

Beauchamp, D.E., and Steinbock, B. 1999. *New Ethics for the Public Health.* New York: Oxford University Press.

Bell, P.A., and O'Connell, J. 1997. *Accidental Justice: The Dilemma of Tort Law.* New Haven, CT: Yale University Press.

Bentham, J. 1780. *An Introduction to the Principles of Morals and Legislation.* Reprint. Oxford: Clarendon Press.

Binding, C. and Hoche, A.E. 1920. Die Friegabe der Vernichtung lebensunwerten Lebens (Authorization for the Destruction of Life Unworthy of Life).

Broder, J.M. 2006. Smoking Ban Takes Effect, Inside and Out. *New York Times,* March 19.

Burris, S. 1997. The Invisibility of Public Health: Population-Level Measures in Politics of Market Individualism. *American Journal of Public Health* 87 (10):1607–10.

Burris, S., Wagenaar, A.C., Swanson, J., Ibrahim, J.K., Wood, J., and Mello, M.M. 2010. Making the Case for Laws that Improve Health: A Framework for Public Health Law Research. *Milbank Quarterly* 88 (2):169–210.

Calabresi, G. 1970. *Cost of Accidents: A Legal and Economic Analysis.* New Haven, CT: Yale University Press.

Caldwell, B.J. 1994. *Beyond Positivism: Economic Methodology in the 20th Century.* New York: Routledge.

Cameron, L. 2006. *Environmental Risk Management in New Zealand*: Is Scope There to Apply a More Generic Framework? Wellington: New Zealand Treasury Policy Perspectives Paper.

CDC (Centers for Disease Control and Prevention). 1999. Ten Great Public Health Achievements—United States, 1900–1999. *Morbidity and Mortality Weekly Report* 48 (12):241–43.

———. 2008. Smoking-Attributable Mortality, Years of Potential Life Lost, and Productivity Losses–United States, 2000–2004. *Morbidity and Mortality Weekly Report* 57 (45):1226–28.

———. 2009. Federal and State Cigarette Excise Taxes: United States, 1995–2009. *Morbidity and Mortality Weekly Report* 58 (19):524–27.

Chaloupka, F.J., and Davidson, P.A. 2010. *Applying Tobacco Control Lessons to Obesity: Taxes and Other Pricing Strategies to Reduce Consumption.* St. Paul, MN: Tobacco Control Legal Consortium.

Corbett, A. 2006. Regulating Compensation for Injuries Associated with Medical Error. *Sydney Law Review* 28 (2):259–96.

Cranor, C.F. 2004. Toward Understanding Aspects of the Precautionary Principle. *Journal of Medicine and Philosophy* 29 (3):259–79.

Daniels, N. 1979. Wide Reflective Equilibrium and Theory Acceptance in Ethics. *Journal of Philosophy* 76 (5):256–82.

DHEW (U.S. Department of Health, Education and Welfare, Public Health Service, Office of the Assistant Secretary for Health and Surgeon General). 1979. *Healthy People: The Surgeon General's Report on Health Promotion and Disease Prevention.* Washington, DC: DHEW.

DHHS (Department of Health and Human Services). 2000. *Healthy People 2010.* Washington, DC: DHHS.

Dobbs, D.B. 2000. *The Law of Torts.* St. Paul, MN: West Group.

Elbel, B., Kersh, R., Brescoll, V., and Dixon, L.B. 2009. Calorie Labeling and Food Choices: A First Look at the Effects on Low-Income People in New York City. *Health Affairs* 28 (6):w1110–w1121.

Etzioni, A. 2002. Public Health Law: A Communitarian Perspective. *Health Affairs* 21 (6):102–4.

———. 2011. Authoritarian Versus Responsive Communitarian Bioethics. *Journal of Medical Ethics* 37 (1):17–23.

Farley, T.A. 2009. New York City's Fight over Calories Labeling. *Health Affairs* 28 (6):w1098–w1109.

FDA (Food and Drug Administration). 2003. Food Labeling: Trans-Fatty Acids in Nutrition Labeling, Nutrient Content Claims, and Health Claims. *Federal Register* 68 (41):433.

———. 2010a. Regulations Regarding the Sale and Distribution of Cigarettes and Smokeless Tobacco to Protect Children and Adolescents. *Federal Register* 75 (13):225.

———. 2010b. FDA Issues Statement on IOM Sodium Report. Available at http://www.fda.gov/NewsEvents/Newsroom/PressAnnouncements/2010/ucm209155.htm, accessed June 13, 2011.

Feinberg, J. 1984. *The Moral Limits of the Criminal Law: Harm to Others.* New York: Oxford University Press.

———. 1986. *The Moral Limits of the Criminal Law: Harm to Self.* New York: Oxford University Press.

———. 1988. *The Moral Limits of the Criminal Law: Harmless Wrongdoing.* New York: Oxford University Press.

Flegal, K.M., Carroll, M., Ogden, C., and Curtin, L. 2010. Prevalence and Trends in Obesity among U.S. Adults, 1999–2008. *Journal of the American Medical Association* 303 (3):235–41.

Francisco, J. 2006. Smokers' Old Refuge Is Now No Man's Land. *Chicago Tribune,* April 9.

Gavagan, T.F., Du, H., Saver, B., Adams, G., Graham, D., McCray, R., and Goodrick, G. 2010. Effect of Financial Incentives on Improvement of Medical Quality Indicators for Primary Care. *Journal of the American Board of Family Medicine* 23 (5):622–31.

GHSA (Governor's Highway Safety Association). 2010. Highway Safety Law Charts. Available at http://www.ghsa.org/html/stateinfo/laws/index.html, accessed June 13, 2011.

Glendon, M.A. 1991. *Rights Talk: The Impoverishment of Political Discourse.* New York: Free Press.

Gostin, L.O. 2000. *Public Health Law: Power, Duty, Restraint.* Berkeley: University of California Press and Milbank Memorial Fund.

———. 2002. Public Health Law in an Age of Terrorism: Rethinking Individual Rights and Common Goods. *Health Affairs* 21 (6):79–93.

———. 2003. When Terrorism Threatens Health: How Far Are Limitations on Personal and Economic Liberties Justified? *Florida Law Review* 55 (5):1105–70.

———. 2005. Law and the Public's Health. *Issues in Science and Technology* 21 (3).

————. 2010. Mapping the Issues. In L.O. Gostin, Ed., *Public Health Law and Ethics: A Reader* (pp. 1–22). Berkeley: University of California Press.

Gostin, L.O., and Gostin, K. 2009. A Broader Liberty: J.S. Mill, Paternalism and the Public's Health. *Public Health* 123 (3):214–21.

Gostin, L.O., Jacobson, P.D., Record, K.L., and Hardcastle, L.E. 2011. Restoring Health to Health Reform: Integrating Medicine and Public Health to Advance the Population's Wellbeing. *University of Pennsylvania Law Review*, 159(1): 101–147.

Gostin, L.O., and Taylor, A.L. 2008. Global Health Law: A Definition and Grand Challenges. *Public Health Ethics* 1 (1):53–63.

Haile, A.J. 2009. Sin Taxes: When the State Becomes the Sinner. *Temple Law Review* 82 (4):1041–70.

Hyman, D.A., and Silver, C. 2005. The Poor State of Healthcare Quality in the United States: Is Malpractice Part of the Problem or Part of the Solution? *Cornell Law Review* 90 (4):893–993.

IIHS (Insurance Institute for Highway Safety). 2011. State Law Facts. Available at http://www.iihs.org/laws, accessed June 13, 2011.

IOM (Institute of Medicine). 1988. *The Future of Public Health*. Washington, DC: National Academy Press.

————. 2002. *The Future of the Public's Health in the 21st Century*. Washington, DC: National Academy Press.

————. 2010. *Strategies to Reduce Sodium Intake in the United States*. Washington, DC: National Academy Press.

————. 2011. For the Public's Health: Revitalizing Law and Policy to Meet New Challenges. Washington, DC: National Academy Press.

IRS (Internal Revenue Services). 2010. Indoor Tanning Services; Cosmetic Services; Excise Taxes. *Federal Register* 75:33683–88.

Jacobson, P.D., and Warner, K.E. 1999. Litigation and Public Health Policy: The Case of Tobacco Control. *Journal of Health, Politics, Policy and Law* 24 (4):769–804.

Jennings, B. 2009. Public Health and Liberty: Beyond the Millian Paradigm. *Public Health Ethics* 2 (2):123–34.

Jones, M.M., and Bayer, R. 2007. Paternalism and Its Discontents: Motorcycle Helmet Laws, Libertarian Values, and Public Health. *American Journal of Public Health* 97 (2):208–17.

Koh, H., and Sebelius, K.G. 2010. Promoting Prevention through the Affordable Care Act. *New England Journal of Medicine* 363 (14):1296–99.

LaFrance, A.B. 2000. Tobacco Litigation: Smoke Mirrors and Public Policy. *American Journal of Law and Medicine* 26 (2–3):187–202.

Lappe, M. 1986. Ethics and Public Health. In J.M. Last, Ed., *Public Health and Preventive Medicine* (pp. 1867–77). Norwalk, CT: Appleton-Century-Crofts.

Leonard, E.W. 2010. Tort Litigation for the Public's Health. In J.G. Culhane, Ed., *Reconsidering Law and Policy Debates: A Public Health Perspective* (pp. 187–220). New York: Cambridge University Press.

Let's Move. 2011. Available at http://letsmove.gov, accessed June 13, 2011.

Loewenstein, G., Brennan, T., and Volpp, K., 2007. Asymmetric Paternalism to Improve Health Behaviors. *Journal of the American Medical Association* 298 (20):2415–17.

Magnusson, R. 2009. Book Review. *Medical Law Review* 17 (3):477–91.

Meier, B.M., Phil, M., Gebbie, K., and Hodge, J. 2007. Contrasting Experiences of State Public Health Law Reform Pursuant to the Turning Point Model State Public Health Act. *Public Health Reports* 122 (4):559–63.

———. 2009. Transitions in State Public Health Law: Comparative Analysis of State Public Health Law Reform following the Turning Point Model Statute. *American Journal of Public Health* 99 (3):423–30.

Mello, M., Studdert, D., and Brennan, T. 2006. Obesity: The New Frontier of Public Health Law. *New England Journal of Medicine* 354 (24):2601–10.

NAAG (National Academy of Attorney Generals). 1998. Master Settlement Agreement. Available at http://www.library.ucsf.edu/tobacco/litigation/usa.pdf, accessed June 13, 2011.

NCSL (National Conference of State Legislatures). 2010a. State Cigarette Excise Taxes: 2010. Available at http://www.ncsl.org/default.aspx?tabid=14349, accessed January 30, 2011.

———. 2010b. Tanning Restrictions for Minors: A State-by-State Comparison. Available at http://www.ncsl.org/default.aspx?tabid=14394, accessed June 13, 2011.

———. 2011. Trans Fat and Menu Labeling Legislation. Available at http://www.ncsl. org/default.aspx?tabid=14362, accessed June 13, 2011.

NHTSA (National Highway Traffic Safety Administration). 2009. 2008 Traffic Safety Annual Assessment: Highlights. Available at http://www-nrd.nhtsa.dot.gov/ Pubs/811172.pdf, accessed June 13, 2011.

NIAID (National Institute of Allergy and Infectious Diseases). 2008. *NIAID: Planning for the 21st Century: 2008 Update.* Washington, DC: DHHS.

Nolte, R., Franckowiak, R., Crespo, C.J., and Andersen, R.E. 2002. U.S. Military Weight Standards: What Percentage of U.S. Young Adult Males Meet the Current Standards? *American Journal of Medicine* 113 (6):486–90.

Nuffield Council on Bioethics. 2007. *Public Health: Ethical Issues.* London: Nuffield Council on Bioethics.

Oberlander, J. 2006. Who Pays? Who Benefits? Distributional Issues in Health Care: The Political Economy of Unfairness in U.S. Health Policy. *Law and Contemporary Problems* 69 (4):245–64.

Ogden, C.L., Carroll, M., Curtin, L., Lamb, M., Flegal, K. 2010. Prevalence of High Body Mass Index in U.S. Children and Adolescents 2007–2008. *Journal of the American Medical Association* 303 (3):242–49.

Owen, D.G. 2005. *Products Liability Law.* St. Paul, MN: West Group.

Parmet, W. 2009. *Populations: Public Health and the Law.* Washington, DC: Georgetown University Press.

Parmet, W., and Daynard, R.A. 2000. The New Public Health Litigation. *Annual Review of Public Health* 21:437–54.

Pope, T.M. 2000. Balancing Public Health against Individual Liberty: The Ethics of Smoking Regulations. *University of Pittsburgh Law Review* 61 (2):419–92.

———. 2005. Is Public Health Paternalism Really Never Justified? A Response to Joel Feinberg. *Oklahoma City University Law Review* 30 (1):121–207.

PPACA (Patient Protection and Affordable Care Act). 2010. H.R. 3590 (2009) (Rangel, D-N.Y.), enacted as Pub. L. No. 111–148.

Pulos, E., and Leng, K. 2010. Evaluation of a Voluntary Menu-Labeling Program in Full Service Restaurants. *American Journal of Public Health* 100 (6):1035–39.

Roberto, C.A., Larsen, P., Agnew, H., Baik, J., and Brownell, K. 2010. Evaluating the Impact of Menu Labeling on Food Choices and Intake. *American Journal of Public Health* 100 (2):312–18.

Rose-Ackerman, S. 1994. Product Safety Regulation and the Law of Torts. In J.R. Hunziker and T.O. Jones, Eds., *Products Liability and Innovation: Managing Risk in an Uncertain Environment* (pp. 151–58). Washington, DC: National Academy Press.

Rudd Center (Rudd Center for Food Policy and Obesity, Yale University). 2011. Legislation Database. Available at http://yaleruddcenter.org/legislation, accessed June 13, 2011.

Schroeder, C.H. 2002. Lost in the Translation: What Environmental Regulation Does that Tort Cannot Duplicate. *Washburn Law Review* 41 (3):583–606.

Schuck, P.H. 1988. *Agent Orange on Trial: Mass Toxic Disasters in the Courts.* Cambridge, MA: Belknap Press.

Schwartz, G.T. 1997. Mixed Theories of Tort Law: Affirming Both Deterrence and Corrective Justice. *Texas Law Review* 75 (7):1801–34.

Shavell, S. 1987. *Economic Analysis of Accident Law.* Cambridge, MA: Harvard University Press.

Siegel, A. 2001. Jurisprudence of Public Health: Reflections on Lawrence O. Gostin's Public Health Law. *Journal of Contemporary Health Law and Policy* 18 (1):359–72.

Tandon, P.S., Wright, J., Zhou, C., Rogers, C., and Christakis, D. 2010. Nutrition Menu Labeling May Lead to Lower-Calorie Restaurant Meal Choices for Children. *Pediatrics* 125 (2):244–48.

Thaler, R.H., and Sunstein, C.R. 2009. *Nudge: Improving Decisions about Health, Wealth, and Happiness.* New York: Penguin Group.

Thomas, M., and Buckmaster, L. 2010. Paternalism in Social Policy: When Is It Justifiable? *Parliament of Australia, Department of Parliamentary Services* Research Paper No. 8, 2010–11.

Wagner, W. 2007. When All Else Fails: Regulating Risky Products through Tort Law. *Georgetown Law Journal* 95 (3):693–732.

Wallace, R.B. 2008. *Public Health and Preventive Medicine.* New York: McGraw-Hill.

Weiner, J.B., and Rogers, M.D. 2002. Comparing Precaution in the United States and Europe. *Journal of Risk Regulation* 5 (4):317–49.

Winterfield, A., Morandi, L., and Shinkle, D. 2010. *Promoting Healthy Communities and Preventing Childhood Obesity: Trends in Recent Legislation.* Denver: National Conference of State Legislatures.

11

Should the Value of Future Health Benefits Be Time-Discounted?

PAUL T. MENZEL, PhD ■

INTRODUCTION

What is the value of a year of life lived 10 years from now compared to the value of a year of life that starts now? Different contexts in which the question is asked can greatly influence the answer. It is clear the answer health economists and health policy decision makers typically give: *the current value of a future year of life is less than the current value of a year of life lived now.* Put more generally, their answer is that the further into the future a health benefit is temporally located, the less value that health benefit has compared to an otherwise identical benefit occurring earlier. The answer applies to all future health benefits: additional years of life, improvements in health-related quality of life, and, indeed, people's very lives (their "whole lives").

In the standard methodology of cost-effectiveness analysis (CEA), the practice of calculating the value implied by this answer is referred to as "discounting back to present value." Whatever rate health policy analysts use to discount future *monetary* expenditures and savings back to present value, they typically use the same rate to discount future *nonmonetary health benefits*—therefore the term "uniform discounting" (Severens and Milne 2004). The debate is about both whether to discount future nonmonetary items such as health benefits at all, and if so, whether to practice *uniform* as distinct from *differential* discounting. In the latter, future health benefits would be discounted at a lower rate than monetary items.

Regardless of which form the debate is pursued, the matter is important in estimating the relative value of prevention compared to treatment. Typically, treatment's health benefits occur sooner than prevention's health benefits. A secondary prevention such as routine screening for prostate cancer may produce benefits, but many of them emerge years down the road. Although routine screening will discern some tumors amenable to treatment early on, most gains for a given cohort of patients come from maintaining the screening over several decades. The effects of radiation and surgical treatment of prostate tumors, even if they may not be immediate, are usually seen to occur more quickly. Similarly, although a lifestyle influencing measure such as prediabetes counseling may yield equal or greater health benefit outcomes at a lower cost, those benefits typically lie further into the future than the likely results of disease-delaying drugs or ameliorative treatments (DPP Research Group 2009).

When the anticipated results are then discounted back to present value, the calculated cost-effectiveness of prevention typically slips compared to the cost-effectiveness of treatments for the same eventual condition. By how much? At a 3.0% discount rate over 20 years, for example, which is at the low end of the typical 3.0–7.0% range, the present value of 10 years of future life drops to less than 6 years.[1]

Many well-known studies of preventive measures provide specific illustration. Comparison of mobile coronary care units (MCCU) with a prevention program of screening children for elevated cholesterol and following it up with recommended dietary changes found a cost-effectiveness advantage for MCCU of over 2:1 when costs and added life were uniformly discounted at 5.0%. It found an opposite 3:1 advantage for screening, however, when the years of added life were not discounted (Cretin 1977; Keeler and Cretin 1983, 301). A well-known study of Pap smears to screen for cervical cancer revealed that if costs and benefits were uniformly discounted at 5.0%, then, begun at age 20, they had a relatively modest cost of $10,000 per added year of life done every 4 years. They caught more cancers if done every 3 years, but at a marginal cost of $185,000 per year of life. If those added years of life were not discounted, however, even screening at 3-year intervals on average saved at the relatively modest marginal cost rate of $20,000/year of life (Eddy 1990, 218).

As of 2008, the U.S. government recommended uniform discounting with rates of 3.0–7.0% (Zeckhauser and Viscusi 2008). In 1996 an influential panel

1. This chapter almost exclusively uses relatively short time spans as the context for controversies about health-related discounting. There the effects of discounting are relatively modest, as in the change over 20 years just cited from 10 units of benefit to six. The effects of discounting for longer periods, however, are huge: at 5% over 425 years, for example, one billion becomes one (Frederick 2006, 672). Even for the longest time spans within a lifetime (50 years, say) at 5% eleven becomes less than one.

appointed by the U.S. Public Health Service recommended uniform discounting between 3.0% and 5.0%, with sensitivity estimates to be done over a 0–5.0%
range (Lipscomb, Weinstein, and Torrance 1996). Before 2003 the United
Kingdom, by contrast, had been discounting differentially—future health benefits at 1.5–2.0% and future monetary costs and savings at 6.0%.[2] Then the
National Institute of Clinical Effectiveness, acting on recommendations from
the UK Treasury, urged that both be discounted 3.5% (Severens and Milne
2004). Analysts often debate what rate should be used, but rarely in the health
policy world is there debate about the necessity of discounting future nonmonetary benefits at some rate (Morrall 2003, 227; Brazier et al. 2007, 275).[3] Such
homogeneous views are reflected in actual practice; the almost universal prescription by government bodies and regulatory institutions is to discount health
effects and costs at the same rate (Claxton et al. 2011, 13).

My aim in this chapter is to provide a comprehensive normative assessment[4]
of the practice of uniform discounting in health economics, and in cost-
effectiveness analysis in particular. In the end I will conclude that even when the
often powerful reasons of economists are taken into account, the moral case for
a general practice in CEA of uniform discounting is weak. My route to this conclusion will involve (1) drawing a distinction between two fundamentally different kinds of time preference judgments, about individual utility and social value;
(2) comparing money and health in respect to characteristics that generate

2. Brouwer et al. (2005) note how much difference a 6.0/1.5% differential in discounting
makes compared to a uniform 6% discounting. Meningococcal C vaccine costs £15,710/
Quality Adjusted Life Year (QALY) with uniform discounting, but only £3,845/QALY with
differential discounting. With uniform discounting hormone replacement therapy costs
£42,374/hip fracture prevented but only £7,362/hip fracture prevented with differential
discounting.

3. Illustrative is a terse sentence in Corso and Haddix (2003, 94). Having noted that "some
prevention-effectiveness practitioners argue that health outcomes should be discounted at a
lower rate than costs," they simply observe that "*there is no theoretical basis for this approach*"
(emphasis added).

4. By "normative" assessment here I mean *ethical* (moral, philosophical). Economists' sense
of the term is often different. For them, as for me, a "descriptive" or "empirical" critique of
discounting focuses on whether the discount rates used match the actual time preferences
people have, but then economists often use "normative" to connote a contrasting theoretical perspective, not necessarily a moral one. Given the alleged consistency problems that
differential discounting encounters in the theory of discounted utility, for example, many
economists say we *ought* to practice uniform discounting regardless of whether it matches
actual time preference. See Redelmeier and Heller (1993, 216) and Weinstein (1993, 219) for
this sense of normative assessment. By contrast, in the morally normative approach I pursue,
I critique the economist's theoretical justification for discounting along with its empirical
basis.

change in value over time; (3) summarizing and examining some particularly relevant segments of the empirical data on time preference; (4) assessing two moral arguments that ground the practice of discounting in individual utility time preferences; and (5) addressing the so-called Keeler–Cretin paradox that differential discounting encounters. Finally, (6) I will address the degree to which a moral justification of discounting can rely on empirical preferences.

TWO PERSPECTIVES AND A FURTHER CLARIFICATION OF THE ISSUE

Contrast the widespread and typically unquestioned practice of uniform discounting in health economics with looking at the issue intuitively as a matter of value, without the influence of an academic discipline's constructed theoretical framework. We immediately find ourselves torn by two sharply different judgments about discounting future health benefits.

Take lives and life extension, for instance. On the one hand, in any sense of either the moral value or the subjective value of lives to the people who live them, it seems plainly false to say that the value of future lives is less than the value of present ones. Do we really want to claim that the very life of a person living from 2010 to 2090, for example, is less valuable than the life of a person living 5 years earlier, from 2005 to 2085? *Of course not.* The very value of different people's lives, including the subjective value to the respective persons whose lives they are, does not vary by temporal location.

On the other hand, if we ask ourselves an *intra*personal question, the answer seems to be the opposite. Will you do more (pay more now, for example) to gain an immediate 10-year life extension for yourself than you will now pay to gain a 10-year extension of life 20 years from now? *Of course you will.* Not for a moment would you agree to have a coin flipped, after you paid, to determine which 10-year span of life would be preserved, as if the two spans were equally valuable. If your life doesn't get extended now, you won't be around in 20 years to begin to experience any later 10 years!

We might object to the way this last trade-off is stated. Part of what causes the quick "of course" response is that without the earlier of these two life extensions, a person does not get the 20 years between now and the later life extension. Call this the disruptive factor of "Intervening Years," which is clearly present in intrapersonal comparisons of later with earlier life extensions.[5] If the Intervening Years factor is not present, however, it is unclear what the attraction of the 10 earlier

---

5. The factor of Intervening Years might be related to what Gafni (1995) has called "sequence-preference" as distinct from "time preference." Gafni uses his distinction to raise serious

years really is over the 10 later ones. It is very difficult, however, to remove the influence of the Intervening Years factor from people's thinking, or even to construct a hypothetical choice that could eliminate it.[6] The tendency to prefer a nearer life-extending benefit to a later one within our own lives is stubborn, though we should note that it may not hold nearly as strongly for nonlifesaving health benefits, where there is little if any factor analogous to Intervening Years.[7]

This short exercise, eliciting sharply different responses about time preference, points to the fact that we make two fundamentally different kinds of choices about intertemporal value. *Within our own lives* we face trade-offs between obtaining a lifesaving or other health benefit sooner rather than later; in this case we usually prefer the sooner. This preference certainly holds for life itself, in part because of the Intervening Years factor, and it seems likely to hold, though perhaps to a lesser degree, for many health benefits short of life itself. We would generally expect 20 years of severe chronic illness in our 30s and 40s, for example, to have a more pervasively devastating effect on our whole life than an illness of similar severity in our 60s and 70s. When we are expressing such relative valuations about health benefits within our own lives, we are expressing *individual utility* judgments.

Such evaluations are very different, and respond to very different questions, than *social value* judgments (Menzel 1999). The latter, like individual utility judgments, can be made by individuals, but they are *about* something different: *interpersonal* trade-offs. For example, should a program that would prevent

questions about whether we really know what constitutes "time preference," as well as to raise problems about its empirical measurement.

6. One such possible choice involves a comparison of insurance contracts. Imagine that one of two situations will develop in your life. Either (1) you will contract a life-threatening disease a week from now that can be treated with a high likelihood of extending your life another 10 years (10 years only, but with good daily function—"normal health") or (2) you will contract an equally life-threatening disease 20 years from now that can be treated with an equally high likelihood of extending your life for 10 years (10 years only, and with the same good daily function as in the first situation). It cannot be known which of these two situations will develop, though you do know that *the probability of each is equal.* You can buy an "advance treatment contingency contract" for either or for both, but to get any life-extending treatment in either prospective situation, you must pay now. *Are you willing to pay more for the first contract than for the second?* With the choice thus revised, it is not so clear that people will pay more for life-extending treatment for the first development than they will for the second. Perhaps many will pay more for the first, but without the Intervening Years factor present, it is not clear what the attraction of 10 earlier years really is over 10 later ones.

7. Redelmeier and Heller (1993) found fairly low individual-utility time preference in comparing present nonlifesaving health benefits with similar benefits 5–10 years in the future: a mean of 0.25% as an annual discount rate. Also, 62% of their respondents expressed a zero discount rate, and 10% had *negative* time preference (preference for a later benefit).

kidney failure in persons A–M over the decade 2010–2020 take precedence over a similar program for persons N–Z effective in 2020–2030?

I will come back to this distinction between individual utility (IU) and social value (SV) in later discussion of the relevance of individual time preference to the normative debate about uniform discounting.[8] Before pursuing the overall issue in detail, though, a subtle aspect of the claim that is being made about intertemporal values by defenders of discounting warrants attention.

The claim behind discounting based on time preference is *not* that the value of a year of life 10 years from now is, *at that time*, less than the current value of a year of life now. That value—the value *then*—is the full normal value of a year of life. It is the same as the value of a year of life lived presently. Discounting does not deny this. The claim behind the practice is subtly different. It is that to *compare* the value of goods accurately *across time, all values have to be expressed in the common terms of value at one particular time*. Value at one time is not the same as value at another time.

The need for expressing value as value at a particular time is very easy to see in the case of money. The value of year-2020 dollars and the value of year-2010 dollars, if they are to be accurately and fairly compared with each other, need to be put in terms of exclusively either 2010 dollars or 2020 dollars. There is no such transtemporal thing as a temporally unallocated value of a dollar. And a 2020 dollar's value *in 2010—that is, as seen from and used in 2010*—is less than that 2020 dollar's value seen from and used in 2020.

Then the first reason that there can be legitimate debate about discounting, despite its overwhelmingly standard use, becomes apparent: the difference between money and nonmonetary goods. Despite the fact that translation of intertemporal values is clearly needed for money, it is not easy to see, intuitively, that it is appropriate for many nonmonetary goods. It is especially difficult to see that it is appropriate for SV as opposed to IU judgments about health benefits.

To assess whether the typical insistence in health policy analysis on uniform discounting makes sense, including moral sense, I turn to an examination of how monetary items and health outcomes compare in the characteristics most relevant to time preference.

---

8. Frederick (2006) thinks it highly relevant to distinguish discounting "one's *own* future utility" from "discounting the utility of *others* who will be alive in the future." That is not exactly the distinction between IU and SV preferences that I use; SV preferences are not necessarily about others' *utility*, but about (for example) distributive relationships. The essential thrust of the two distinctions, however, is the same: about myself vs. about something beyond myself. Earlier Bonneaux and Birnie (2001) contrasted the standard economic model using individual utility preferences with what they referred to as "societal preference."

MONEY AND HEALTH BENEFIT COMPARED

Any defense of uniform discounting is anchored in the unchallenged legitimacy of discounting future monetary costs and savings. Before taking up several compelling reasons for that discounting, it would be best to discuss and eliminate two reasons that are *not* part of the basis in economics for the practice of discounting monetary items, though these reasons are likely to occur quickly to any lay-person. One is *uncertainty*: possible intervening events (death, loss of important capacities, opportunity-blocking world events, etc.) make it less than certain that with any money I would hold onto I could later engage in consumption that would have the same value to me as it does now. A second is *inflation*: a given dollar will likely buy less in the future than it buys now.

Both are important considerations, but when we are working within the analytical framework of CEA, both of these factors are already accounted for *before* anything referred to as "discounting" is applied. In regard to uncertainty, suppose that a future additional 10-year span of life has only a 90% chance of coming about. In reputable CEA that future 10-year benefit will already be calculated as a statistically likely 9 years (Zeckhauser and Viscusi 2008).[9] Similarly, inflation is already included in an accurate estimation of the future actual costs of care, or the future actual savings from avoiding that care. This prior accounting for inflation may look like discounting, but it is not what economists refer to by the term. Accounting for inflation is aimed at *accurately predicting* what the real future costs and savings are likely to be. Discounting, by contrast, constitutes a *revaluation* of those savings and expenses in light of time preference.[10]

9. In addition to uncertainty itself, which in an accurate estimation of the costs and benefits before any revaluation to present value is supposed to be accounted for already, *aversion to* uncertainty may enter as a factor creating time preference. In the numerical example used here, a 90% chance of a 10-year benefit is statistically equivalent to 9 years. The "90% chance," though, still has its own separate character: a range between no fewer than 6 years and no more than 12 years, for example. An aversion to *the range that one would be risking* in going for the statistically likely 9 future years could reduce its value further, compared to a more definite number of earlier years. I owe this observation to Erik Nord.

10. George Miller (Altarum Institute) has articulated an alternate version of what economists are doing in discounting as distinct from accounting for inflation. In cost analysis economists typically express future costs in constant (e.g., 2010) dollars; then they use a discount rate that is *net* of inflation, expressing the rate at which constant dollars will grow over time. The alternative would be to express future costs in real dollars and add an inflation rate to the discount rate; to be sure, that is a possible alternative, equivalent in final result to the constant dollar approach. But it is messier, requires estimating future inflation rates, and complicates the issue of how (or whether) to discount future health benefits in order to account for inflation as well as time value.

To be sure, health benefits may experience something parallel to monetary inflation, but that, too, should already be included in accurate discernment of benefits. I might not expect to value full restoration of athletic-level mobility 20 years into the future (in my 70s, say) as much as I value such restoration now, but those differences should already be accounted for in quality adjustments to the value of a given objective increment of health. This is the "quality adjusted" part of a QALY (quality-adjusted life year—see Chapter 1 of this volume, note 10).[11]

The appropriate reasons for economists' practice of discounting future costs and savings back to a different present value are not, then, uncertainty or inflation. The appropriate reasons are two other factors: the fact that "money makes money" (capital capacity), and time preference.

1. *Capital capacity*. Money, used as capital, makes money. Just as trees can be left to grow and produce more wood to harvest 10 years from now, similarly money, if its use for current consumption is passed over, can be invested to increase productive capacity (Broome 1994, 53). Running forward, money thus earns interest. The underlying reality, seen in reverse, requires arithmetically the opposite, discounting: a given amount of future money is equivalent to a smaller present amount.

2. *Time preference*. "Pure" time preference refers to the inherent preference that people typically have for obtaining goods earlier rather than later. People do not want to postpone experiences and goods if they can just as well have them now. Separate from guarding against uncertainty and inflation, this preference may stem from imprudence, from impatience and demand for relatively instant gratification, or from simple failure to imagine the future vividly enough to make an accurate comparison between a development then and a similar but more immediate one now.[12] It might also, however, be grounded in an arguably more rational factor, what philosopher Derek Parfit

11. This observation is also true for intergenerational future health benefits, outside the context of individual utility judgments. There the proper comparison is not between mobility preservation for a person in their 50s and mobility preservation for that same person in their 70s, but between mobility preservation for one person in their 50s in 2010 and mobility preservation for *another* person in their 50s 20 years later. Inflation in health benefit units from one generation to the next, although possible, does not appear ubiquitous or great enough to require careful "prior" accounting within CEA; even if it were, it would warrant only prior accounting and not further discounting.

12. The last reason is particularly interesting in the context of debating priorities between prevention and treatment. The same lack of accurate imagination of events further into the

observes: is the weak identity connections between our present and our future selves. So much will change in our lives that we do not strongly identify with our future selves, suspecting (correctly, perhaps) that they are not fully *our* (the present "our") future selves (Parfit 1971, 1982; Frederick et al. 2002, 359).

Despite the indubitable fact that people have some such time preference, however, almost every aspect of it is ambiguous. For starters, people sometimes manifest the opposite preference, obtaining enjoyment from anticipation and preferring future enjoyments that they can anticipate in the meantime (Frederick et al. 2002). Complicating the empirical discernment of any pure time preference are great difficulties in separating out the influence of the two practical matters dealt with previously, perceived uncertainty and inflation. When people respond to questions designed to detect time preference, are they unwittingly influenced by everyday assumptions they make about inflation and uncertainty?

In any case, how do gains and losses in health compare to money in respect to capital capacity and time preference?[13]

Capital Capacity

Some goods in addition to money make more of themselves—trees, for example, as noted above. In a certain sense, life does, too: people reproduce. Compare a universe populated by an additional person capable of reproduction in the second decade of the twenty-first century with a universe also populated by an additional person of the same age, but later, whose likely reproduction is instead in the fifth decade of that same century. In the first case procreation has an additional generation in which to work. That will likely yield a net gain, in the history of the human species, of at least one more whole life. Improved health can also be productive in other ways, including careers and creative achievements that health makes possible. Selectively, then, health can indeed "make more of itself." It is still different on this score, however, than money, which has a ubiquitous power to make more of itself. Relatively few of the additional life-years that medicine makes possible result in new lives; most life extension

future that helps to explain time preference is one of the reasons people may regard prevention as less important than treatment.

13. Goodin (1982) discusses somewhat different characteristics, and more of them. His approach in criticizing uniform discounting, though, is fundamentally similar to the structure of this section: directly comparing money with other goods.

accomplished by health care, because of the age of its beneficiaries, results in no additional reproduction. Even when improved health is productive in other ways, the reason for preserving and improving health is seldom that "health makes health." The health benefit itself, independent of its relationship to other health, is the primary locus of value.

In one context, though, "health makes health" can be an apt characterization: in much intrapersonal time preference about health benefits, where the focus is on individual utility. A person who considers great positive versus negative health outcomes, which could occur either sooner or later in her life—not only lifesaving itself but severe disability or chronic illness, say—will often naturally prefer the nearer benefit. If when we get to our future, our opportunity range has already been much narrowed by previous extended illness, future health gain is not worth as much. "Health makes health" may not be quite the right expression to capture this; perhaps "health makes health possible" is a more correct appellation. Thus, although we should be cautious in doing so, we can plausibly refer to health's "internal productivity," its capacity to produce more of itself, a kind of "capital capacity."

It is important to note, however, that much less of this consideration applies to the *interpersonal* social values about health and life that people hold and express. Those values are elicited by asking questions about, say, extending the lives of one group of persons 10 years now compared to 10-year life extensions of a different set of persons decades into the future.[14] The reproductive capacity point, that "lives make lives" and "health makes health possible," is sometimes applicable in the interpersonal context, but it is more at home in intrapersonal judgments of individual health utility.

Time Preference

Do we have any pure time preference in our valuation of health? As with money, imprudence, impatience, and failure to imagine the future fully enough can influence intrapersonal IU judgments. Those factors all appear irrational, however; if they were the basis for discounting future health benefits, the practice would hardly stand on firm and stable societal and moral ground. The problems that Parfit (1971, 1982) perceives with a self-identity that diminishes across time spans may provide a more rational ground for discounting, but that less-of-myself phenomenon may not apply to attitudes toward our own health as

---

14. To make the comparison fair and an accurate gauge of pure time preference, the two respective life extensions need to have more in common than just the same number of years – they also need to occur for people at the same ages in life and for the same quality of life.

much as it applies to the enjoyment of more typical "consumption." In any case, the influence of any of these factors on our SV preferences, which necessarily involve interpersonal comparisons beyond IU judgments, is more dubious. And, as we shall see, it is not only normatively more dubious, but empirically.

The conclusion is that although health benefits manifest some of the same capital capacity and time preference characteristics as money does, they have neither characteristic to the same degree, or as consistently.

EMPIRICAL DATA ON SOCIAL VALUE TIME PREFERENCE

Let me focus the inquiry now on the empirics of time preference. An immediate consideration is whether the discounting debate should take its cue from IU preferences about the relative value of health benefits at different times, or from SV preferences. For decisions about different options within individual patients' lives, it is logical to look to IU preferences. CEA and other economic assessments of health benefits, however, are usually pursued in making judgments about various measures across different potential recipients. The people who would receive a treatment for a certain condition are often not the same people who would receive preventive care. For the former, for one thing, it may be too late for prevention. For the typical interpersonal context in which CEA is used, then, if our moral focus ought to be on empirical preferences at all, it ought to be on SV preferences.[15] The rest of this section, therefore, will concentrate on empirical data on people's SV, not IU, preferences about temporal location.

In a frequently cited study Cropper, Aydede, and Portney (1994) found strong preference for saving a specified number of lives presently over a much greater number of lives 25 or 100 years later. Respondents' average marginal preference point (the point closest to indifference) was to save one person today over saving 45 people in 100 years. For a 5 year horizon, the responses implied a discount rate of 17%; for a 25 year horizon, over 10%; and for a 100 year horizon, 3.7%. On the upper end, 47% of respondents implied a discount rate of

15. This is not to say that IU preferences have no proper role in social valuations. (1) As we shall see later, there is an important argument for the relevance of IU valuations in even interpersonal comparison contexts. (2) A discussion similar to the one here about the respective roles of IUs and SVs in discounting has unfolded in debates about the proper methodology in CEA for health state valuation. Because the results of CEA are most often used to make decisions across different groups of patients, SV preference data derived with "person trade-off" (PTO) questions have risen to some prominence in CEA. Preferences elicited by PTO questions, however, may achieve the greatest moral relevance if the participants responding to them are first informed of the IU preferences of those who actually experience the various health states being evaluated. See Menzel (1999), Ubel, Richardson, and Menzel (2000), and Dolan et al. (2003).

over 4.3% for a 100 year horizon, and 38% implied a rate over 14.8% for a 25 year horizon. Johannesson and Johansson (1997) found even greater discounting: 243 lives to one life for a 100 year time difference.

For purposes of assessing the use of discounting in CEA, one of the strengths of the Cropper et al. (1994, 245) study is that its questions were clearly designed to elicit SV preferences.[16] For example, this question: Which program would you prefer, Program A that will save 100 lives now, or Program B that will save 200 lives 25 years from now? It is highly questionable, however, whether the study's results indicate anything like pure time preference. They are influenced, for example, by respondents' consideration of uncertainty: more than 10% of respondents cited a perception that the "future is uncertain" as their lead reason for preferring to save lives today rather than in the future (Cropper et al. 1994, 250). Other lead reasons given by respondents also seem to contradict the goal of the study to elicit pure time preferences. From 22.8% to 31.3%[17] said that "technological progress provides means to save people in the future." Another reason, "one should live day by day," was cited by 21.2–31.7%, a response that is totally puzzling as a reason for an SV preference. Living "day by day" may be an attitude pointing an individual to benefit his or her own health now rather than invest in measures or activities that will pay off only in the future, but it is no reason for making an interpersonal judgment that 45 lives saved 100 years from now are equal in value to merely one person's life saved now.[18]

A multilayered study by Frederick (2003) is a better candidate for having elicited pure time preferences. It, too, used clearly SV questions. Given all the empirical data of positive time preference commonly cited in the literature to support discounting, it is perhaps surprising that Frederick found something apparently very different: preferences that implied only the tiniest of discount rates, almost zero in fact, and in some cases even negative time preference (favoring the saving of future over present lives). In what Frederick calls the "rating" format question, respondents choose whether outcome A, one person dying next year in the United States from exposure to pollutants, and outcome B, one person similarly dying 100 years from now, are "equally bad" or whether one was "worse" than the other. A total of 64% said A and B were equally bad, 28% said A was worse, and 8% said B was worse. For the 28% who said A was

---

16. Other studies that clearly focus on SV choices include Cairns (1994) on lifesaving and Olsen (1993) on lifesaving and health improvement.

17. The variation range is due to different time horizons: 5 to 50 years.

18. Frederick (2003, 49) similarly has critical things to say about the implications of the respondents' reported reasons in the study by Cropper et al. (1994).

worse, the substitution rate was only three lives 100 years from now to one life next year, reflecting a discount rate of a very small fraction of 1% (Frederick 2003, 43).

In asking, with this question, whether the time-variant outcomes were "equally bad" or one was "worse" than the other, respondents were likely encouraged to think of their preference in moral terms. This kind of question is arguably relevant if the responses are being used in a moral assessment of discounting. Frederick's other questions, though, only asked which of two outcomes respondents "preferred." In his "sequence" format question, for example, respondents were asked which program they preferred, program C that will become more effective over time (saving 100 lives this decade, 200 lives next decade, and 300 lives the third decade) or program D that will become less effective over time (saving 300 lives this decade, 200 the next, and 100 in the third). But these questions, just as those in the previous format, revealed no preference for saving lives earlier rather than later. Program C, for example, which became more effective over time, was preferred by 71% of respondents over program D, which would became less effective over time.[19]

Frederick (2003, 48) summarizes his findings: "many of the alternate elicitation procedures tested [in my study] ... suggest that lives in this generation and lives in future generations are valued about equally," with implied substitution rates "close to 1 to 1." These results appear to reflect careful consideration, in the study design, to elicit something closer to the ideal of pure time preference.[20] In many other choices used to elicit preferences, "respondents can readily express skepticism that the future deaths will actually occur by simply choosing the present-oriented program." The simple stark choice in the "rating" format question, Frederick argues, is more confining than the use of multiple numbers and

19. The responses to the choice between C and D might partially be expressions of a more general preference for "progress," not just time preference. On the other hand, even if the perception of "progress" influences the preferences here, this may illustrate only the more general point made by Frederick, Loewenstein, and O'Donoghue (2002) that the item we have conceptualized as "pure time preference" remains fundamentally and stubbornly ambiguous.

20. Some are skeptical that anyone can ever empirically elicit "pure" time preferences, or even whether such preferences exist. In a lengthy review of the literature on time discounting, Frederick et al. (2002, 389–390) conclude that there seems to be considerable ambiguity about a measurable notion of pure time preference: "the various elicitation procedures... consistently fail to isolate time preference, and instead reflect...a blend of both pure time preference and other theoretically distinct considerations. ... Our discussion...highlights the conceptual and semantic ambiguity about what...properly counts as time preference per se and what ought to be called something else... It is not obvious where to draw the line between factors that operate through utilities [such as uncertainty and inflation] and factors that make up time preference."

thus less likely to permit slippage toward unconscious suspicion of uncertainty about the future. Thus, the responses elicited with the "rating" question are likely indicative of something closer to pure time preference—though with his questions, of course, of an SV sort.

Frederick elicited only time preferences about lifesaving, not other health benefits. Earlier studies by Olsen (1993) and Cairns (1994) that also focused largely on SV time preferences dealt with nonlifesaving health benefits as well as lifesaving ones. They found results similar to those of Cropper et al.—i.e., more time preference. As with Cropper et al., however, Cairns's and Olsen's elicitation techniques did not contain the refinements added by Frederick to sharpen respondents' focus on moral and SV preferences and minimize the unwitting influence of uncertainty. If future studies extend refinements such as Frederick's to nonlifesaving health benefits, keeping an equally clear focus on SV and minimizing the intrusion of practical factors such as uncertainty and inflation, why would we expect the results to be much different? To be sure, more studies are needed, but that shows only that the empirical foundation of uniform discounting remains highly contingent. If most of the uses of CEA are for interpersonal comparison and allocation, and if the most relevant preferences are thus SV preferences, then the ground may already have shifted. Frederick's strong findings of almost zero time preference arguably throw the burden of proof back to those who wish to claim that people manifest enough pure time preference for earlier over later health benefits in their *social value* judgments to justify a practice of uniform discounting.

If carefully elicited preference data continue to bear out the direction Frederick has found, we may face a quite different situation in normative argument about whether discounting is justifiably based on subjective time preference. We began the assessment of the practice of discounting with a strong intuitive moral judgment, that truly equal health benefits have equal *interpersonal* value regardless of their temporal location. That judgment stood in apparently stark conflict with the preferences that people have for earlier over later benefits. Once the distinction between IU and SV time preferences is made, however, and the proper focus of the discounting debate *for CEA* is seen to be SV preferences, the empirical findings of psychology about time preference may well turn out to reinforce typical moral convictions.

(The next two sections concern arguments for uniform discounting that are extremely important in the academic literature. They and their critical analysis, however, may strike many who are not economists or philosophers as particularly difficult to follow. As important as the assessment of these arguments is, some readers may wish to skip over these sections.)

CAN INDIVIDUAL UTILITY STILL PROVIDE AN ARGUMENT FOR DISCOUNTING?[21]

We are not yet done, however, with individual utility. Let us suppose what seems plausible to say on the basis of the empirical literature: people see higher IU in earlier than in later health benefits, but it is highly debatable whether they express much time preference for health benefits in direct SV contexts. At least two strategies remain for building on IU to make a "welfarist" case for discounting future health benefits. (Welfarist approaches use only individual utilities—"welfare"—to build a notion of social value.)

Maximum Aggregate Utility Is Itself a Social Value

Assume both that people express little if any time preference in response to questions clearly focused on interpersonal, social value, and that CEA is typically used to make comparisons between various treatments and preventions for different people. Still, if people can stand back from their time-neutral SV preferences and reflect on the fact that each of them who will be affected likely has his or her own positive IU time preference, why wouldn't each of them say something like this:

> I do not know what my likely specific needs for health care are going to be, but I do know I will likely benefit both from some prevention that has relatively distant future benefits and from some other measures, treatments, whose benefits are likely to come more quickly after the care. My own welfare (IU) is generally higher when otherwise equivalent benefits come earlier rather than later. Therefore, despite the fact that I express little if any time preference in interpersonal situations, it is in my interest that future benefits be discounted at a rate that accords with my IU time preference. But there is nothing confined to myself in such observations: discounting future benefits at a rate that accords with others' IU time preferences would seem to be in their interest, too. Thus, I can universally prescribe the discounting of future health benefits for everyone, including myself, and they can also. It is a justifiable practice from a much wider perspective than just my own interest.[22]

21. I owe to Erik Nord the reminder that despite the other major points in this chapter, a different kind of argument for uniform discounting still needs to be dealt with.

22. This line of argument mirrors an argument used to defend a utilitarian view of moral action in general, far beyond the confines of discounting. See Hare (1997, 147–65).

This view is itself a social value judgment—that aggregate individual utilities make up interpersonal social value. Thus it can hardly be discounted as any less relevant to the interpersonal comparisons and allocations that are the primary focus of CEA than the arguably more intuitive, direct SV judgments expressed in the relatively time-neutral preferences elicited by Frederick, for example.

Such a welfarist utilitarian view is *an argument* for why IUs should be the primary elements taken into account *in discerning SV*, not simply a dogmatic insistence that only IU, not SV, matters. The question, though, is whether this view should be accorded any more weight than opposite SV judgments that manifest little time preference. It is not necessarily more reflective or sophisticated just because it emerges as a conclusion from a complex argument. Frederick's "rating" format question, for example—are one person's death next year and another person's death in the same manner at the same age but 100 years from now both equally bad?—provokes responses about the value of different lives at different times that are no simpler or more glib than the welfarist view just articulated.

In any case, although people may indeed find utility maximizing views of SV attractive, they are also drawn to value strongly other distributive relationships. A dialogue between the advocate of maximum utility and a defender of equal value across different persons in different times will perhaps come down to this case put by the egalitarian:

Once we are focused on *two* individuals who gain their similar benefits at different times, how can we privilege one over the other? Sally, say, gains her extra life through prevention that takes longer to gain its equally assured (or equally unassured) and later effect. Joe gains his through treatment whose effect comes with the same likelihood but earlier. To be sure, Sally, too, would prefer her benefit earlier if that were possible, but that hardly puts Sally in a position in which she should admit that Joe's treatment should take precedence over her prevention. They are two different people. Sally's later benefit is no less valuable *to her* than Joe's earlier benefit is *to him*.[23]

Moreover, even taken on its own terms, there is arguable slippage in the welfarist argument for discounting. Within Joe's life, for example, treatment and

---

23. This point is very similar to the argument that is made for the equal value of two people realizing their health potential even when that potential is less for one than for the other. See Menzel et al. (1999, 10–11) and Ubel et al. (2000). Note, also, that for Sally and Joe in my example, we could use the John and Bill of the thought experiment described in the Introduction to this volume.

prevention *for a given problem* (and with presumably equivalent health gains) will have to begin at different times—the prevention earlier than the treatment. The benefit that he receives from treatment will not occur any earlier than the benefit he would receive (or would have received) from prevention, so by the inherent nature of the situation he cannot have a *time preference* for the treatment. To be sure, at a given point in time, he may still have a time preference for a fast acting treatment of a health problem over a slow acting preventive approach to a *different* health problem. Insofar as CEA is used to compare curative with preventive approaches *to the same problem*, however, people will not have time preferences for the benefits of treatment over the benefits of prevention.[24]

A Savings Rate Implies a More General Time Preference

This second welfarist argument, unlike the previous one, aims directly at *uniform* discounting, not the discounting of future health benefits per se. The argument starts with the observation that the time preference that drives the savings rate that underlies the discount rate for money is likely to be mirrored in a similar time preference for health benefits. Nord elucidates the argument as follows (2011, 23–24):

> The rational consumer is willing to save up to a point at which the utility loss he suffers from delaying a marginal unit of consumption a year is exactly compensated by the increase in consumption that he/she achieves through the interest obtained on the saved money. ... [For] goods in general...all individuals' degree of discounting of future consumption is... approximated by the market rate of interest to which they all have adjusted their saving at the margin... Assume furthermore that over time, individuals value health relative to other goods at a constant rate, i.e., the individual willingness to pay for health, or the "dollar value of health," is constant. Then it seems reasonable to assume that individuals at the margin discount health benefits at the same rate as they discount other goods. The latter is...observable...in the market rate of interest. ... So the appropriate rate for discounting health benefits is the same as the appropriate rate for discounting costs.

---

24. Admittedly, this critique of the welfarist utilitarian argument is not telling against the use of CEA to make decisions across different conditions. It also still leaves differential discounting vulnerable to the postponement problem discussed in the next section.

As Nord notes, the argument is transparently dependent on the empirical question of whether individuals do in fact value health relative to other goods at a constant rate over time, and whether, for that or for other reasons, their time preferences for health really are consistent with the monetary savings rate.[25] Perhaps they are not. Therefore this argument becomes entirely dependent on certain empirical questions and cannot be made on theoretical grounds.

In any case, societal decision makers, as Nord (2011, 24) among others has noted, are not necessarily IU maximizers. Why should they be, when the SV preferences of the population they represent differ markedly from the SV judgment made by welfarist utilitarians?

THE POSTPONEMENT PROBLEM (KEELER–CRETIN PARADOX)

Even if IU does not provide an adequate normative foundation for uniform discounting, however, the basic debate has still not been settled. One of the most powerful arguments for uniform discounting is that nonuniform discounting runs into an "indefinite postponement" problem, commonly referred to as the "Keeler–Cretin paradox" (Keeler and Cretin 1983). This problem is critical to the debate regardless of whether the issue's proper focus is on IU or on SV.[26]

The alleged problem is that if nonmonetary benefits are discounted at a lower rate than money, cost and benefit calculations point toward continually postponing spending on lifesaving and health and instead invest financial resources for their later use. If health benefits stay the same in value whenever they occur, then 10 lives saved in 2020, for example, have no less value than do 10 lives of the same age saved in 2010. However, the money needed to save the 2010 lives ($100,000, say) would grow more than 30% by 2020 if invested at a conservative 3% annual interest. If we wait until 2020, we could then save not only the

25. Others in addition to Nord (e.g., Claxton et al. 2011, 13–14; Paulden and Claxton 2009) have noted this same importance of whether, empirically, the consumption value of health relative to the consumption value of other goods is constant over time. An increase in health's relative value points toward discounting future health benefits at a lower rate than money and other goods. Many believe that the weight of empirical study points toward such a greater relative value of health over time.

26. Keeler and Cretin (1983, 302) acknowledge the interpersonal context for most CEA of health care and therefore the relevance of SV preferences.

originally anticipated 10 lives, but another three as well (Donohue 1999, 1905).[27] Not discounting future health benefits at the same rate as money favors future over present lifesaving.

But then note that it is actually the failure to discount the value of a life (or any form of nonuniform discounting) that is inequitable. A zero discount rate on the value of life only *appears* to represent equity in the valuation of different lives located at different times. The Keeler–Cretin paradox is not just a technical, analytically theoretical argument for uniform discounting. It is also a moral argument: the postponement encouraged by any form of differential discounting would be unfair to present persons.

This argument has been a powerful factor reinforcing economists in their typical practice of discounting. Is it the devastating argument for uniform discounting it is usually taken to be? I will argue it is not. To grasp why, we first need to use a distinction between *expenditure-start* and *benefit-receipt* times clarified by Nord.[28]

Sometimes comparisons between health programs involve different expenditure-start times. Suppose the program that will save lives in 2020 does not require us to expend money until 2020. In this circumstance, the comparison with a program whose expenditure starts in 2010 and whose benefits still occur in 2020 triggers Keeler and Cretin's point, that the later program gets favored by cost–benefit calculation. These are similar receipt-time/different start-time cases. But many (perhaps even most) of the cases in which people raise objections to discounting future health benefits the same as money are the opposite; they involve similar expenditure-start times but different benefit-receipt times: spending in 2010 on prevention and not reaping benefits until 2020, say, compared with spending on treatment in 2010 and getting the benefits much sooner.

Then note that comparison cases involving different benefit-receipt times are much more common when treatments are compared to preventive measures. *In these more typical situations, not discounting health benefits does not disadvantage treatment or favor prevention.* Because expenditures on prevention start at

27. In such examples cost-inflation is above and beyond the interest rate, which is time preference based.

28. Nord (2011, 17–18) uses "program start time" and "benefit time." His and my conceptions of the distinction are equivalent. I prefer the additional clarity of "expenditure-start time" and "benefit-receipt time," but for brevity I will often use "start time" and "benefit time." Frederick (2006, 672) also notices the case of comparative programs with similar start-times but different benefit-times. Nord (2011, 19) pursues the implications of the distinction not only for putting aside the Keeler–Cretin problem as ultimately "a small tail wagging a big dog" but for rejecting the alleged logical consistency arguments for uniform discounting that emerge from Keeler–Cretin.

the same time as they do for treatment, no additional money from financial investment will become available for expanding lifesaving capacity if we shift resources from prevention to treatment. There is thus no need to compensate for any advantage of enlarged assets from investment by discounting the value of later health benefits back to present value.

A more general practical point about comparison cases with similar expenditure-start times can then be made. Indeed we can expand financial resources and save more lives by postponing the start of a prevention program—from 2010 to 2020, say (with its benefits then postponed another 10 years, too, of course). But this opportunity to expand resources and increase benefits applies also to any treatment program: gain the same expansion of resources by postponing its start (from 2010 to 2020, say). *Not discounting future health benefits while discounting monetary elements creates incentives to postpone all programs,* those with near-term benefits as well as those with longer term ones.

Keeler and Cretin's argument does not necessarily deny this point, and some will observe that the point even makes the case for uniform discounting more powerful: the postponement problem afflicts all health care programs, treatment as well as prevention. In a narrow sense, that is correct. But the incentive to invest in order to do or have more financial resources later is true for many, many activities in addition to health care. Generally human beings do not unduly give in to such incentives to postpone. There are many practical and moral reasons for this. In health care, for one thing, there are people all around us whose lives and health are at stake. We have self-interested reasons in not wanting them to take a back seat to future beneficiaries. Moreover, people are arguably not just utility maximizers.[29] Equity convictions, too, have influence. Nonutilitarian grounds for allocations within a contemporaneous time frame— reasons of fairness, for example—apply also to allocations across time.

Frederick (2003, 45–46) has found precisely such equity preferences across time. In one of his formats respondents were asked which they would prefer, program A that saves 300 lives in their generation, none in their children's generation, and none in their grandchildren's generation, or program B that saves 100 lives in each of these three generations. Overall, 80% preferred program B. Surprising? Hardly, once a moral distribution question providing a visible equity option was asked.[30]

29. Ganiats (1994, 298) and Nord (2011) make this point as a basic criticism of the Keeler–Cretin objection to differential discounting.

30. Frederick (2003, 46) notes that the question formats used by Cropper et al. (1994) and Johanneson and Johansson (1997) did not provide respondents any "opportunity to express concerns for equity."

We can thus put the Keeler–Cretin "paradox" in its proper place. First, it correctly calls attention to the fact that differential discounting will create an incentive to postpone expenditures. This is hardly, though, a *paradox* implying some sort of contradiction.[31] It is more accurate to speak of the Keeler–Cretin *effect*.

Second, it is not accurate to say that differential discounting would create an advantage for prevention over treatment. In the typical cases in which people see a dilemma in the comparison between prevention and treatment, the benefit times of programs are different though the expenditure start times are the same. But in that situation the Keeler–Cretin effect constitutes an equal incentive to postpone *both* programs.[32]

Third, the incentive that constitutes the Keeler–Cretin effect hardly boxes anyone in. People and societies have ample practical and equity-focused reasons for not postponing programs at the expense of the current generation. They should also, of course, properly save for their own future, and future generations. Determining a justified savings rate is a much greater challenge that applies to all consumption and investment. In fact a critic might be rightfully dismissive in responding to the Keeler–Cretin effect by wondering why anyone would ever think it so important and powerful an argument in the debate about uniform discounting. Incentives to maximize utility by postponing expenditure are rather ubiquitous in life. In observing human behavior generally we do not seem to lament those incentives much. More likely, we lament the fact that they are often so weak.[33]

---

31. If one's preconceptions are of a certain sort, the incentive to postpone to which Keeler and Cretin call attention may strike one as "odd," but why call it "paradoxical"? There is no statement that contradicts itself (one sense of paradox—"this sentence is false," e.g.). Nor is there any seemingly contradictory statement that is nonetheless true (another sense of paradox; e.g., "standing is more tiring than walking"). The only thing paradoxical about the Keeler–Cretin effect is surprise on the equity front: a zero discount rate on the value of life that initially seems driven by convictions about the equal value of lives at different times will *not* end up representing equity *if* differential discounting is allowed to have as one of its consequences the strong favoring of future over present lives. Perhaps the fact that economists have so routinely referred to the Keeler–Cretin effect as a "paradox" reflects the fact that it seldom occurs to them that a distributive value such as equity would be used by societal decision makers to block the straightforward pursuit of maximum aggregate utility.

32. There is another, technically verbal reason for thinking that differential discounting should not be seen as creating an advantage for prevention over treatment. Relative to uniform discounting, yes, it would help prevention, but the alternative, uniform discounting, is itself the thing that initially created a disadvantage for prevention. It is perhaps straining language (as well as unfair) to refer to removing a disadvantage to prevention as "giving an advantage" to it.

33. Generalizations are always dangerous, of course. In some cases we lament not how weak the incentives for saving are but that they are too strong or misplaced. Halley Faust noted to

MONETARIZING THE VALUE OF LIFE

Whether or not the previous analysis of the postponement problem is correct, and even as important as Keeler and Cretin's argument based on it is, we still have not dealt fully with why uniform discounting has such a powerful hold in economics. One reason is a set of alleged logical inconsistencies that differential discounting is alleged to encounter.[34] Another reason, reflected in the discussion of previous sections, is the fact that economics as a discipline has been prone to focus more on individual utility than on social value, and when it has focused on social value, it has tended to hold a welfarist utilitarian view of it. There is likely a third important reason as well, revealed by Lisa Heinzerling in a vigorous dialogue with John Donohue (1999). Heinzerling (1999, 1913) attributes the practice to "an unstated normative assumption that lives are fungible with dollars." Heinzerling's core insight is simple: once we think of the value of lives and other health benefits as a *monetary value*, it becomes perfectly natural to discount the value of future health benefits in the same way we discount monetary items themselves.

A fundamental question in the discounting debate then becomes whether the value of lives and health benefits can and should be rendered as monetary. There are very strong reasons for thinking that lives and health benefits *have* monetary value—in earnings potential, for example, or in people's willingness to pay to reduce risks to life and health. That is far, though, from saying that the whole value of a life can be adequately captured by a monetary surrogate. Heinzerling (1999, 1913) notes the many differences between money and lives (italics added):

me that when someone dies without having enjoyed their wealth we may lament that they should have known that "you can't take it with you."

34. I will not pursue those here, on prohibitive grounds of space. The reader can consult the clear, consistent, and concise argument by Claxton et al. (2006, 2): we obtain one cost/QALY ratio running the calculation forward in the time that a measure needs to take effect, but then, if we do not use uniform discounting, we obtain a very different ratio when the calculation is run in the reverse direction. This inconsistency may also be at the heart of the Keeler–Cretin problem (as it particularly appears to be in the treatment by Nord 2011), in which case, insofar as differential discounting can defend itself effectively in the face of Keeler–Cretin, the apparent inconsistency may be resolved. In any case, Gravelle et al. (2007) defend differential discounting against it. Another consistency argument is presented by Weinstein and Stason (1977) and by Lipscomb, Torrance, and Weinstein (1996); this is the one that Lipscomb et al. explicitly label "the consistency argument." A third is Viscusi's (1995, 133) "equivalence argument." Nord (2011, 19–22) gives cogent criticisms of the last two arguments. I do not pursue these important disputes here, but only make this observation: given the counterarguments by critics such as Nord, the *normative moral* power of these consistency arguments is questionable.

The person who "invests' in her future by quitting smoking or exercising regularly will be disappointed if she expects that by doing so she will gain more than one life to live. *Lives do not compound the way money does. Nor do they disaggregate the same way.* Discounting lives the way we discount money implies that a death in the future is not a whole death, but only a part of one.

Defenders of uniform discounting can reply that they do not claim that lives themselves compound or disaggregate. They claim only that *the value* of lives compounds and disaggregates. Heinzerling's insight, though, can be put more cautiously to be correct: by thinking of the value of life as a monetary value, uniform discounting comes to seem natural, even obvious. If so, it is not surprising that uniform discounting came to dominate in a whole enterprise, CEA, situated within the larger field of economics. This helps us to understand the stark contrast between the uniform discounting that is so unquestioned a part of health economics practice and the stubborn moral observation that it is plainly false to claim that the value of a future life is less than the value of a present one. Both are "correct" within their own perspectives—the former where the value of life is represented in monetary terms and the latter where it is not.

Should we be compelled by this point to take a highly tolerant stance toward health economics' established practice of uniform discounting? Not at all. Yes, uniform discounting does follow naturally if all benefits are seen in monetary terms. But *health* economics does *not* typically monetize the value of life and other health benefits; CEA is a much more central activity in health economics' impact on health policy than is cost–benefit analysis (CBA).

The distinction between CEA and CBA is well known (Drummond et al. 1997, 3–4; Warner and Luce 1982, 46–50). CEA does not place a monetary value on life; it only compares the ratio of expense to size of benefit. CBA goes a critical, controversial step further: it puts a monetary value on any health benefit, including life, so as to compare all possible benefits, even if seemingly incommensurable. CEA for a particular area of life such as health care must adopt some common metric for expressing the "size" of all health benefits (for example, QALYs), but it never needs to express the value of any health benefit as an amount of money. CBA does, and by doing so and expressing the value of *all* benefits in a common metric, gains the power to make judgments of efficiency across life as a whole. That power comes at the price of having to make the debatable move of representing the value of everything, even life and health, in monetary terms.

In the common practice of *health* economics, CEA is the order of the day. CBA plays a relatively secondary role, relevant only when health care resources compete with nonhealth needs. In most of the activity of health economics, therefore, the values of life and health do not need to be expressed in monetary terms.[35] But if they do not, then we can get skeptical about the need for uniform discounting. If the Keeler–Cretin effect creates no compelling argument for uniform discounting, if IU is radically incomplete as a normative basis for uniform discounting, if SV-eliciting questions reveal distinctly less time preference for health benefits than IU-eliciting questions reveal for monetary items, and if the practice of health economics routinely holds CBA at arms length and does not monetarize the value of life and health, then why should uniform discounting continue to be a standard practice in health economics?

NORMATIVITY AND PREFERENCE

We have seen that when we do try to discern accurately the value of lifesaving and improvements in health that can be achieved by various measures and policies, strong, though perhaps not compelling, arguments can be made for an equal-value-at-any-time answer. Also, as a matter of empirical fact, people's direct SV judgments do not reveal much preference for near-term benefits once practical factors such as uncertainty and inflation are pulled out. Moreover, even if people in their preferences, whether about interpersonal social value or intrapersonal individual utility, strongly favor near-term over more temporally distant lives benefits, we would be hard pressed to defend discounting nonmonetary benefits over generations. Consider, for example, a point made by Page (1977, 169–70) that I construct as a hypothetical here:

> Suppose that in a thousand years, 3010, the world is shortly about to end or massively degrade, when that development could have been prevented by our generation's action now in 2010. Discounting, however, had showed in 2010 that any catastrophic events in 3010 had only a minuscule negative present value. The residents of 3010, faced with catastrophe, find a note for future generations left in 2010: "We took a vote of all those present and decided to follow our own time preferences."

We tend to recoil. Preferences are such a thin reason, hardly capable of determinant moral force when such large stakes are involved. They need to be backed

---

35. An important exception is a context such as the British National Health Service and its attendant National Institute for Clinical Excellence (NICE), in which a global budget spurs the use of a specific cost-effectiveness ratio (e.g., £15,000/QALY). NICE's 2005 adoption of uniform discounting has been defended, in fact, by precisely the observation that QALYs get a monetary value in NICE's NHS context (Claxton et al. 2006, 2).

by some sort of moral reason. It is wrong for future persons to have their prospects doomed or greatly harmed by previous generations' mere time preference.

Fortunately, we may not need to mediate a battle between normative convictions of relative equity between generations and time preference. We have seen that when people are asked clearly SV preference questions, not IU questions, and especially when they are given choices that offer them the opportunity to express concerns for equity, they express little if any preference for saving present over future lives. We do not need expanses of anything like 1000 years to find lack of time preference, either; 25 years suffices (Frederick 2003, 46–47). Admittedly, we have mediocre data on shorter spans such as 10 years, but if people express little if any preference for saving some people's lives now over saving others' lives 25 or 100 years from now, why would we expect them to show SV preference for current lifesaving over lifesaving 5 or 10 years from now?

Individual utility questions do show significant time preference, but as previously explained, the moral relevance of these for decisions in which various measures and programs have different recipients is dubious. My overall conclusion is that time preferences do not provide an adequate normative basis for uniform discounting.

CONCLUSIONS

In their comprehensive review of the literature on time discounting and time preference, Frederick, Loewenstein, and O'Donoghue (2002, 351) note that the founder of the discounted-utility model, Paul Samuelson (1937), had "manifest reservations about the normative and descriptive validity of the formulation he had proposed."[36] Nonetheless, the model was accepted almost instantly. Its manifestation in contemporary health economics, the practice of uniformly discounting health benefits at the same rate as monetary effects, is part of an elegant model of the value of goods over time.

Critically examined, the moral case for uniform discounting as an almost universal practice in health economics and health policy is unpersuasive. (1) Time preference itself is difficult to separate from other factors such as

36. Robinson (1990) provides fascinating details about the history of suspicion against discounting in earlier economic theory. He also notes the central role of the IU/SV distinction to that discussion (p. 259) and the relevance of an intrageneration as opposed to an intergeneration context (p. 260). The critique of discounting as a social policy practice by Goodin (1982) has considerable affinity with these earlier reservations.

uncertainty that are already accounted for in the estimation of future health benefits. (2) Only some of the characteristics of money that make discounting future monetary effects compelling are shared by health benefits, and then only sometimes. (3) The distinction between individual utility and social value must be carefully appreciated since discounting health benefits usually has implications for the relative value of measures and programs that affect *different* people. In that circumstance intrapersonal time preference is much less relevant than interpersonal, social value preference. (4) Welfarist arguments do not create a persuasive case for grounding social value in aggregate individual utilities, even if people show significant time preference in individual utility. (5) The empirical evidence for interpersonal time preference is thin, at best, once social value is made the focus of elicitation questions, the reasoning of respondents is examined to test for their understanding of the question, and options concerning intertemporal equity are introduced. (6) Even if there is good evidence for positive time preference about life and health, the moral reach of preferences in normative matters faces significant questions and counterexamples. (7) The highly regarded Keeler–Cretin "paradox" is not a persuasive argument against differential discounting. (8) Uniform discounting can make sense if the value of all effects is expressed in monetary terms, but in cost-effectiveness analysis, a central activity within health economics in which uniform discounting is common practice, the value of health benefits is generally not monetarized.

The one circumstance in which lifesaving and health improvement benefits in the future are, in general, arguably less valuable than those benefits closer to the present is life extension *within* a person's own life. One of the most powerful influences here is what I have called the factor of Intervening Years: without lifesaving (or lower risk to life) in the present and near future, there will (or may) not even be a further future in which people could have the same benefits later. For many comparisons of benefits at different times within a person's life, future benefits should be discounted. Yet this circumstance is seldom the context for the sorts of allocations of resources between preventive services and treatments that are influenced by CEA. Moreover, even for allocations that represent trade-offs within given persons' own lives, time preference varies. It appears weaker for non-life-extending health benefits than it is for money, and some people even value anticipated future benefits more than apparently equivalent benefits enjoyed earlier.

ACKNOWLEDGMENTS

I am indebted to Charles Roehrig and George Miller of Altarum Institute (Ann Arbor) and to Erik Nord of Folkehelsa (Oslo) for extensive conversation and communication about the topic and many of my claims. James Dwyer and the Center for Bioethics and Humanities at Upstate Medical University (Syracuse, NY) provided a valuable opportunity for presentation at a colloquium. Halley Faust gave invaluable feedback on all dimensions of the chapter over many months.

REFERENCES

Bonneaux, L., and Birnie, E. 2001. The Discount Rate in the Economic Evaluation of Prevention: A Thought Experiment. *Journal of Epidemiology and Community Health* 55 2(Feb):123–24.

Brazier, J., Ratliffe, J., Salomon, J.A., and Tsuchiya, A. 2007. *Measuring and Valuing Health Benefits for Economic Evaluation*. Oxford, UK: Oxford University Press.

Broome, J. 1994. Discounting the Future. *Philosophy and Public Affairs* 23:128–56. Reprinted in J. Broome, *Ethics Out of Economics* (pp. 44–67). Cambridge, UK: Cambridge University Press, 1999.

Brouwer, W.B.F., Niessen, L.W., Postma, M.J., and Rutten, F.F.H. 2005. Need for Differential Discounting of Costs and Health Effects in Cost Effectiveness Analyses. *British Medical Journal* 331 (20–27 Aug):446–48.

Cairns, J.A. 1994. Valuing Health Benefits. *Health Economics* 3:221–29.

Claxton, K., Paulden, M., Gravelle, H., Brouwer, W., and Culyer, A. 2011. Discounting and Decision Making in the Economic Evaluation of Health-Care Technologies. *Health Economics* 20 1(Jan):2–15.

Claxton, K., Sculpher, M., Culyer, A., McCabe, C., Briggs, A., Akehurst, R., Buxton, M., and Brazier, J. 2006. Discounting and Cost-Effectiveness in NICE—Stepping Back to Sort Out a Confusion. *Health Economics* 15:1–4. Available online as DOI:10.1002/hec.1081.

Corso, P.S., and Haddix, A.C. 2003. Time Effects. In A.C. Haddix, S.M. Teutsch, and P.S. Corso Eds., *Prevention Effectiveness: A Guide to Decision Analysis and Economic Evaluation* (pp. 92–102). New York: Oxford University Press.

Cretin, S. 1977. Cost/Benefit Analysis of Treatment and Prevention of Myocardial Infarction. *Health Services Research* 12:174–89.

Cropper, M.L., Aydede, S.K., and Portney, P.T. 1994. Preferences for Life Saving Programs: How the Public Discounts Time and Age. *Journal of Risk and Uncertainty* 8:243–65.

Dolan, P., Olsen, J.A., Menzel, P.T., and Richardson, J. 2003. An Inquiry into the Different Perspectives That Can Be Used When Eliciting Preferences in Health. *Health Economics* 12 7(Jul):545–51.

Donohue, J.J., III. 1999. Why We Should Discount the Views of Those Who Discount Discounting. *Yale Law Journal* 107:1901–10.

DPP [Diabetes Prevention Program] Research Group. 2009. Ten-Year Follow-Up of Diabetes Incidence and Weight Loss in the Diabetes Prevention Program Outcomes Study. *The Lancet*, October 29. Available online at DOI: 10.1016/S0140-6736(09)61457-4.

Drummond, M.F., O'Brien, B., Stoddart, G.L., and Torrance, G.W. 1997. *Methods for the Economic Evaluation of Health Care Programmes,* 2nd ed. New York: Oxford University Press.

Eddy, D.M. 1990. Screening for Cervical Cancer. *Annals of Internal Medicine* 113 3(Aug):214–26.

Frederick, S. 2003. Measuring Intergenerational Time Preference: *Are* Future Lives Valued Less? *Journal of Risk and Uncertainty* 26 (1):39–53.

———. 2006. Valuing Future Life and Future Lives: A Framework for Understanding Discounting. *Journal of Economic Psychology* 27:667–80.

Frederick, S., Loewenstein, G., and O'Donoghue, T. 2002. Time Discounting and Time Preference: A Critical Review. *Journal of Economic Literature* 40 (Jun):351–401.

Gafni, A. 1995. Can We Measure Individuals' 'Pure Time Preferences'? *Medical Decision Making* 15:31–37.

Ganiats, T.G. 1994. Discounting in Cost-Effectiveness Research. *Medical Decision Making* 14:298–300.

Goodin, R.E. 1982. Discounting Discounting. *Journal of Public Policy* 2 (1):53–72.

Gravelle, H., Brouwer, W., Niessen, L., Postma, M., and Rutten, F. 2007. Discounting in Economic Evaluations: Stepping Forward Towards Optimal Decision Rules. *Health Economics* 16:307–317.

Hare, R.M. 1997. *Sorting Out Ethics.* Oxford, UK: Oxford University Press.

Heinzerling, L. 1999. Discounting Life. *Yale Law Journal* 108:1911–15.

Johannesson, M., and Johansson, P.-O. 1997. Saving Lives in the Present Versus Saving Lives in the Future—Is There a Framing Effect? *Journal of Risk and Uncertainty* 15:167–76.

Keeler, E.B., and Cretin, S. 1983. Discounting of Life-Saving and Other Nonmonetary Effects. *Management Science* 29:300–6.

Lipscomb, J., Weinstein, M.C., and Torrance, G.W. 1996. Time Preference. In M.R. Gold, J.E. Siegel, L.B. Russell, and M.C. Weinstein, Eds., *Cost-Effectiveness in Health and Medicine* (pp. 214–46). New York: Oxford University Press.

Menzel, P.T. 1999. How Should What Economists Call 'Social Values' Be Measured? *The Journal of Ethics* 3 (3):249–73.

Menzel, P.T., Gold, M., Nord, E., Pinto-Prades, J.-L., Richardson, J., and Ubel, P. 1999. Toward a Broader View of Cost-Effectiveness in Health Care. *Hastings Center Report* 29 (3):7–15.

Morrall, J.F., III. 2003. Saving Lives: A Review of the Record. *The Journal of Risk and Uncertainty* 27 (3):221–37.

Nord, E. 2011. Discounting Future Health Benefits: The Poverty of Consistency Arguments. *Health Economics* 20 1(January):16–26. Available online as DOI:10.1002/hec1687.

Olsen, J.A. 1993. Time Preferences for Health Gains: An Empirical Investigation. *Health Economics* 2:257–65.

Page, T. 1977. *Conservation and Economic Efficiency.* Baltimore: Johns Hopkins University Press.

Parfit, D. 1971. Personal Identity. *Philosophical Review* 80 (1):3–27.

———. 1982. Personal Identity and Rationality. *Synthese* 53:227–41.

Paulden, M., and Claxton, K. 2009. *Budget Allocation and the Revealed Social Rate of Time Preference for Health* (CHE Research Paper 53). York, UK: Centre for Health Economics, York University.

Redelmeier, D.A., and Heller, D.N. 1993. Time Preference in Medical Decision Making and Cost-Effectiveness Analysis. *Medical Decision Making* 13 3(Jul-Sep):212–17.

Robinson, J.C. 1990. Philosophical Origins of the Social Rate of Discount in Cost-Benefit Analysis. *The Milbank Quarterly* 68 (2):245–65.

Samuelson, P. 1937. A Note on Measurement of Utility. *Review of Economic Studies* 40:1–33.

Severens, J.L., and Milne, R.J. 2004. Discounting Health Outcomes in Economic Evaluation: The Ongoing Debates (editorial). *Value in Health* 7 (4):397–401.

Ubel, P., Gold, M., Nord, E., Pinto-Prades, J.-L., and Richardson, J. 2000. Improving Value Measurement in Cost-Effectiveness Analysis. *Medical Care* 38 (9):892–901.

Ubel, P., Richardson, J., and Menzel, P. 2000. Societal Value, the Person Trade-Off, and the Dilemma of Whose Values to Measure for Cost-Effectiveness Analysis. *Health Economics* 9:127–36.

Viscusi. W.K. 1995. Discounting Health Effects for Medical Decisions. In F. Sloan, Ed., *Valuing Health Care* (pp. 125–148). Cambridge, UK: Cambridge University Press.

Warner, K.E., and Luce, B.R. 1982. *Cost-Benefit and Cost-Effectiveness Analysis in Health Care*. Ann Arbor, MI: Health Administration Press.

Weinstein, M.C. 1993. Time-Preference Studies in the Health Care Context. *Medical Decision Making* 13:218–19.

Weinstein, M.C., and Stason, W. 1977. Foundations of Cost-Effectiveness Analysis for Health and Medical Practices. *New England Journal of Medicine* 296:716–21.

Zeckhauser, R.J., and Viscusi, W.K. 2008. Discounting Dilemmas: Editors' Introduction (to special issue). *Journal of Risk and Uncertainty* 37:95–106.

PART THREE

Religious and Cultural Perspectives

12

Prevention vs. Treatment

How Do We Allocate Scarce Resources from Jewish Ethical Perspectives?

ALAN JOTKOWITZ, MD, AND SHIMON GLICK, MD ■

THE METHODOLOGY OF JEWISH MEDICAL ETHICS

Currently the most commonly used criteria in secular ethics are the four basic principles emerging from the Georgetown group—autonomy, beneficence, nonmaleficence, and justice (Beauchamp and Childress 1994). Each dilemma is evaluated by these four criteria, with the obvious difficulty being that there are no clear guidelines for how to solve the many dilemmas in which these principles may conflict. Stephen Toulmin talks about the "tyranny of principles" and defends the system that he calls case-based ethics (Toulmin 1981). This phrase essentially characterizes the bulk of the Jewish literature on medical ethics. It is based to a large extent on a long history of responsa in which a person facing a dilemma turns to a Jewish religious and legal scholar and asks for guidance. The collection of responsa over the years is integrated to form a corpus of religious law. In most of the cases the decisor gives not only his (we chose the masculine form because for historical and sociological reasons up until the modern age decisors have traditionally been men) final opinion but describes in detail the sources in the legal literature that preceded him, and on which his decision is based. Provision of the detailed discussion enables any subsequent scholar to evaluate the logic of the decision and to either accept it or offer an alternative interpretation.

The development of the system is fascinating because since the destruction of the Jewish Temple some 2000 years ago we have neither a single authority such as the Pope nor a single judicial body, such as the Supreme Court, which can render a universally binding and authoritative decision. The decisions as to which responsa are ultimately accepted and which are rejected are not taken by a convocation of rabbis who vote, but somehow over the years the Jewish community, as it were, reaches a consensus. Rabbi Moshe Feinstein, when asked how he came to be recognized as one of the foremost Jewish legal decisors of the twentieth century, responded tellingly, "You can't just wake up in the morning and decide that you are an expert. If people see that one answer is good, and another answer is good, gradually you will be accepted," (Shenker, 1975) attesting to the role the community plays in establishing normative behavior.

Much of the above-mentioned responsa literature is based on the principles of casuistry using analogical case analysis to render decisions, in contrast to reasoning from theoretically derived principles. Casuistry, as championed by Jonsen and Toulmin (1988), has been suggested as the optimal methodology to analyze modern bioethical dilemmas. This methodology was used extensively during Jonsen's tenure on the National Commission for the Protection of Human Subjects of Biomedical and Behavioral Research. The members of the committee, instead of beginning by developing a set of principles that could then be applied to problematic cases, started immediately by analyzing the cases in order to reach a consensus on practical guidelines. According to Arras (1991), "the new casuistry insists that our moral knowledge must develop incrementally through the analysis of concrete cases." Bioethical principles emerge from the responses to particular cases. In fact, the Committee's statement of principles was written only after the Committee reached consensus on many of the difficult issues. This method seems very similar to Rabbi Joseph B. Soloveitchik's contention that a true Jewish theology can come only from a legal perspective (Soloveitchik 1986, 101). Rabbi Immanuel Jakobovits (1990), the father of modern Jewish medical ethics, also endorses this view:

Secular medical ethics is the effort to turn ethical guidelines or rules of conscience into law i.e., into legislation. Attempts are made constantly to choose ethical insights and then to gradually distill these into legislative laws adopted by different legislatures, Jewish medical ethics does the reverse. We determine law or legislation, distill it, and then come to the conclusion that it contains certain ethical guidelines. Thus Jewish medical ethics derives from legislation. It does not lead to legislation. We look at legislation as rulings of law that have been given i.e., halakha, which means law or legislation, and then try and extrapolate ethical rules from the legislation.

Therefore the Jewish concept of medical ethics is the very reverse of that commonly accepted in civilized countries of the world (Jakobovits 1990).

Jewish law is determined through the use of casuistry, and ethical principles are derived from a thoughtful analysis of precedent cases. In this system, the decisor analyzes the ancient sources, primarily the Mishnah (compiled c. 200 C.E.), the Talmud (compiled c. 500–600 C.E.), the medieval codes, and the responsa literature to find similar relevant cases and precedents from which a judgment may be rendered. As has been pointed out by Newman and other critics of the system, the reasoning from the various analogies at times may seem forced and inconclusive (Newman 1990).

With respect to the relative priority of prevention over treatment the difficulties are even more severe. In the absence of an independent Jewish state the kinds of questions with which we are dealing, on a country or state level, were rarely if ever posed to Jewish legal authorities. Thus the cases upon which to base a casuistic body of ethical decisions are almost nonexistent. In fact, the monumental *Encyclopedia of Jewish Medical Ethics* devotes only 3 pages out of 1191 to the Jewish perspective on the allocation of scarce resources (Steinberg 2003). This paucity reflects the lack of responsa on the subject. Interestingly, in the English edition of the encyclopedia, published several years after the Hebrew edition, significantly more pages appear, reflecting the result of increasing interest and discussion of the subject.

PREVENTIVE MEDICINE IN JUDAISM

In the Jewish tradition G-d is the ultimate healer and the physician is merely his agent. The Jew is commanded to strive to emulate the Almighty, *imitatio dei*. When we seek a definition of G-d's role as physician in the text of the Bible, the "job description" is clearly one of prevention, rather than one of merely treating the disease after it has already appeared:

> And He said: "If you will diligently hearken to the voice of the L-rd, your G-d, and will do that which is right in His sight, and will give ear to His commandments, and keep all His statutes, I will put none of these diseases upon you which I put on the Egyptians; for I am the L-rd, your healer (*rofecha*)."[1]

1. Exodus, 15:26.

The classic Biblical commentator, Rashi, is explicit in his explanation:

I am the Lord, your healer, and I teach you the Torah and the command-ments in order that you may be saved from these diseases–like a physician who says to a man: do not eat this thing lest it will bring you into danger from this illness.

It is tempting to assign preventive medical motivations for many Biblical commandments, including circumcision, laws of family purity, dietary laws, ritual ablutions, and many others, as many secular historians have done over the centuries. But in our view the guiding overall *raison d'être* for the myriad of Biblical admonitions is spiritual and not medical. Nevertheless we believe that G-d in His infinite wisdom has prescribed behaviors that are simultaneously health promoting. The Bible tells us expressly, "You shall therefore keep my statutes and ordinances, which if a man do he shall live by them."[2]

A number of Biblical precepts are clearly life and health promoting. These include the law forbidding the putting of others at risk, mandating constructing a parapet around your roof to prevent individuals from falling,[3] and the law forbidding the placing of a stumbling block in front of a blind person, inter-preted very broadly to mean preventing foreseeable mishaps, physical or other, to any individual.

The Talmud is full of specific public measures to protect people's health, again interpreted quite broadly to include not only specific health hazards, but also pollution by foul smells and excessive noise. Streets and market areas are to be kept clean. Scholars are advised not to dwell in a city without a public bath. An illustration of the importance attached to personal hygiene is the following folktale about the famous Talmudic scholar, Hillel:

Once when Hillel was leaving his disciples, they said to him: "Master, where are you going? He replied: "To do a pious deed." They asked: "What may that be?" He replied: "To take a bath." They asked: "Is that a pious deed?" He replied: "Yes. If in the theaters and circuses, the images of the king must be kept clean by the man to whom they have been entrusted, how much more is it a duty of man to care for the body, since man has been created in the divine image and likeness."[4]

2. Leviticus, 18:5.

3. Deuteronomy, 22:8.

4. Leviticus Rabbah, 34:3.

Maimonides in his classic compendium of Jewish Law, *Mishne Torah*, goes into great detail about the aspects of health-promoting behaviors that he recommends with respect to diet, sleep, exercise, bathing, blood letting, and sex. He concludes by promising that those who follow these recommended behaviors will be guaranteed good health, unless they have a genetic disorder, have an accident, or are caught in a severe plague epidemic. He also concludes that we do not have the right to ignore admonitions against self-endangerments, but if we do so, claiming that it is no one's affair other than his own, the individual is subject to punishment by a court (Maimonides). This is a rather stringent and coercive attitude toward the violation of health-promoting behaviors.

The late Benjamin Freedman in his unique monograph, *Duty and Healing*, emphasizes the role of man as a guardian of his body, which has been given to him in stewardship by the L-rd (Freedman 1999). Man is thus commanded to be vigilant in preventing damage in the form of ill health to his body.

With respect to treatment, when a physician or any other individual is confronted with a sick or suffering individual seeking help, the Jewish tradition places an impressive array of immediate demands upon the prospective provider of services. This is in striking contrast to American law, which, except for four states (Vermont, Rhode Island, Minnesota, and Wisconsin), imposes no obligation of provision of medical care by physicians (Hendel 2001). A moral obligation does seem to exist, but it is not backed by legal sanction.

The Biblical imperative of "do not stand idly by your neighbor's blood" imposes powerful demands upon the individual. Not only must the individual offer assistance at the cost of personal inconvenience, but even at a significant financial cost. To what extent we must do so, at risk to our lives, is a subject of considerable discussion among the legal authorities. Does this demand take precedence over competing demands such as long-term health promotion or disease prevention? When dealing with the individual confronted with a request for assistance we believe that Al Jonsen's "rule of rescue" (Jonsen 1986) describes the Jewish attitude perfectly. In a discussion of this rule Hadorn (1991) wrote:

> any plan to distribute health care services must take human nature into account if the plan is to be acceptable to society. In this regard there is a fact about the human psyche that will inevitably trump the utilitarian rationality that is implicit in cost-effectiveness analysis: people cannot stand idly by when an identified person's life is visibly threatened if rescue measures are available.

This statement is an almost direct quote of the biblical admonition, and may be applied by the treating physician in his daily life. In keeping with this tradition an Israeli law (Laws of State of Israel 1998) is actually entitled "do not stand idly by your neighbor's blood," requiring any citizen to come to the aid of individuals who are under threat of death or severe injury.

But aside from strictly moral and legal considerations, Jewish and Israeli societies have been deeply affected by the past century's Holocaust experience. One of the most profound messages that has impacted on the Jewish consciousness resulted from what was perceived as the unwillingness of the nations of the world to come to the assistance of the Jews being tortured and murdered by the Nazis. Refugees fleeing certain death were denied asylum and perished. As a result there has developed a heightened sensitivity to the plight of even a single suffering individual; the possibility of denial of life-saving therapy, even at exorbitant cost, is anathema to the Jewish society. Paradoxically this "rescue" mentality extends even to the recovery and burial of body parts of soldiers and civilians killed by terrorists, where Israeli society is willing even to endanger lives in order to recover body parts. We may relate that extreme behavior to assure future soldiers and their families of the great efforts that will always be made to ensure proper burial in the case of death.

In another area of endeavor, the laws of charity may give us some guidance. When we are confronted with a myriad of competing demands for assistance, Jewish law is clear: the poor of our city take priority over others. Were this not the case none of us in the developed world would be able to sit down to a sumptuous meal knowing that the money spent on our indulgences could save the life of an infant dying of starvation in Africa. Similarly the patient presenting in our office asking for assistance takes unquestionable priority over another whose needs are more distant either in time or in place.

In dealing with triage Rabbi Dichovsky, one of Israel's leading *halakhic* authorities, rules that we should treat our closest relatives first, before others in need of help.[5] His ruling is in keeping with the recognition that the demands of the Torah are meant for human beings and not for angels. To expect an individual to bypass his next of kin at the scene of a major public disaster is not reasonable and therefore it is not demanded of the individual. Saintly behavior is supererogatory and encouraged, but not mandatory. The emotional impact of an immediate need for treatment would thus carry weight even if faced by a more weighty demand in the preventive medicine area.

In this context, Avishai Margalit suggests that there is a difference between morality and ethics (Margalit 2002). Morality deals with the universal principles we use in our relationships with strangers. Ethics refers to our relationship with those with whom we hold a special bond such as families and friends.

---

5. Dichovsky, S. Personal communication (2008).

According to Jonathan Sacks, this distinction explains the difference between the Jewish concepts of *tzedek* (justice) and *hessed* (caring). In his own words:

> The beauty of justice (*tzedek*) is that it belongs to a world of order constructed out of universal rules through which each of us stands equally before the law. *Hessed*, by contrast, is intrinsically personal. We cannot care for the sick, bring comfort to the distressed or welcome a visitor impersonally. If we do so, it merely shows that we have not understood what these activities are. Justice demands disengagement. *Hessed* is an act of engagement. Justice is best administered without emotion. *Hessed* exists only in virtue of emotion, empathy, and sympathy: feeling-with and feeling-for. (Sacks 2005)

We would argue that the doctor–patient relationship should be grounded in the worlds of *hessed* as opposed to *tzedek*. This formulation mandates giving priority to the patient with whom you have developed a personal therapeutic relationship. Although some of these conclusions might seem to be in conflict with attempts to deal rationally with utilization of health care resources in an era of skyrocketing health care costs, we cannot ignore emotions in ethical decision making. Recent research in neuroethics strongly suggests that there are some almost universal basic ethical principles, and it has revealed that the locale in the brain for "emotional" decisions in the case of ethical dilemmas is distinctly separate from that for the so-called "rational" decisions (Hauser 2006). The amount of weight that should be given to these deeply seated ethical intuitions is a subject of some controversy, but it is hard to ignore the almost universal societal identification with the "rule of rescue." We find striking concordance between those who support evolutionary wisdom for these attitudes and those who base their conclusions on the G-d-given Biblical-based traditions.

BROADER HEALTH RESOURCE ALLOCATION IN JEWISH TRADITION

Thus far we have dealt with the individual confronted with a call upon his services in an acute situation, and have stated that this call may not be ignored. But can the same guidelines be applied to societal decision making when budgetary allocations need be made for society or an institution at large? Here Jewish law expects the "elders" of society to set priorities that go beyond the immediate heart-rending demands of the suffering individual, and the elders must allocate the resources in a rational and responsible manner. They are responsible not only for priorities within the health care field but also for setting priorities for other community needs, such as security, education, and transportation. They have the luxury of time for analysis and discussion and are expected to act more rationally, being concerned not just for immediate life saving but for guidance of a society, balancing the just health needs with the multitudes of other societal needs.

Benjamin Freedman in his article defending the priority of treatment over prevention in the Jewish tradition (Freedman 1977) is undoubtedly correct in stating that saving a person's life has priority over preserving an individual's health, but saving one life should not have priority over preserving the health of multitudes. And these are the kind of decisions that responsible community leaders must make. The issue is not one or the other, prevention or treatment; obviously a society needs both. The issue is what is the proper balance between the resources devoted to each of these programs. The enthusiastic advocates of preventive medicine programs may be no less subjective and prejudiced about the primacy of their priorities than the vocal demanders for the latest and most expensive new diagnostic equipment. In an era of evidence-based medicine the precise budgetary allocations to each program must be determined by objective data, in keeping with the ethical values of the society.

THE THOUGHT EXPERIMENT

In analyzing the thought experiment proposed by Faust and Menzel in this volume the physician is to choose between treating a patient with an acute coronary syndrome, treating a patient with risk factors for coronary disease, or participating in a teleconference to approve a community-wide heart attack prevention program. In all three scenarios, $250,000 will be spent to save 12 years of life. In analyzing a Jewish response to the question of who should be seen two classic Jewish sources are relevant. Our subsequent discussion also illustrates the use of casuistry in Jewish ethical decision making.

THE PRINCIPLE OF "BEFORE YOU"

According to Jewish law a body must be buried immediately undisturbed because of the holiness of the corpse, having been the repository of the soul. The question has been raised over the generations of whether an autopsy, which has the potential to save future lives, can be performed. The dilemma is based on the Jewish legal principle that all the commandments may be violated excerpt three (murder, illicit sexual relations, and idol worship) to save a life. However, it is important to define how connected to potential life saving the autopsy must be. For example, may medical students perform an autopsy based on the rationale that what they learn may help them care for patients in the future. Rabbi Landau, the renowned eighteenth-century Chief Rabbi of Prague, formulated the legal principle that only if the patient whose life may be saved is "before you" may the sanctity of the corpse be violated.[6] How do we define "before you?" This has been the subject of much rabbinic controversy. Many authorities have taken a strict definition requiring a "here and now" benefit and maintain that a patient dying of a similar disease must be literally "before you." Other decisors believe that if a disease is very common it fulfills the definition of "before us," whereas others maintain that a modern hospital filled with many patients automatically fulfills the necessary criterion.[7] Rabbi Immanuel Jakobovits pointed out that modern methods of communication between physicians across the globe can have the effect of putting many more patients "before you" (Jakobovits 1974). Rabbi Ben-Zion Uziel, a twentieth-century Chief Rabbi of Israel, argued with Rabbi Landau's claim, and held that every autopsy for the study of illness represents the possibility of saving future life.[8] How literally we interpret "before you," and Rabbi Uziel's inclination to look forward to future benefits, can have an impact on the question of spending for acute care versus preventive care. But even those who are willing to broaden the "before you" definition would almost certainly still give priority to an identifiable patient who is actually "before us" over others further removed in time or space, in line with the "rule of rescue."

Laurie Zoloth has developed a Jewish ethics based on a close reading of the biblical story of Ruth that places great emphasis on the encounter with the other (Zoloth 1999, 193–220). In this paradigm intimacy/family is seen as an obligation beyond justice and law and would also necessitate treating the patient "before you," especially if there exists a prior doctor–patient relationship. This would also be in keeping with Levinas' emphasis on the "other" facing us (Levinas 1969), particularly when someone is in acute distress.

---

6. *Noda B'Yehuda* II, YD 210.

7. For a comprehensive discussion see A. Steinberg (2003) section on Autopsy.

8. *Mishpetai Uziel YD*, 28, 29.

TWO TRAVELERS LOST IN THE DESERT

The Talmud[9] records the argument between the sages on what is the proper behavior in the following case. Two people are lost in the desert and one of them has a canteen that contains just enough water for one of them to survive until they reach another source of water. Ben Petura rules that both should drink in spite of the high certainty that both will die. Rabbi Akiva is of the opinion that the owner of the canteen should drink because his own life comes first. Normative Jewish law follows Rabbi Akiva. There are a myriad of explanations for what is the precise point on which Ben Petura and Rabbi Akiva disagree, but two have relevance to our discussion. Rabbi Abraham Karelitz interprets the dispute as revolving around the question of whether saving two lives for a short time is preferable to saving one life for an extended period of time.[10] Ben Petura maintains that saving two lives even for a short time is preferable; therefore they should share the water. Rabbi Akiva believes that it is more important to save the one life. Applying Rabbi Akiva's logic to the allocation of scarce resources, it would follow that resources should preferably be used where many lives can be saved long-term, as opposed to the short-term extension of a single life. This argument could then possibly justify spending more for prevention than for acute hospital care that has no hope of providing long-term extension of life.

Rabbi Chaim Ozer Grodzinski, the preeminent decisor of twentieth-century European Jewry, maintained that the central issue revolves around ownership of the water.[11] Rabbi Akiva believed that the reason you do not have to share the water is that it belongs to you. Ben Petura believed that in the context of life saving ownership is irrelevant. The logical conclusion that follows from Rabbi Akiva's position is that if the water belongs to a third party then it must be shared. As the modern question of allocation of resources is more akin to a case of third-party ownership, this would imply that acute care, even if it can provide only short-term extension of life, should be favored over prevention that has the potential for long-term extension of life. These two interpretations of the rationale behind Rabbi Akiva's ruling could lead to differing conclusions regarding whether acute or preventive care should take preference in the allocation of scarce resources, illustrating a not infrequent problem in using casuistry to resolve ethical dilemmas. As is common in Talmudic discussions the logic behind the decision is not always readily accessible and is open to sometimes contentious debate.

---

9. *Baba Metzia*, 72a.

10. *Hoshen Mishpat, Bava Me'tzia Likutim* 20, p. 62a.

11. *Achiezer, Yoreh Deah*, 16:3.

THE ROLE OF THE COMMUNITY

Until this point we have focused on the choice of an individual (i.e., the physician); however we need to ask whether, according to Jewish law, a community or society is required to act differently when allocating scare resources and developing priorities. Two Talmudic sources are relevant to the discussion.

1. The Talmud[12] discusses whether a community is required to share its limited water resources with another community even if it needs the water only for laundry while the other community needs the water to drink. Rav Yosi stated that the community's own laundry needs have priority even over the drinking needs of the neighboring community. The reason for this is because if the community does not do laundry it might later lead to illness and possible danger to life.

Moshe Tendler is disturbed by this conclusion. Why should the community not be required to share its water in order to save the neighboring community at immediate risk? He explains that a community is different from an individual because it is required to consider future risks (Tendler 1984). Apparently, the doctrine of "before you" applies differently to an individual than a community. An individual is required to do whatever is in his or her power to save a person at immediate risk. A community, however, is required to think in broader terms, either because the future needs of its own citizens take precedence over the immediate needs of another community's citizens or because when dealing with a community the principle of "before you" should be interpreted broadly, along the lines of Rabbi Uziel's reasoning for permitting autopsies in a modern society. Jewish law requires the leaders of society to take into account future needs when allocating resources.

2. The Talmud[13] teaches that you are not allowed to redeem captives for an exorbitant sum for one of two reasons.
   a. Doing so might encourage future hostage taking.
   b. A community does not have to impoverish itself for the sake of one individual.

The first answer (2a) takes a teleological approach to the question. Life is an ultimate value, but by saving the hostage's life, other lives will be put in danger.

---

12. *Nedarim*, 80b.

13. *Gitin*, 45a.

We can infer from this answer that a community should take into account future considerations even when dealing with immediate life and death questions.

The second answer (2b) has obvious relevance to our question and again Tendler is disturbed by its implications (Tendler 1984). Even if paying the ransom will not lead to future hostage taking, the community does not always have the obligation to pay the ransom. However, isn't saving a life an ultimate and priceless value in Judaism? Again, the answer is that the perspective of an individual and the perspective of the community are different. He explains that a community does not have to exhaust its resources to save an individual. Although this case is not completely analogous to our situation, it does teach us that a society does not have to impoverish itself to save an individual life. The case is therefore relevant to our question of how to distribute a fixed health care budget among different health care priorities and suggests that for a community there are limitations to the "law of rescue."

Shabtai Rappaport suggests another possible source that is found in the responsa literature. A medieval scholar was asked about a case in which the government has ordered the Jewish community to hand over a number of Jews for royal servitude (which was considered a life-threatening situation). In this case can you use personal connections to save your friend? He answers that if the friend was already selected by the kidnappers you are not allowed to save him at the expense of others, but if there was only a general decree before the actual selection you are allowed to do whatever is in your power to save your friend.[14] According to Rappaport it follows from this responsum that if a patient is already hospitalized or has a date for surgery or treatment you cannot deny him or her the necessary care because of rationing, but you may, and perhaps must, decide for future patients to limit this level of care and instead use the resources for other health care priorities. But the question remains how we should decide between competing health care needs. Rappaport answers, "it is obvious that the community should attempt to save the many before the individual" (Rappaport 1993). He thus justifies using the limited resources available and applying them for preventive health care such as smoking cessation and screening programs. Noam Zohar (1997) explains that, as opposed to the individual, the responsibility of the collective regarding life saving is not only to respond to immediate needs but also to prepare for future needs. Elliot Dorff (1998) maintains that it is not fair to ask individual physicians to decide who should receive scarce medical resources; it is a decision that society as a whole should make (of course with physician input). The physician's primary

14. *Responsa of Mahari ben Lev*, volume 2, number 9.

therapeutic role is being an advocate for the patient in order to gain the patient's trust and confidence.

However, the physician is also a member of society and if the community decides on a set of rational health care priorities that limit treatment to the patient "before him" the physician is obligated to follow these guidelines and not attempt to circumvent the system.

A NEW THOUGHT EXPERIMENT

We would respectfully like to suggest a variant of the thought experiment. What would be the ethically appropriate behavior in a case in which the equivalent sum of money could save one patient immediately or 10 people in the future? For example, in the scenario envisioned by Faust and Menzel, what would be the most ethically appropriate action if by taking the conference call from the local health department you could save 10 lives in the future for the same amount of money needed to save the patient currently in the office with an acute myocardial infarction? We suggest that from a Jewish ethical perspective an individual physician should use the resources to treat the patient "before him" but that society could decide to spend the scarce resources where it will save the most patients in the future. For example, where the local health department is debating whether to invest in a new catheterization laboratory that would save an additional 10 patients a year at the cost of one million dollars or in a smoking cessation program that will save 100 patients a year at the cost of one million dollars, the representatives of the community should choose the program that will save the most lives. Thus Jewish ethics has a two-tiered response to the problem of allocation of scarce resources. The individual should treat the sickest first because similar to the secular response typified in the words of Jonsen "our moral response to the imminence of death demands that we rescue the doomed" (Jonsen 1986). This perspective is consistent with an ethical perspective that impresses on man the value of caring for the patient "before him" and not turning a blind eye to tangible suffering. However, the community has the difficult and often unpopular obligation to rise above these understandable emotional responses and plan for the most for the long run.

REFERENCES

Arras, J.D. 1991. Getting Down to Cases: The Revival of Casuistry in Bioethics. *The Journal of Medicine and Philosophy* 16:29–51.

Beauchamp, T.L., and Childress, J.F. 1994. *Principles of Biomedical Ethics*, 4th ed. New York and Oxford: Oxford University Press.

Dorff, E.N. 1998. *Matters of Life and Death: A Jewish Approach to Modern Medical Ethics.* Philadelphia and Jerusalem: Jewish Publication Society.

Freedman, B. 1977. The Case for Medical Care, Inefficient or Not. *Hastings Center Report* 31–39.

———. 1999. *Duty and Healing: Foundations of a Jewish Bioethic.* New York: Routledge.

Hadorn, D.C. 1991. Setting Health Care Priorities in Oregon: Cost-Effectiveness Meets the Rule of Rescue. *Journal of the American Medical Association* 265:2218–25.

Hauser, M.D. 2006. *Moral Minds; How Nature Designed Our Universal Sense of Right and Wrong.* New York: Harper Collins Publishers.

Hendel, N. 2001. Law of Do Not Stand Idly By Your Neighbor's Blood–Inspiration and Reality. *Bar Ilan Law Studies (Mechkarei Mishpa)* 16:229–75. [Hebrew.]

Jakobovits, I. 1974. The Problem of Dissection of the Dead in the Halakhic Literature and in Light of Current Conditions. *Torah u'Mada* 4:55–66.

———. 1990. The Role of Jewish Medical Ethics in Shaping Legislation. In Fred Rosner, Ed., *Medicine and Jewish Law* (pp. 1–18). Northvale,NJ: Jason Aronson.

Jonsen, A.R. 1986. Bentham in a Box: Technology Assessment and Health Care Allocation. *Law, Medicine and Health Care* 14:172–74.

Jonsen, A.R., and Toulmin, S. 1988. *The Abuse of Casuistry: A History of Moral Reasoning.* Berkeley: University Press.

Laws of State of Israel. 1998. Jerusalem. Israel Government Printing Office, 245.

Levinas, E. 1969. *Totality and Infinity: An Essay on Exteriority.* A. Lingis, trans. Pittsburgh, PA: Duquesne University Press.

Maimonides. *Mishne Torah, Deot* 4:1–19.

Margalit, A. 2002. *The Ethics of Memory.* Cambridge, MA: Harvard University Press.

Newman, L.E. 1990. Woodchoppers and Respirators: The Problem of Interpretation in Contemporary Jewish Ethics. *Modern Judaism* 10:17–42.

Rappaport, S.A. 1993. Priorities in the Allocation of Public Resources for Healthcare. *Asia* (51–52) 13:46–53. [Hebrew.]

Sacks, J. 2005. *To Heal a Fractured World: The Ethics of Responsibility.* London: Continuum.

Shenker, I.L. 1975. Responsa: The Law as Seen By Rabbis for 1,000 Years. *New York Times*, May 5, pages 33 and 61.

Soloveitchik, J.B. 1986. *The Halachic Mind.* New York: Simon & Schuster.

Steinberg, A. 2003. *Allocation of Scarce Resources in Encyclopedia of Jewish Medical Ethics.* Jerusalem: Feldheim Publishers.

Tendler, M. 1984. *Problems in Triage: Public Expenditures and Saving One Life versus Another. Sefer Hayovel in Honour of Rabbi J.B. Soloveitchik.* New York: S.O.Y. [Hebrew.]

Toulmin, S. 1981. The Tyranny of Principles. *Hastings Center Report* 11:31–38.

Zohar, N.A. 1997. *Alternatives in Jewish Bioethics.* Albany, NY: State University of New York Press.

Zoloth, L. 1999. *Health Care and the Ethics of Encounter.* Chapel Hill: University of North Carolina Press.

13

Cure vs. Prevention

Catholic Perspectives

NUALA KENNY, OC, BA, MD, FRCP(C) ∎

INTRODUCTION

Developed nations are clearly enamored of medical science and technology. The love affair is no passing fancy but rather a deep devotion akin for many to religious belief.

The powerful dominance by acute, high-technology, fix-oriented medicine over the full spectrum of health need seems to be so obvious as to require no explication. Disease prevention and health promotion, chronic illness management, long-term and rehabilitative care, and palliative care are clearly far behind in the public imagination, media headlines, and arguably in resource allocation.

This dominance is highlighted in all media accounts of the crisis in health care. Worldwide health systems are "in crisis." In the developed world, especially in North America, it is a crisis of equitable access; efficient, efficacious response to medical need; and sustainability. This crisis is, in no small part, due to this belief in technology, especially in health care and medicine. In the developing world the crisis is one of providing minimal health and preventive care even as the pull of high technology beckons.

In their introductory first chapter in this volume, Faust and Menzel focus our attention on a particular aspect of this dominance in the privileging and prioritizing of acute medical care over disease prevention and health promotion. They identify issues regarding the apparent intrinsic valuing of the cure focus over prevention and the practical confirmation of such valuing in resource allocation. They demonstrate some of the perverse power of this cure-fix dominance in bringing to our attention the illogic of preferring treatment of established conditions to the prevention of suffering, disability, illness, and premature death. Using the example of Avastin they identify the myriad choices we make day in and day out in health care to expend thousands of dollars and hours of human effort for minimal health gain to individuals.

Disease prevention and health promotion are given the expected politically correct lip service. However, under careful scrutiny, they are not understood to be crucial elements of basic health care but, rather, elite extras. Faust and Menzel describe the well-known reality that, in economic hard times, programs that have focused on prevention are the first to go, leaving prevention to the affluent to pursue as a "mania."

The crucial questions asked in this volume are why are we so fixated on cure, and why does the prevention of health harm not occupy a higher place in our thinking and policy development? In looking for answers to these questions, the lead authors turn to a number of sources, and religious perspectives are, not surprisingly, among them. After all, the roots of modern health care are found in the responses of faith traditions to those with health need. The shaping of priorities regarding health and health care is highly dependent on foundational beliefs and values.

Catholicism has a long and strong tradition in the provision of health care. That care is understood to be a continuation of the healing ministry of Jesus Christ Himself and is shaped by a commitment to ameliorate physical pain and suffering and to restore the whole person. The form of response to health need has changed over the years but the motivation remains the same, that is, a duty to continue the healing ministry of Christ.

Disease prevention and health promotion, in the formal sense, receive no comparable prominence in the Catholic health care tradition. Although there is a general obligation of prudent care for our health, there is no robust tradition of disease prevention and health promotion comparable to the tradition of health care. In fact, there are some beliefs and ascetic practices that have historically generated ambiguity regarding care of the body.

However, there is also an important, more recently developed social justice teaching of the Church. In this teaching we find some powerful motivations for addressing risks to human health and well-being. Here, issues of primary prevention with attention to the reduction of risk factors related to poverty, lifestyle, the environment, and globalization are addressed in the notions of the dignity of the human person, social interdependence, the common good, and the "preferential option for the poor." There has been little rigorous and sustained attention to the relationship between these two traditions.

Although Catholic health care facilities provide a range of services from primary care, especially to the poor and marginalized, long-term care to the elderly and handicapped, and hospice and palliative care, hospitals have dominated the landscape and the moral imagination. Indeed, the hospital has its roots in the Christian tradition of care for the sick and dying (Guinan 2004). Catholic hospitals have assumed obligations for both excellent medical care and attention to the spiritual dimensions of care and illness in their mission statements. They focus on health care as a ministry of healing, rather than a business. As complex regulatory and financial arrangements become essential components of all health care systems, increasing dependence on third-party payers has eliminated "charity hospitals." Some question the role of Catholic hospitals and acute care facilities in this milieu (McCormick 1987; Cochran 1999; Brodeur 1999). Many want closer alignment of health care with social justice teaching (Bernadin 1995; McCann 2000; Cahill 2005; McDonough 2007). Increasing awareness of the justice issues presented by individually focused medical care generates serious questions as to how priorities and practices in acute health care have consequences for the health and well-being of all, but especially for the poor and disadvantaged. All of this raises some challenging questions for the prioritizing of disease prevention and health promotion.

In this chapter I will (1) describe some features of a "Catholic perspective" on this prioritizing, (2) review the tradition of health care and some contemporary concerns, (3) identify some elements of Catholic teaching and practice regarding health promotion and disease prevention with particular attention to the social justice teaching, (4) assess implications for the "thought experiment" introduced in Chapter 1 of this volume, and (5) suggest a future vision.

WHAT CONSTITUTES A CATHOLIC PERSPECTIVE?

Over two millennia, the Christian/Catholic tradition has developed robust teachings and practices on health, happiness, and the good life. Some of these have been core theological dogma; others have been more personal pieties or time-bound customs. All of these have had an influence on the shaping of values and practices regarding health and health care.

To reflect on priorities from a Catholic perspective, we need to understand its central or foundational beliefs and approaches to moral actions. The central reality of Christianity is in the Paschal Mystery, that is the life, death, and resurrection of Jesus Christ, Son of God. This reality is central to the foundational beliefs described by Charles Curran (1999, 33) as the "fivefold Christian mysteries of creation, sin, incarnation, redemption and resurrection destiny." In addition, the notion of sacrament or sign of God's presence and action is a crucial element in Catholic life.

In the Roman Catholic tradition, morality is concerned with norms and actions consistent with this faith. Insight into the formal and informal Catholic contributions to the prioritizing of cure versus disease prevention and health promotion will be found in these beliefs and in the sources of moral wisdom in the Catholic tradition: scripture, tradition, especially Magisterial teaching, reason, and experience (Curran 1999). The New Testament with its *good news* of the healing and reconciling ministry of Jesus Christ is a unique and powerful source of inspiration. Tradition, especially Magisterial teaching, plays an important role in shaping Catholic understandings of the right and the good. Magisterial teaching is the formal teaching authority of Bishops and the Pope. Faith and reason are understood as mutually reinforcing, not contradictory, in the Catholic tradition. Appeals to reason are commonly found in the natural law tradition in which humans, attending to patterns of meaning in creation, can discern good and evil. Natural law is at the core of human moral reasoning, which achieves conformity with nature by discerning and working out the implications of four essential goods in human existence—life, procreation, knowledge and reason, and sociability. This emphasis on natural law emphasizes the significance of the physical and biological in much of Catholic moral thought. Finally, experience is also an essential component of moral reasoning in another way as it takes into account the particularities of persons and situations and the importance of compassionate response. The church's experience in the healing ministries shapes and reflects belief in the sacredness of life and the duty to care for and protect others, especially the poor and marginalized. So, "Tradition, in its best theological sense, refers to a living reality…A living tradition includes the formative effects of the past. It is instructed by the past, but… not paralyzed by it" (McCormick 1987, 3–4).

Each of these sources of moral wisdom is properly understood in light of the others. As we look for insights into the Catholic valuing and prioritizing of health care and disease prevention and health promotion these sources will provide valuable clues. Some representative ideas from these sources will be utilized here to provide a sense of the relative importance of health care and disease prevention from the Catholic perspective. However, Catholics start with no clear, formal authoritative teaching on this prioritization.

HEALTH CARE AND THE HEALING MINISTRY OF CHRIST

The foundation of Catholic commitment to health care is found in the healing ministry of Jesus Christ. Although the theme of Jesus as the Divine Physician develops early in the tradition, Jesus is not portrayed in the Gospels as a physician. Rather, his healing is part of his ministry of reconciliation and service. Healing is a sign of the coming of the Kingdom.

The Gospels tell of many dramatic physical cures by Jesus. Luke, reputed to be a physician himself, recounts many healings including the cure of the Centurion's servant (Luke 7:6–10),[1] the healing of Simon's mother-in-law (Luke 4:38–39), the cleansing of a leper (Luke 5:12–16), and the curing of a woman with hemorrhage (Luke 8:40–48). Matthew tells of the healing of the paralytic (Matthew 9:1–8). John recounts the cure of the man born blind (John 9:1–10) and the raising of Lazarus (John 11:1–45), among others. A remarkable one-fifth of the Gospels together is devoted to Jesus' healing miracles (Latkovic 2008). It is characteristic that these physical cures are accompanied by a healing that is both a restoration of personal wholeness and a restoration of the person to the community.

Jesus also tells parables of healing most paradigmatically, perhaps, in the story of the Good Samaritan. Jesus identifies himself with the Samaritan (Luke 10:25 37). Even more dramatically, Jesus identifies himself with the sick: "I was sick and you visited me" (Matthew 25:36); "He took our infirmities and bore our diseases" (Matthew 8:17).

So, from the earliest days of Christianity the apostles imitated and continued Jesus' healing work as recounted in Peter and John's cure of the lame man (Acts 3:4–9). Care of the sick is of inestimable value in Catholic thought:

> Health care is a ministerial instrument of God's outpouring love for the suffering person, and, at the same time, it is an act of love for God shown in the loving care for the person. (Catholic Church and *Pontificium Consilium de Apostolatu pro Valetudinis Administris* 1995: no. 4)

CATHOLIC HEALTH CARE SYSTEMS

It has been said, "The Catholic Church is possibly the most institutionally focused Christian tradition" (Cochran 1999, 31). Institutionally based health care in hospitals, clinics, nursing homes, and hospices is a major part of the ongoing response to health need. In addition, the health care needs of the poor and marginalized have been a crucial element in the history of Catholic institutions. This institutional focus has not been by accident. The Catholic sacramental understanding situates institutions as signs of God's presence and action. Catholic health care is itself a "sign of hope" (Bernardin 1995).

As early as the fourth century rudimentary hospitals developed under the local bishop. Healing shrines devoted to prayer for relief of suffering often had priests with a range of medical skills to offer. The hospital, as we know it, did not

---

1. All citations from scripture are taken from *The Jerusalem Bible* (Jones 1980).

exist prior to 330 when Constantinople was named capital of the Eastern Roman Empire. The modern disease-oriented, scientifically based hospital owes much of its development to at least three Christian contributions: an understanding of health care as the following of Christ's example; the reconciliation of early Christian theologians, notably Origen, of pagan science with Christian asceticism; and the Greek Fathers of the Church synthesis of Christian agape with care of the sick (Guinan 2004).

The scientific revolution of the seventeenth century created a new worldview and new possibilities for medicine. Even as Cartesian dualism overtook society, Christianity cautiously accepted empirical science because of belief that God is in all reality, including human ingenuity and scientific progress. Scientific inquiry is part of the fundamental natural good of knowledge and reason. The modern hospital has been shaped more by advances in medical science and technology than by these explicitly religious and spiritual understandings. With the dramatic advances of the last half of the twentieth century—the portable ventilator, cardiopulmonary resuscitation, immunology and transplantation, and modern genetics—the modern hospital has focused on the provision of increasingly sophisticated technological care to individuals. The Catholic hospital strives to be a credible deliverer of this sophisticated technological care and to continue to witness to the healing ministry of Christ. Per Bernardin (1996):

> Our distinctive vocation in Christian health care is not so much to heal better or more efficiently than anyone else; it is to bring comfort to people by giving them an experience that will strengthen their confidence in life. The ultimate goal of our care is to give those who are ill, through our care, a reason to hope.

In keeping with the importance of experience and reason in the moral tradition, and to maintain the moral integrity of Catholic facilities in light of medical advances, a set of moral and ethical directives has been developed. These are powerful influences in setting the sense of Catholic priorities. The *Ethical and Religious Directives for Catholic Health Care Services (ERDs)* (United States Conference of Catholic Bishops and Catholic Church 2005) in the United States and the *Health Ethics Guide* (Catholic Health Association of Canada 2000) in Canada respond to the moral issues of modern health care. However, Catholic health care ethics has been focused on dilemma ethics with particular attention to sexual and reproductive ethics and, more recently, end of life care. Neither the U.S directives nor the Canadian ethics guides devote specific attention to disease prevention and health promotion. Their focus has emphasized life and death issues and acute, high technology care dilemmas; they have mostly neglected larger issues of global justice (Cahill 2005).

Flowing from this duty to respond to medical need and a sacramental under-standing of organizations and systems, Church teaching has addressed the issue of societal response to health need. Pope John XXIII's 1963 Encyclical *Pacem in Terris* (1963: no. 11) proclaims:

> We see that every man has the right to life, to bodily integrity, and to the means which are suitable for the proper development of life…Therefore, a human being has the right to security in sickness.

Exactly how to ensure this "security in sickness" is not specified. Different structural responses to the funding and provision of health care have developed in Western nations. Callahan and Wasunna's (2006) general review of international attempts at health system organization and reform concluded that the approach ultimately chosen by a country fosters either equity or choice. McDonough's (2007) specifically faith-based analysis of health system crises sees nations turning either to creative market approaches to deal with the acute care demand issue, such as the focus in the United States on managed competition and consumer-driven health care, or to a fundamental rethinking of basic values such as Canada's commitment to equity or Western Europe's commitment to solidarity. Although Catholic thinking is not totally in agreement on the details of health system organization, as the Obama health reforms of 2010 demonstrated dramatically, the Catholic approach to questions of system development is consistent with perspectives on dignity and justice. In Canada, for example, the Canadian Conference of Catholic Bishops (CCCB) has been very active in giving direction to public debate regarding health care:

> Specifically, health-care justice obliges a society to provide all its citizens with an appropriate level of health care. Maintaining both universality and the accessibility of comprehensive health care remains a prime objective of health-care justice. The grounds for deciding who gets health care cannot be based on merit, social worth, or the ability to pay. Everyone has the right to health care. (The Permanent Council of the Canadian Conference of Catholic Bishops 2005: no. 5)

In the United States ethical issues in health system funding and organization have dominated the debate (Kaveny and Keenan 1995; Keane 1993). A set of Catholic values that should guide U.S. health care reform has been proposed (Place 1999, 249):

- Every person enjoys an inalienable human dignity.
- Health care is an element of the common good.

- Health care is a service to people.
- There is a special duty to care for the poor.
- There must be responsible stewardship of resources.

Subsidiarity means that to the greatest degree practicable, administration must be carried out at the level of organization closest to those to be served.

Interestingly, these values, which were not always apparent in the recent U.S. reforms, come not from the long tradition of health care but from Catholic social teaching. So mapping them in any coherent fashion to the actual organization and focus of Catholic health care is challenging.

The general issue of disease prevention and health promotion has not been totally lacking in reflections on health systems and their reform. In their influential health ethics text, Ashley and colleagues (Ashley, DeBlois, and O'Rourke 2006, 221) suggest that

> the type of health care program that Catholics can consistently support must be economically sound yet aim at preventive medicine, at achieving healthier people who can care for themselves, rather than an ever-increasing dependence on technical medical care and professional help.

The U.S. Bishops (1993, 100) "Resolution on Health Care Reform" contained a criterion of "comprehensive benefits" defined as those benefits "sufficient to maintain and promote good health, to provide preventive care, to treat disease, injury, and disability appropriately and to care for persons who are chronically ill or dying." However, the focus of concern in the U.S. and Canadian health reform debates remains access to acute health care. There is a concern for many that the Catholic focus on hospital-based health care has reinforced the technological medical paradigm (Brodeur 1999, 9).

DISEASE PREVENTION AND HEALTH PROMOTION

Compared with the long, strong, and even sanctifying tradition of health care, disease prevention and health promotion have not been given much attention in Catholic thought. Some insight into this lack can be found in Catholic teaching regarding care of our health and bodies. Some lessons can be learned in reviewing a few examples of conflict between public health practices and Catholic moral thought.

Faust and Menzel in the introduction to this volume (Chapter 1) ask that our reflection focus on primary and secondary disease prevention. They limit the discussion here to born and live human beings. Thus, they avoid a few areas of deep-seated controversy from Catholic morality such as some prenatal preventive strategies that include abortion and preimplantation genetic diagnosis. Although explicitly excluded from discussion here, Catholic sensitivity on these issues may be adversely affecting enthusiasm for prevention more generally. Faust and Menzel also state that some illness develops from identifiable threats to health created by smoking, high sodium intake, lack of physical activity, etc. These threats are *risk factors* to health, which may be personal, communal, or global. If, as Evans says, "What prevention treats—if treat be the word—is a set of conditions under which disease may arise" (Evans 1998), then we need a deep and wide understanding of all relevant conditions determining the health of individuals and populations. That would include the social determinants of health, rendering the scope of prevention enormous (see Wallace in Chapter 4 of this volume).

Here, we are concerned with the somewhat more limited scope of classic primary prevention in public health measures, including harm reduction and immunization and promotion of health behaviors, and with secondary prevention such as screening for disease. Because there is no clear, continuous tradition regarding disease prevention and health promotion in Catholicism, we need to look for insight into their value and priority in other areas.

CONCERN FOR THE BODY AND HEALTH

The Christian Scriptures demonstrate some ambiguity and contradiction regarding human bodies and health. On the one hand, the New Testament is very concerned with the body and bodily integrity. The Incarnation of Jesus Christ is essential here because, for the Christian, "The Word was made flesh, he lived among us" (John 1:14). In doing so, all flesh becomes holy. In the writings of St. Paul the dignity of the body is emphasized "always, wherever we may be, we carry with us in our body the death of Jesus, so that the life of Jesus, too, may always be seen in our body" (2 Corinthians 4:10). The body is "the temple of the Holy Spirit" (1 Corinthians 6:19).

On the other hand, the physical body can be controlled by the flesh, that is, by the sinful impulses of the body (1 Corinthians 15:43). Different authors of Scripture used the body and the flesh in different ways so that confusion developed early regarding the holy body and the sinful flesh. In the third century Origen and others developed an early *anthropological dualism* that emphasized the gap between body and soul and posited an active war between them (Ammicht-Quinn 2008). As a result of Origen's dualism, from late antiquity in Western Christianity there arose a fear of primal drives located in the body because these are a source of sin. Some of these fears were captured in the teachings regarding the "deadly sins" of gluttony and sloth. The soul is imprisoned in the body. Ambivalence regarding the body and the flesh becomes a powerful theme. This notion of a battle with the body underlies much of Christian asceticism. Flagellation, mortification, and fasting were practices aimed at taming the body and its desires for the life of the soul. Manichean and Gnostic heresies, which taught that the body/flesh was evil, were ultimately condemned, but their influence has lingered on in attitudes and pious practices.

Recent Magisterial teaching has clarified a more authentic Catholic understanding of the body (Pope Paul VI 1965):

> Man, though made of body and soul, is a unity. Through his very bodily condition he sums up in himself the elements of the material world... For this reason man may not despise his bodily life. Rather he is obliged to regard his body as good and to hold it in honor since God has created it.

Precisely because the body is good, the Catholic tradition requires persons to take care of their health and life. As the Catechism of the Catholic Church teaches (Vatican 2009: no. 2288), "Life and physical health are precious gifts entrusted to us by God. We must take reasonable care of them, taking into account the needs of others and the common good." It is important to note here the mutuality of the needs of individuals and the common good, a concept conspicuously absent from most reflections about priorities.

Some explicit teaching about behaviors that promote health and prevent some diseases is found in teaching and preaching about the importance of virtues such as temperance and the avoidance of excess of food, alcohol, and tobacco (Vatican 2009: no. 2290). The abusive use of nonprescription drugs with their corrosive effects on health and relationships is clearly condemned (Vatican 2009: no. 2291). The avoidance of excess and its consequences rather than positive action for health seems to be the theme. Interestingly, although prudent care of life and care of health are important duties, discrimination and exclusion from needed services for lifestyle-related conditions such as those caused by alcohol and tobacco are unacceptable in the Catholic tradition. As stated by the Catholic Health Association of the United States (1991, 25), "When people are in need of health care services, the way they contracted their disease and the extent to which they may be held personally responsible must play no part in decisions to withhold health care services." In other words, the duty to provide care prevails. Once a person is ill, care is unconditionally warranted, regardless of any previous deficiencies in the individual's prudent preventive care of his or her health and body.

In this tradition care of the body and health is understood prudently. This is definitely not the fixation on the ideal body or Godlee's virtual mania of prevention (Godlee 2005). The modern "body project" with the exercise studio as temple of worship aims at bodily perfection—ascetic or functional—for its own sake. This worship of the body is very different from an asceticism that focuses on the body for the sake of the life of the soul (Ammicht-Quinn 2008). The Catechism sums it up this way (Vatican 2009: no. 2289):

> If morality requires respect for the life of the body, it does not make it an absolute value. It rejects a neo-pagan notion that tends to promote the *cult of the body*, to sacrifice everything for its sake, to idolize physical perfection and success at sports.

Although care of life and health is an important duty, little attention has been given to it in preaching and official teaching. Even in the landmark *Theologies of the Body* by the eminent moral theologian Benedict Ashley, there is no discrete section devoted to care of the body or to disease prevention and health promotion (Ashley 1995). The widely used *Health Care Ethics: A Catholic Theological Analysis* by Ashley, DeBlois, and O'Rourke (2006) has no special section on public health or disease prevention and health promotion.

CATHOLIC SOCIAL JUSTICE AND COMMUNAL RESPONSIBILITY FOR HEALTH

In the Judeo-Christian story God relates to and makes covenants with a people, an *ecclesia*. The notion of community is thus central to Catholic thought. Although individuals have clear responsibility for their own health, the community has a reciprocal responsibility to individuals in need. We have seen that in the New Testament, cures are important, but more important is healing of the whole person and restoration of the person to the community. This restoration to the community was particularly important when illness and disability were seen as judgments of God making the victims ritually unclean.

Central to the community of the faithful is the notion of justice. At the beginning of Jesus' public ministry he proclaims, using the words of the prophet Isaiah, "I have come to bring good news to the poor, to proclaim liberty to captives…to set the downtrodden free" (Luke 4:18). These themes are complementary to the theme of response to the sick. Both care of the sick and attention to the social determinants of health are elements in Jesus' ministry. Some explicit obligations for continuing this ministry of care and justice have been spelled out over the past one hundred years in Catholic social teaching. "Formally speaking, Catholic social teaching is a social vision, morally based, theologically grounded, publicly argued, and institutionally embodied" (McCann 2000, 233).

Central to this vision of the good society is the Catholic conception of social justice (Coleman and Ryan 2005) with the following fundamental themes:

- Dignity of the human person
- Social interdependence and social solidarity
- Commitment to the common good
- Special obligation to the poor and vulnerable
- Stewardship of resources
- Subsidiarity decisions should be made at level of those most affected.

This tradition is rooted in the dignity of individual persons who are understood to be in community and socially interdependent. The notion of the common good is crucial here. The common good "is the sum total of those conditions of social life which allow social groups and their individual members, relatively thorough and ready access to their own fulfillment" (Pope Paul VI 1965: no. 26). All conditions for human flourishing are important. Moreover, stewardship of resources is a fundamental requirement if we are to serve the common good.

Rose (1992) observes the "prevention paradox" in which "a preventive measure that brings large effects to the community offers little to each participating individual." In the highly individualistic societies of today, motivating for the common good is essential for the development of public health measures focused on the community. The commitments of Catholic social teaching can be a powerful source for theorizing about and advocating a transformative stance toward the prioritizing of disease prevention and health promotion for individuals and communities.

SOME CATHOLIC CONTROVERSIES IN DISEASE PREVENTION

Before this transformation can take place we need to recognize some problematic history. Primary prevention is compatible with Catholic concerns for prudent care of the body; positive health behaviors are consistent with the virtues of prudence and temperance. Mitigating health risks to communities and populations is consistent with issues of justice and concern for the poor and marginalized. And public health's historic attention to women, children, and workers resonates with social justice. So, we might expect that disease prevention and health promotion would have a prominent place in Catholic teaching.

However, there have been conflicts between some standard public health practices and strategies and Roman Catholic moral theology. These suggest that some of the failure to value disease prevention and health promotion highly is not only because of the importance of health care in the Catholic tradition, but also from some controversial experiences with disease prevention. Some examples from harm reduction and immunization can illustrate this situation.

Harm Reduction Strategies

Harm reduction strategies recognize that legal and moral prohibitions are not sufficient to eliminate harmful activities. Although not condoning these activities, they aim not at preventing a condition resulting from choices and behaviors, but at ameliorating their negative consequences. These strategies have been particularly important in public health policies concerning injected drug use and the use of condoms for disease prevention. Churches have had reservations about these strategies because of concerns that they might be condoning or facilitating immoral behavior. It has been suggested that Catholics can offer at least conditional support for harm reduction based on four main sources: "the biblical example of Jesus, the historical example of the Christian community in its practice of hospitality, theological reflection on the ethics of mercy, and the wisdom of the Catholic moral tradition embedded in the long established concepts of the counseling of the lesser of two evils, and the principle of cooperation" (Vogt 2004, 318).

Scriptural witness to Jesus' concern for the poor and marginalized, and the Church's response for merciful outreach to the vulnerable and strangers, supports a compassionate commitment to outcasts. So it is not surprising to hear that Church support has been crucial in harm reduction programs focusing on drug addiction in the U.K. (O'Hare 2007), Australia (Norden 2008), and Canada (Kerr et al. 2006). Needle exchange programs and safe injection sites have received at least tacit support.

The use of condoms for disease prevention is more complex. Despite the fact that Catholic resources provide health care for a large number of the victims of HIV/AIDS victims, especially in Africa, many have accused the Catholic Church of lacking compassion because of its position regarding the promotion of abstinence and monogamy as the real answers to the crisis, and its prohibition against condom use for prevention. The Church has a clear opposition to the use of condoms for contraceptive purposes. However, theologians have argued on both sides of the issue regarding the use of condoms for disease prevention and containment (Fuller 1996; Keenan 1999, 2000; Grisez 2008). "For many decades, theologians have admitted that it is sometimes permitted to *counsel* the lesser of two evils" (McCormick 2006, 322). To counsel the lesser of two evils two conditions are given: the person being counseled is determined in the pursuit of the greater evil, and there is no other way of preventing the greater evil.

In 2010 Pope Benedict's remarks in a book with Peter Seewald on the use of a condom to prevent HIV infection "as a first step in the direction of a moralization" received mixed responses (Seewald 2010). Some applauded this traditional use of the principles of the lesser of two evils and material cooperation in evil; others were appalled that the pope seemed to be affirming condom use. The Congregation for the Doctrine of the Faith (CDF) then issued a magisterial statement affirming the Church's position that condoms do not constitute the real or moral solution to the problem of AIDS. However, in the context of putting others at risk of HIV infection, "it cannot be denied that anyone who uses a condom in order to diminish the risk posed to another person is intending to reduce the evil connected with his or her immoral activity" (Congregation for the Doctrine of the Faith 2010, 2). The CDF then goes on to state "that some commentators have interpreted the words of Benedict XVI according to the so-called theory of the 'lesser evil' but 'this theory is, however, susceptible to proportionalistic misinterpretation. An action which is objectively evil, even if a lesser evil, can never be licitly willed" (Congregation for the Doctrine of the Faith 2010, 2). Following this strict interpretation a definitive pronouncement on the issue was made on June 10, 2011 by Archbishop Francis Assisi Chullikatt, Permanent Observor of the Holy See to the United Nations during the high-level plenary on HIV/AIDS: The Holy See does not endorse the use of condoms/commodities as part of HIV and AIDS prevention programmes or classes/programmes of education in sex/sexuality. Prevention programmes or classes/programmes of education in human sexuality should focus not on trying to convince the world that risky and dangerous behavior forms part of an acceptable lifestyle, but rather should focus on risk avoidance, which is ethically and empirically sound. (Chullikatt, 2011).

While Catholics have been involved in the development of some important harm reduction strategies, there ha been a certain resistance to the morality of these approaches. The 2011 clarification has stated explicitly that "The Holy See does not accept so-called "harm reduction" efforts related to drug use…as they do not treat or cure the sick person, but instead falsely suggest that they cannot break free from the cycle of addiction." (Chullikatt, 2011) This formal teaching will present new difficulties for fostering Catholic attention to general disease prevention policies.

At issue, as well, is the principle of moral cooperation which has a long history in Catholic morality. It helps determine whether an individual's or institution's participation in the illicit action of another is justified for a greater good, using a set of criteria regarding intent: the nature of the cooperation, the reason for the cooperation, and the role of cooperation, i.e., is it indispensable. This principle too is under scrutiny as different approaches to moral decision making, different understandings of intrinsically evil acts, and differing applications of the use of these principles in practice characterize the contemporary Catholic debate regarding the acceptability of public strategies. So, contemporary moral priorities create ongoing tensions for Catholic participation in general harm reduction and disease prevention policies and practices.

Immunization

Immunization and vaccination against infectious disease would seem to be far from issues of sexual and reproductive ethics. However, here too Catholic moral concerns have affected support for some infectious disease prevention programs such as human papilloma virus (HPV) immunization and vaccines derived from aborted fetuses.

In Ontario, Canada a Catholic school district voted to disallow within their schools a publicly funded vaccination program for HPV, a sexually transmitted virus associated with the majority of cases of cervical cancer. The program was targeted at Grade 8 girls. The school board decision was based on concerns regarding vaccine safety and on the conviction that vaccinating against a sexually transmitted disease in a school system teaching abstinence before marriage was hypocritical (Kirkwood 2008). The Ontario Conference of Bishops affirmed the right of parents to decide regarding the vaccination of their daughters but made nonempirically validated claims regarding the vaccination and promiscuity. The public perception was that Catholics had damaged the effectiveness of a public health program, especially for the poorest girls whose parents could not afford vaccine.

Vaccines derived from aborted fetal tissue, particularly rubella, have also been the source of concern (Pontifical Academy for Life 2006). Recognizing the devastating effects of the disease *in utero* and the difficulty of avoidance of the infection, eliminating congenital rubella has been a public health priority. For Catholics the moral concern here is not related to the use of the vaccine but rather to its production. Because of its preparation in cells coming from voluntarily aborted fetuses it raises the concern of material cooperation in the evil of abortion. Although theological opinion allows the use of these vaccines, using the principle of material cooperation, there is again a linkage of public health practice and Catholic suspicion.

These examples serve to demonstrate that some standard public health practices aimed at disease prevention have come into conflict with Catholic sexual ethics and principles of the lesser of two evils and material cooperation in evil. These experiences have surely contributed to the gap between public health disease prevention and health promotion activities and Catholic priorities in health.

THE THOUGHT EXPERIMENT AND CATHOLIC CHOICE

How has this cure versus prevention priority been answered in the Roman Catholic tradition of health care? Clearly, the priority has been given to a duty to the alleviation of pain and suffering in persons in need of immediate care. Forced to make a choice, the general Catholic response in the situations described in this volume's thought experiment (see Chapter 1) would be to attend to Bill, the person in immediate need of care. There would be some resistance to the forced choice because of what has been described as the "both/and" (McBrien 1994) quality of Catholicism: *both* health care *and* disease prevention are important human goods. However, even in this brief reflection we see the powerful dominance of response to individual medical need in the Catholic moral imagination and tradition.

The option to see John for preventive care, rather than Bill who is now suffering a likely life-threatening condition, would be an extraordinary response of any Catholic. If forced to a consideration of the options, Catholic thought might push for a more holistic attention to all patients in which the treatment versus prevention distinction would not be so sharp, and all patient interactions would include both treatment and preventive actions.

Finally, the option to take a call regarding a community-wide heart attack prevention program would also be unlikely. Although disease prevention and health promotion have force in the social justice tradition, it is not in this individual medical benefit sense. The Catholic social justice tradition focuses not only on individuals but also on the common good. Its focus has been more on community and population benefits from understanding and responding to the socioeconomic determinants. As crises in health systems force us to fundamental rethinking of our priorities, many Catholic commentators are asking how to better integrate this social justice tradition with that of health care.

Although responsible stewardship is an element of Catholic social justice, it would be resistant to some of the "bottom line" thinking that might be furthered in cost-effectiveness analysis (CEA). The duty of care seems to regularly trump conversations about effectiveness in Catholic discussions regarding resource allocation (Engelhardt, Tristram, and Cherry 2002). Some of the limits of CEA, especially in QALY assessments, have been identified in the general ethical and policy literature (Menzel et al. 1999). Moreover, CEA neglects a number of important values such as maintenance of hope, assurance of care, lifesaving treatment in the face of imminent death, etc. We've seen that Catholic thought often trades off health benefit or effectiveness of health outcomes for other goods and values such as assurance of care in need, maintenance of hope, and the preservation of human life. Generally, Catholics reject quality of life arguments, understood as a judgment of lives not worth living; because of the belief in inherent dignity and that each person is created in the image of God (Walter 1990; Walter and Shannon 1990; Wildes 1996). As a result, any methodology that contains the concept of quality of life judgments is met with suspicion.

CONCLUSIONS

What might health priorities look like and how might health systems be organized if there were more integration between the Catholic tradition of health care and Catholic social teaching? There is a tendency in today's secular pluralism to exclude the claims of particular communities, especially religious ones, from public policy debate. The reality is that religions have shaped contemporary culture and still have an important role to play in promoting informed, civil discourse. In this reflection it is clear that Roman Catholic commitments to health care have strongly reinforced the contemporary privileging of medical care over prevention and promotion. Precisely because "religions share a drive toward coherence, resistance to exploitation, and a transcendent framework for evaluating human projects" (Cahill 2005, 3), religious voices have an important role in rethinking and reshaping priorities in health and health care.

Gustafson (1990) analyzes four modes of discourse necessary to sustain communities:

- Ethical—microfocused on specific choices
- Prophetic—providing a broad vision of large cultural trends and sins
- Narrative—inspirational stories of belief and character
- Policy—working within the constraints of culture and history and the "art of the possible."

To these, theologian and bioethicist Lisa Cahill (2005) adds a "participatory discourse," which commits to dialogue and civil discourse. In each of these areas of discourse better integration of Catholic social teaching and health care can lead to a much needed reprioritizing.

In ethics discourse there is a clear imperative to move beyond the important but narrowly conceived focus on acute health care ethical dilemmas of life and death regarding individuals and the almost exclusive focus on beginning and end of life issues. As Cahill (2005, 3) has claimed:

A new item on the agenda of both theology and public bioethics is examining critically the connections among individual decisions and social practices, with the aim of showing how practices that favor the privileged and enable their free choices and access to resources carry a negative impact for global health patterns and the choices and resources of the poor.

The prophetic dimension to Catholicism calls for it to be a voice for the voiceless and an agent of transformation. That prophetic voice needs to ask larger, more visionary questions about our approaches to health and health care. Many of these questions regarding personal responsibility for health, the inordinate demand for individual benefit from health technology with no consideration of stewardship or resources or the common good, and our failure to include disease prevention appropriately find the beginning of answers in social justice.

The powerful narrative stories from Scripture and from the proud history of the Catholic healing ministry need to be reimagined, with a new focus on preventing harm and protecting the vulnerable. This is not to abandon acute health care but rather to rethink what needs to be prevented or promoted in order to continue the healing ministry of Jesus. Some, like Cochran (1999, 38), are already imaging a new vision:

> Although some Catholic hospitals should continue to exist, it may be time for the Church to focus on other forms of healthcare that better model the sacramental encounter. These might be neighborhood clinics for abused children and battered wives, hospices for the dying, AIDS ministry, inner city clinics for those without health insurance, clinics in immigrant labor camps, rehabilitation centers, addiction treatment facilities, and outpatient mental health centers.

Policy discourse needs to make more clear and explicit the interests and values embedded in present approaches and priorities. The root causes of treatment priority in modern society need careful and courageous attention to social and economic forces.

The setting of new priorities in health care and disease prevention seems to be a critical first step in this examination. For Catholics, participation in a kind of communal examination of conscience is needed to integrate more fully the priorities of health care with the commitment to social justice, stewardship of resources, and the common good. If the Catholic vision could be more clearly and intentionally aware of the balance between health care and disease prevention and health promotion, it could be a powerful force for real transformation.

REFERENCES

Ammicht-Quinn, R. 2008. Body Culture. In W. Schweiker, Ed., *The Blackwell Companion to Religious Ethics* (527–535). Malden, MA: Blackwell.Ashley, B.M. 1995. *Theologies of the Body: Humanist and Christian,* 2nd ed. Braintree, MA: Pope John Center.

Ashley, B.M., DeBlois, J., and O'Rourke, K.D. 2006. *Health Care Ethics: A Catholic Theological Analysis,* 5th ed. Washington, DC: Georgetown University Press.

Bernardin, J. 1996. What Makes a Hospital Catholic—A Response. *America* 174 (15): 9–11.

———1995. A Sign of Hope—Pastoral Letter on Health Care. Office of Communications, Archdiocese of Chicago.

Brodeur, D. 1999. Catholic Health Care: Rationale for Ministry. *Christian Bioethics* 5 (1):5–25.

Cahill, L.S. 2005. *Theological Bioethics: Participation, Justice, and Change.* Washington, DC: Georgetown University Press.

Callahan, D., and Wasunna, A.A. 2006. *Medicine and the Market: Equity vs. Choice.* Baltimore, MA: Johns Hopkins University Press.

Catholic Church and Pontificium Consilium de Apostolatu pro Valetudinis Administris. 1995. *Charter for Health Care Workers.* Ikeja, Nigeria: Paulines Publications Africa.

Catholic Church and Pope John XXIII. 1963. *Pacem in Terris—Encyclical Letter of His Holiness Pope John XXIII on Establishing Universal Peace in Truth, Justice, Charity, and Liberty.* London: Catholic Truth Society.

Catholic Health Association of Canada. 2000. *Health Ethics Guide.* Ottawa: Catholic Health Association of Canada/Association Catholique Canadienne de la Santé.

Catholic Health Association of the United States. 1991. *With Justice for All? The Ethics of Healthcare Rationing.* St. Louis, MO: Catholic Health Association of the United States.

Chullikatt, F.A. 2011. Defending the Dignity of Human Life from Concepts which Stand against the Natural Law. L'Osservatore Romano (June 28).

Cochran, C.E. 1999. Institutional Identity; Sacramental Potential: Catholic Healthcare at Century's End. *Christian Bioethics* 5(1):26–43.

Coleman, J.A., and Ryan, W.F. 2005. *Globalization and Catholic Social Thought: Present Crisis, Future Hope.* Maryknoll, NY: Orbis Books.

Congregation for the Doctrine of the Faith. 2010. *Note on the Banalization of Sexuality: Regarding Certain Interpretations of "Light of the World."* Available at http://www.vatican.va/roman_curia/congregations/cfaith/documents/rc_con_cfaith_doc_20101221_luce-del-mondo_en.html, accessed June 9, 2011.

Curran, C.E. 1999. *The Catholic Moral Tradition Today: A Synthesis.* Washington, DC: Georgetown University Press.

Engelhardt, J., Tristram, H., and Cherry, M.J., Eds. 2002. *Allocating Scarce Medical Resources: Roman Catholic Perspectives.* Washington, DC: Georgetown University Press.

Evans, H.M. 1998. The Limits of Preventative Medicine. *International Journal of Moral and Social Studies* 3 (3):255–66.

Fuller, J. 1996. AIDS Prevention: A Challenge to the Catholic Moral Tradition. *America* 175:13–20.

Godlee, F. 2005. Editor's Choice: Preventive Medicine Makes Us Miserable. *British Medical Journal* 330: 7497 (April 25).

Grisez, G. 2008. Moral Questions on Condoms and Disease Prevention. *National Catholic Bioethics Center* 8 (3/Autumn):471–76.

Guinan, P. 2004. Christianity and the Origin of the Hospital. *National Catholic Bioethics Center* 4 (2/Summer):257–63.

Gustafson, J. 1990. Moral Discourse about Medicine: A Variety of Forms. *The Journal of Medicine and Philosophy* 15 (2):125–42.

Jones, A. 1980. *The Jerusalem Bible, Reader's Edition*. Garden City, NY: Doubleday.

Kaveny, M.C., and Keenan, J. 1995. Ethics Issues in Health Care Restructuring. *Theological Studies* 56 (1):136–50.

Keane, P.S. 1993. *Health Care Reform: A Catholic View*. New York: Paulist Press.

Keenan, J.F. 1999. Applying the Seventeenth-Century Casuistry of Accommodation to HIV Prevention. *Theological Studies* 60 (3):492–512.

———, Ed. 2000. *Catholic Ethicists on HIV/AIDS Prevention*. New York: Continuum.

Kerr, T., Small, W., Peeace, W., Douglas, D., Pierre, A., and Wood, E. 2006. Harm Reduction by a "User-Run" Organization: A Case Study of the Vancouver area Network of Drug Users (VANDU). *International Journal of Drug Policy* 17 (2): 61–69.

Kirkwood, K. 2008. Catholic Bioethical Perspectives on Ontario's HPV Vaccination. *Open Medicine* 2 (4). Available at http://www.openmedicine.ca/article/viewArticle/177/209 accessed June 9, 2011.

Latkovic, M.S. 2008. The Vocation to Heal. Health Care in the Light of Catholic Faith: Scriptural, Theological, and Philosophical Reflections. *Linacre Quarterly* 75 (1): 40–55.

McBrien, R.P. 1994. *Catholicism*. San Francisco, CA: Harper.

McCann, D.P. 2000. Catholic Social Teaching and the Economics of Health Care Management. *Christian Bioethics* 6 (3):231–50.

McCormick, R.A. 1987. *Health and Medicine in the Catholic Tradition: Tradition in Transition*. New York: Crossroad.

———. 2006. *The Critical Calling: Reflections on Moral Dilemmas Since Vatican II*. Washington, DC: Georgetown University Press.

McDonough, M.J. 2007. *Can a Health Care Market Be Moral? A Catholic Vision*. Washington, DC: Georgetown University Press.

Menzel, P., Gold, M.R., Nord, E., Pinto-Prades, J.L., Richardson, J., and Ubel, P. 1999. Toward a Broader View of Values in Cost-Effectiveness Analysis of Health. *Hastings Center Report* 29 (3):7–15.

Norden, P. 2008. Keeping them Connected—Reducing Drug-Related Harm in Australian Schools from a Catholic Perspective. *Drug and Alcohol Review* 27 (4):451–58.

O'Hare, P. 2007. Merseyside, the First Harm Reduction Conferences, and the Early History of Harm Reduction. *International Journal of Drug Policy* 18 (2):141–44.

Place, M.D. 1999. Health Care as an Essential Building Block for a Free Society: The Convergence of the Catholic and Secular American Imperative. *Kennedy Institute of Ethics Journal* 9 (3):245–62.

Pontifical Academy for Life. 2006. Moral Reflections on Vaccines Prepared from Cells Derived from Aborted Fetuses. *National Catholic Bioethics Quarterly* 6:541–50.

Pope Paul VI. 1965. *Pastoral Constitution of the Church in the Modern World.* Available at http://www.vatican.va/archive/hist_councils/ii_vatican_council/documents/vat-ii_cons_19651207_gaudium-et-spes_en.html, accessed June 9, 2011.

Rose, G. 1992. *The Strategy of Preventive Medicine.* New York: Oxford University Press.

Seewald, P. 2010. *Light of the World: The Pope, the Church and the Signs of the Times: An Interview with Peter Seewald.* San Francisco, CA: Ignatius Press.

The Permanent Council of the Canadian Conference of Catholic Bishops. 2005. *The Catholic Health Ministry in Canada.* Available at http://www.cccb.ca/site/eng/bishops/list-of-bishops, accessed June 9, 2011.

United States Bishops. 1993. Resolution on Health Care Reform. *Origins* 23:98–102.

United States Conference of Catholic Bishops and Catholic Church. 2005. *Ethical and Religious Directives for Catholic Health Care Services.* Washington, DC: National Conference of Catholic Bishops.

Vatican. 2009. *Catechism of the Catholic Church.* Available at http://www.vatican.va/archive/ccc_css/archive/catechism/p3s2c2a5.htm, accessed November 3, 2009.

Vogt, C. 2004. Recognizing the Addict as Neighbour; Christian Hospitality and the Establishment of Safe Injection Facilities in Canada. *Theoforum* 35:317–42.

Walter, J.J. 1990. The Meaning and Validity of Quality of Life Judgments in Contemporary Roman Catholic Medical Ethics. In J.J. Walter and T.A. Shannon, Eds., *Quality of Life: The New Medical Dilemma* (pp. 78–88). Mahwah, NJ: Paulist Press.

Walter, J.J., and Shannon, T.A. 1990. *Quality of Life: The New Medical Dilemma.* Mahwah, NJ: Paulist Press.

Wildes, K.W. 1996. Ordinary and Extraordinary Means and the Quality of Life. *Theological Studies* 57 (3):500–12.

14

Loving God and the Neighbor

Protestant Insights for Prevention and Treatment

AANA MARIE VIGEN, PhD ■

Thus says the LORD: "Act with justice and righteousness, and deliver from the hand of the oppressor anyone who has been robbed. And do no wrong or violence to the alien, the orphan, and the widow, or shed innocent blood in this place."

JEREMIAH 22:3[1]

"Do not store up for yourselves treasures on earth, where moth and rust consume and where thieves break in and steal; but store up for yourselves treasures in heaven… For where your treasure is, there your heart will be also."

MATTHEW 6:19–21

FRAMING THE QUESTIONS

As a Lutheran social ethicist lending her voice to this interdisciplinary conversation, I begin not with questions of allocation, but of values. The scriptural passages above address distinct, yet interlinked values for Christian living: serving others, seeking justice, and keeping God as the orienting love that informs all others. I begin here because it is my sense that what a Protestant perspective most constructively offers is not specific ratios or finalized public

---

1. *The New Revised Standard Version* (NRSV).

policy recommendations, but rather a unique way for thinking about such questions that differs significantly from predominant U.S. medical and societal worldviews. These worldviews, as Kenny concurs in Chapter 13 of this volume, are generally characterized by weighty emphases on individualism, advanced treatments, and medical technologies.

Prominent Protestant ethicists (e.g., Allen Verhey, Stanley Hauerwas, Bruce Birch, Larry Rasmussen, Dennis Sansom) all emphasize that what marks Christian faith communities are the dynamic ways in which they read, interpret, and attempt to live as a "people of the book," meaning that Christians share a common story and seek to live in a manner that is faithful to it in particular times and places. Birch and Rasmussen explain that instead of asking abstract questions about a "universal good," early Jews and Christians asked:

> "What character and conduct is in keeping with who we are as a people of God?" ... There was very little interest in "morality" per se. ... [Morality] and ethics were dimensions of community life in which the concern was how a people of God were to live with one another and with those outside the faith community. The broader interest was faithfulness toward God as the way of life of a people. (Emphasis in the original, Birch and Rasmussen 1988, 19–20)

Of particular relevance for medical ethics, Sansom elucidates how Christian identity, forged in concrete communities, can make sense of mortality:

> We learn what is a "natural life span" and a "tolerable death" by living in a community in which we see and learn from others who have discovered their own narrative unity through their faith in God. By living in a community of faithful people who are shaped by the life, teaching, death, and resurrection of Jesus Christ, we see how people integrate their lives, how they deal with sickness and dying. (Sansom 1998, 265)

For Christians, then, the aim is to juxtapose the best scientific, medical, and public health information available with sacred scriptures and religious traditions so as to discern how to live (and die) in light of our professed confession of belief in something far greater than human medicine or power.

To illustrate the significance of this orientation, consider two existential questions as framed by the particular lens of Christian theology and ethics:

1. Given the divine promise of accompaniment and redemption, how should people make sense of the inescapable realities of mortality and

suffering? Said differently, given that all will die one day, for what
ought human beings to strive and hope?

2. In light of scriptural accounts of God's prophetic, grace-filled acts of
   compassion and healing—often enacted with special attention to the
   poor, vulnerable, and suffering—what constitute contemporary
   Christian obligations with respect to health and medicine?

Such questions, rooted in Christian traditions and faith communities over
the centuries, shift the starting point for a discussion of priorities between prevention and treatment in important ways. For Christians, the most critical and
fundamental challenges human persons face involve more than cost-effectiveness comparisons. They encompass the larger, life-long task of perceiving reality adequately and responding with vibrant moral and spiritual imagination.

My thesis in this chapter is two-fold. First, a Protestant perspective offers a
distinctive framework that can nuance and expand moral imagination for the
sake of public dialogue and policy formation. Second, we arrive at adequate
ethical adjudications of the relationship between prevention and treatment
within particular contexts (e.g., social, economic, political, historical, racial-
ethnic, gender) without postulating a universalized resolution to the tension
between them.

As other contributors demonstrate, the United States has invested a great
deal in treatment, perhaps to the detriment of prevention. However, elsewhere
millions of people with chronic disease have been too easily written off in favor
of prevention strategies. Indeed, in some global contexts, arguments prioritizing prevention have amounted to little more than circumspect rationalizations
for doing little to treat the world's poor who are already infected with tuberculosis, malaria, malnutrition, pneumonia, or HIV/AIDS. Thus, although overall
I favor investment in primordial prevention, I would caution against such a
focus if it justifies a stance that contends it is not worthwhile to treat people
with disease who, in life's arbitrary lottery, were born into impoverished and
at-risk contexts. Instead, dynamic combinations of prevention and treatment
most often offer the most effective, and the most moral, responses to human
need.

After clarifying two terms, the chapter is divided into three sections. First, it
highlights three themes prominent in Christian thought related to health, illness, and obligations to others. Second, it shows why social analysis and social
contexts matter for assessing how to prioritize prevention and treatment in particular times and places. Third, it underscores implications for prevention and
treatment in the twenty-first century—synthesizing the insights from Protestant
ethics and social analysis.

Clarifying Terms: Health/Healing and Prevention

Christian understandings of health and healing have been multifaceted throughout history. Here, I wish only to echo the definition put forward by Protestant womanist ethicist, Emilie Townes:

> Health is not simply the absence of disease—it comprises a wide range of activities that foster healing and wholeness. In this view, health is a cultural production in that health and illness alike are social constructs and dependent on social networks, biology, and environment. As it is embedded in our social realities, health also includes the integration of the spiritual (how we relate to God), the mental (who we are as thinking and feeling people), and the physical (who we are biologically) aspects of our lives. (Townes 1998, 2)

For Christians, health does not fall under the sole purview of medical professionals and is not limited to physiological or mental well-being. Instead, similar to the World Health Organization's (WHO) understanding, health is both individual and corporate; a matter of mind, emotions, body, and relationships.[2]

In the introduction, Faust and Menzel note that health care forums typically identify three kinds of prevention (primary, secondary, and tertiary) and ask contributors to include the first two meanings in our operating use of the term. In this vein, I wish to emphasize the "background" aspects of primary prevention that are not always made explicit: e.g., clean drinking water; healthy and affordable food sources; well-developed public education, sanitation, and social network infrastructures; safe parks and playgrounds; effective violence prevention programs; and the promotion of gender equality. A robust notion of primary prevention as "assuring that all persons are able to live in safe, clean houses and neighborhoods; eat healthy foods; socialize with family and friends; get exercise; rest and manage stress" (Blacksher 2009) complements the Christian perspective of health noted above. It focuses needed attention on questions of how to create the larger social conditions that promote overall human flourishing (physiologically, socially, and emotionally).

---

2. http://www.who.int/suggestions/faq/en/index.html, accessed May 8, 2010.

WHERE DO YOU STORE UP YOUR TREASURE? — THREE PROMINENT CHRISTIAN THEMES

Three theological insights deeply embedded within Christianity merit attention because, together, they serve as a corrective lens for how many of us in the United States conceive of the pertinent questions related to prevention and treatment. They are a radical encounter with divine grace and human finitude; a holistic understanding of health, healing, and illness; and the demanding call to love God and neighbor. These themes are certainly found in Roman Catholicism and resonate within Judaism and other religions as well. In what follows, I merely offer distinctive Protestant accents.

Ultimate Meaning: Divine Grace and Human Finitude[3]

Over the centuries, Christians (along with others) have searched for and crafted meaningful answers to existential questions: What is the ultimate meaning and purpose of life? For what and in what do we hope and trust? Who and what is worthy of love? How do we "order" our various, sometimes competing, loves? These questions grow out of concrete experiences of being human and of suffering, both individually and communally. Christianity's answer to each— expressed with many differing metaphors and emphases—consistently has God in Christ at its heart.[4] Martin Luther is illustrative.

For Luther, human beings radically depend upon God and are intrinsically related to one another. In this pivotal relationship with God, human beings are beloved and embraced *precisely as* imperfect creatures—simultaneously "saint and sinner." In fact, Luther doggedly rails against anyone who claims that human beings, by our own power alone, can bring themselves closer to God and/or perfection. Salvation does not depend on our merits; God bridges the distance we cannot. Our responsibility then is to try, throughout our lives, to accept this gift—this grace—and cling to it with our whole beings. Any quest to save or perfect ourselves will only serve to drive us away from God and from genuinely attending to the pressing needs of our neighbors.[5]

3. For a fuller history of this and other Christian themes related to health/healing, see the chapters by Marty, Amundsen, Ferngren, Numbers, and Sawyer in Marty and Vaux (1982).

4. I elaborate a Lutheran feminist theological anthropology that addresses these questions in Vigen (2006, Chap. 3). "God in Christ" refers to the Christian claim that God was incarnate in the enfleshed, human person of Jesus.

5. For discussions of Luther's worldview/ethics see Moe-Lobeda (2002, 2004), Althaus (1972), and Lazareth (2001).

In a related vein, for Luther (and other theologians) suffering is understood to be a part of life and impossible to root out. In fact, if it serves to draw us closer to God, then it is not entirely unwelcome. Christians are to find solace in remembering that Jesus suffered—and still suffers with those in pain. Christians, especially preceding the nineteenth century, are profoundly aware of the fragility of all human life. Contemporary Christian feminists, womanists, and liberation theologians[6] rightly signal the deep flaws in any romanticizing of suffering. Yet a deep encounter with it may offer a corrective to those who take power, privilege, and medical advances for granted.

Indeed, Luther's view of the human being represents a strong contrast to the one offered by much of western, post-Enlightenment thought that celebrates human rationality, autonomy, and the ability to improve both individuals and society. Luther was not against medicine or technological discoveries per se, but he was skeptical about their abilities to change the basic facts of human existence—mortality, fragility, dependence on God—and he was concerned that achievements would lead to a false confidence in human acumen and power.

Since the emergence of western bioethics as a field in the 1960s, prominent Protestant medical ethicists (e.g., Ramsey, Verhey, Hauerwas) have repeatedly called into question what they see as an idolatry of medicine and science prevalent in U.S. society.[7] From a Protestant perspective, even as advanced medical treatments can often significantly extend and improve our lives, they are not a "cure" for mortality, nor should they be. Part of responsible human living—and good medical care—is confronting this biological and existential reality. At its best, faith in Jesus Christ offers not a flight from death, but a powerful spiritual and moral movement through it.

Holistic View of Health, Healing, and Illness

Given the inability to escape suffering and death, a pressing question for the Christian becomes: "What kind of healing should we seek?" For early Jewish and Christian communities, and even later up to the Reformation and early modernity, the health and healing of mind, body, and soul were integrated (Marty and Vaux 1982). This sense is most clearly seen in their understanding of illness, which signaled that a person or community's relationship with the

6. For example, James Cone, Gustavo Gutiérrez, Beverly Harrison, Delores Williams, Katie Cannon, Kwok Pui Lan, Traci West, and Miguel de la Torre.

7. Ramsey (1970a, 1970b), Ramsey et al. (2002), Hauerwas (1986, 1994, 2001), Lammers and Verhey (1998), and Verhey (2003).

divine had gone amuck. Consequently, the Hebrew Scriptures exhort believers who are ill to seek cures or healing through prayer, repentance, and supplication.[8] Undeniably, this counsel also speaks to the fact that hopes for cures were incredibly fewer than today.

Moreover, disease/infirmity, both because it was connected to sin/being unclean/impurity and for fear of contaminating the community (spiritually and biologically), interrupted an individual's relationship to the larger community. Those with chronic disease were often ostracized. During menstruation, women were expected to separate themselves from everyone else. Thus, when Jesus healed lepers, the blind man, or the hemorrhaging woman, he accomplished more than restoring their physical health. He restored them to families, synagogues, and networks of social relations.

It is important to acknowledge that Christian thought on healing, illness, and the body—found in the New Testament and up through the Middle Ages—is full of ambiguity. Physical disease, disfigurement, infertility, etc. were often perceived as signs of the larger problem of sin and evil—spiritual problems, a sign of God's punishment. Similarly, many Church fathers elevated the spirit over the body and thus regarded physical healing or illness as less important than spiritual union with God, while a few notable others did more to affirm the body and physical health.[9] Consequently, Christians in these eras were sometimes urged to seek healing through practices we might now refer to as preventive or curative measures, and sometimes they were advised instead to seek healing through prayer and repentance.[10]

What is important in scriptural and later historical accounts of a Christian ethos is two-fold. First, physical health and healing were important as far as they served the greater purpose of fostering our relationship to God, which was primary, followed by our relationship to the community. Second, health and illness were not viewed solely, or even primarily, in biological or physiological terms. Illness disrupted not only our physical life; it also profoundly affected our emotional, spiritual, and social well-being. Many contemporary health care professionals, especially those in chaplaincy, social work/case management, hospice, and palliative care roles, carry both of these insights forward.

8. Amundsen and Ferngren (1982, 64).

9. Given his historical context, Luther espoused a radically positive view of the body and an incarnational understanding of God. See Scharen (2000).

10. Amundsen and Ferngren in Marty and Vaux (1982, 100).

The Christian Vocation to Serve Others

The third theme addresses relationships (societal and interpersonal): "How are we called to relate to others in light of who God is and God's relationship to creation?" The answer given by Jesus is: "Love God with all your hearts and minds and love your neighbor as yourself."[11] But who is included in the category "neighbor"?

Noted Protestant biblical scholars (Brueggemann, Long, Wheeler) and Christian ethicists (Lebacqz, Rasmussen, Townes, West) concur with the observation made pointedly by twentieth-century liberation theologians that God's preferential concern is for the poor (also identified as the marginalized, oppressed, sick, vulnerable, outcast, demonized, etc.). Indeed, this emphasis is *not* a modern convention; it is woven throughout scripture. The parable of the Good Samaritan (Luke 10:25–37) may be the most quoted example, but there are notable others, such as Jesus' words recorded in Matthew:

> [F]or I was hungry and you gave me food, I was thirsty and you gave me something to drink, I was a stranger and you welcomed me, I was naked and you gave me clothing, I was sick and you took care of me, I was in prison and you visited me ... Truly I tell you, just as you did it to one of these least of these who are members of my family, you did it to me. (Matthew 25:35–40)

Jesus exhorts his followers to be vehicles of care for the poor, social outcasts, and people in physical, mental, and spiritual anguish. The Gospels overflow with stories of Jesus healing the sick and caring for people in need—not only the fortunate few, but large gatherings of people—hungry masses, gaggles of children, and scores of the infirm or ostracized who trailed after him. Luke records one instance when Jesus healed too many to count or name (Luke 4:40).

Given the prominence of this biblical testimony of Jesus' healing ministry, contemporary Christians have an obligation to ponder seriously how to respond to his command to "cure the sick, raise the dead, cure the lepers, and cast out demons" (Matthew 10:7). Consider also: "You received without payment; give without payment" (Matthew 10:8). That is a rather thought-provoking statement in light of twenty-first century healthcare economics. Theologically, this

---

11. Mark 12:28–34. In his response, Jesus quotes Leviticus 19:17–18. See also Matthew 22:34–40. In Matthew 5:43–48 Jesus commands his followers to love not only our neighbors, but our enemies as well. The point may well be that the stranger, and even the enemy, *IS* the neighbor.

passage reminds us that all people live by the grace of God—given freely. Consequently, Christians are called to embody this grace for others—friends, family, neighbors, and strangers alike.

Undeniably, thorny questions surface when we get down to the details. How much, and what specific kinds, of resources—financial, medical, expert—are we obliged to share with those in need? There were no ICUs or sophisticated medical technologies available in Jesus' time. Still, what *is* clear is that from early Christian communities to the present day, a basic sense of responsibility toward the ill and suffering runs deep. This ethos is found in Jesus' words and examples, but is also evidenced by, as Kenny notes in Chapter 13 compassionate acts of Christian monks and nuns who comprised large numbers of the available physicians and nurses in the Middle Ages and who founded the first hospitals in the West.

At certain times, and for justifiable reasons, Protestants have been accused of complacency and an anemic social ethic. Although this has been the face of some strands of Protestant life, it certainly is not always the case. Indeed, the interpretive key to the distinctive Lutheran motif of "justification by grace through faith" is that out of God's free gift given to all, human beings are *free* to be agents of healing and grace *for* others, and in fact, are *expected* to do so. Consider Luther's interpretation of the fifth commandment, "You shall not kill":

> [T]his commandment is violated not only when a person actually does evil, but also when he fails [*sic*] to do good to his neighbor, or, though he has the opportunity, fails to prevent, protect, and save him [*sic*] from suffering bodily harm or injury. If you send a person away naked when you could clothe him, you have let him freeze to death. If you see anyone suffering hunger and do not feed him, you have let him starve. (Luther 1529, 390–91)[12]

The demands that others make upon us are not limited to a modern notion of negative rights. For Luther, the tangible needs of others make strong, positive claims upon those in a position to help.

In stark language, Luther and subsequent Protestants (e.g., Calvin, Wesley, Bonhoeffer, King Jr.) challenge narrow definitions of "the neighbor" and minimalistic understandings of the obligations to love, serve, and seek justice. Indeed, when we read the poignant theological and social visions of King and Bonhoeffer, we see a vibrant sense of the "common good" that connects well with Catholic Social Teaching, as elaborated by Kenny in Chapter 13.

12. See Vigen (2006), Moe-Lobeda (2002), and Lindberg (1993).

This brief sketch of a theological and ethical framework rooted in Protestant Christianity may contribute to widening the moral vision of public discussions on health/health care; yet it does not make any concrete resolutions obvious. Before we can discern any specific benchmarks, I contend that rigorous social analysis is needed. Thus, I turn now to describe key aspects of the social world(s) in which contemporary decisions about preventive and therapeutic care are made.

THE IRONY OF MEDICAL CARE AND PREVENTION: TOO LITTLE AND TOO MUCH

Why Social Context Matters

Sustained attention to context (e.g., social, economic, political, gender, cultural, and historical) is essential to moral analysis. Blanket equations balancing prevention vis-à-vis treatment are often not as helpful as assessments that attend to specific needs, oversights, and inequalities. In some contexts and for some people, treatment is used excessively. In others, much more effective treatments could be offered. And lamentably, millions of people in impoverished places need more of both.

As I survey U.S. society and the prevalent medical culture, I see two sometimes intersecting but often distinct and paradoxical worlds. In one, the well-insured and relatively affluent are generally able to access the most advanced medical technologies, even if they do not always result in the best or hoped-for health outcomes. Moreover, if they choose to take advantage of them, this population has a full array of prevention strategies at their disposal (e.g., prenatal care, cancer and other early diagnostic screenings, diabetes education and prevention programs, vaccinations). And they have sufficient income, educational resources, and support for eating healthy foods, losing weight, quitting smoking, etc.

In stark contrast, in the other world (sometimes just blocks or neighborhoods away), lower-income and poor people who are disproportionately racial-ethnic minorities are routinely excluded from both the most fundamental and life-enhancing medical treatments that could drastically improve the quality and/or length of their lives. Prevention efforts lag behind here as well. In inner-city and rural poor environments, there is often a dearth of free or affordable clinics, health education programs, healthy and affordable food sources, safe and affordable areas for exercise, and adequate diagnostic technologies such as mammograms.

Because I dwell in the first world, my understanding of Christian responsibility tells me that I have a duty to live with a sharp awareness of the other.

Consequently, I want to highlight two contrasting clusters of stories. Together, they raise critical questions about the appropriate use of medical resources and technologies. And although they do not tell us what the balance of prevention and treatment should be, they place the question of prevention's relationship to treatment in a larger perspective that the Christian ethos demands we not overlook. Through these stories, we glimpse parallel universes on the same planet.

Too Few Prevention and Treatment Options

U.S. Snapshot

Across the nation, middle- and low-income individuals and families are at significant risk for various health problems and premature deaths. In April 2008, Paul Krugman related the story of Trina Bachtel, a pregnant woman who was uninsured and having health complications (Krugman 2008). She sought care at an Ohio clinic, but due to a previous, unpaid balance, the clinic refused to attend her unless she paid $100 per visit. When her condition worsened, she went to a hospital 30 miles from her home. Both she and the fetus died. If she had received consistent preventive and prenatal care, health providers may have been able to avert such a devastating outcome. In another alarming example, "[A] 20 year old inmate named Melissa Matthews chose to turn down parole and stay in prison because that was the only way she could get treatment for her cervical cancer" (Kristof 2009).

Extensive research documents the fact that, overall, U.S. racial-ethnic minorities have a lower health status, are diagnosed with life-threatening diseases later, have higher infant mortality rates and shorter life spans, and receive less adequate care than non-Hispanic whites.[13] Consider breast cancer. One 2009 study found that although "black women are one-third less likely than women of other races to develop [breast] cancer, they are 30 percent more likely than other women to die if they are diagnosed with the disease" (Kaiser Family Foundation 2009a). According to the researchers, black women with breast cancer confront two distinct obstacles to better outcomes: "late presentation associated with the intrinsic characteristic of either the host or the tumor that leads to the additional virulence" and "undertreatment of breast cancer … once a diagnosis is made" (Yang et al. 2009, 864–65). Many black women would

---

13. See Vigen, paperback edition (2011) revised edition Preface, *Women, Ethics, Inequality in U.S. Healthcare* (2006), Siegel (2009), The Commonwealth Fund (2008), The Kaiser Family Foundation (2007, 2009b), Smedley et al. (2003), Rodriguez et al. (2009), and Hicks et al. (2008).

benefit both from more prevention/early detection and from more treatment options following diagnosis.

GLOBAL REALITIES

The dramatic lack of prevention and treatment is even more disconcerting in impoverished nations and merits a bit more illustration than the U.S. context. Consider a 2006 snapshot of Burundi: "an average life expectancy of about thirty-nine years; one in five deaths caused by waterborne diseases or a lack of sanitation; severe malnutrition for 54 percent of children under five; for women, a one-in-nine lifetime risk of dying during childbirth; and fewer than three hundred doctors to serve a population of about seven million" (Kidder 2009, 226). It is unfathomable to conceive of such statistics for the United States, yet millions across the globe confront them daily. Women and girls are at special risk:

At every age, women in high-income countries live longer and are less likely to suffer from ill health and premature mortality than those in low-income countries . . . The most striking difference between rich and poor countries is in maternal mortality—99 percent of the more than half a million maternal deaths every year happen in developing countries . . . [C]omplications of pregnancy and childbirth are the leading cause of death in young women aged between 15 and 19 years old in developing countries. Globally, the leading cause of death among women of reproductive age is HIV/AIDS. (World Health Organization 2009b)

Physician and anthropologist Paul Farmer witnesses the visceral implications of these statistics. In 2008, he visited the largest public maternity ward in Malawi—where "two obstetricians and a handful of nurses were struggling mightily to deliver 12,000 babies each year" (Farmer 2008, 9).[14] The maternal mortality ratio in Malawi is 1,800 per 100,000 live births; it is 17 per 100,000 in the United States (Farmer 2008, 9).

An adamant critique running throughout Farmer's work is that impoverished people too often succumb to what he caustically terms, "stupid deaths," because they are largely prevented and/or effectively treated in wealthier contexts. Children are particularly vulnerable:

- Nearly 9 million children under the age of 5 years die every year, according to 2007 figures.

---

14. This number of deliveries is slightly higher than the annual average for Harvard's Brigham and Women's Hospital. See also Farmer and Kim (2008) and Ivers et al. (2008).

- *Around 70% of these early child deaths are due to conditions that could be prevented or treated with access to simple, affordable interventions* (emphasis mine).
- Leading causes of death in children under 5 years are pneumonia, diarrhea, and health problems during the first month of life.
- Over one-third of all child deaths are linked to malnutrition.
- Children in developing countries are 10 times more likely to die before the age of 5 years than children in developed countries (World Health Organization 2009a).

For Farmer and others, these horrific global health realities call the relatively affluent to account.

Furthermore, they demonstrate why I question the framing of prevention versus treatment questions in oppositional terms. In many developing countries, there is too little of both.[15] Prioritizing one over the other often leads to short-sighted, ineffective, illogical, and draconian policies. For example, malaria "accounts for one in five of all childhood deaths Africa" (World Health Organization 2009c).[16] Yet malaria is highly preventable and curable—and the solutions are relatively low-tech and affordable (insecticidal nets and artemisinin-based combination therapy). Defeating it depends not on choosing prevention over treatment, but on the moral resolve of wealthy nations and citizens.[17]

In short, the searing testimony found in the particular experiences of impoverished, often dark-skinned, communities and glimpsed above is why I cannot offer an abstract rationale for uniformly favoring prevention over treatment. Prevention absolutely merits more serious and sustained investment than it often receives. Indeed, surveying certain segments of the U.S. context, more prevention and less treatment may be what is needed and ethically responsible. Yet in response to international tuberculosis, malaria, and HIV/AIDS, some policy-makers recommend focusing predominately on prevention.[18] Instead, creative and adapting collaborations of prevention and treatment often offer more hope and are more just.

15. See McNeil (2010) on HIV/AIDS.

16. See also the WHO (2010).

17. See Kidder (2003), Farmer (2005), Kim and Farmer (2006), and Walton et al. (2004).

18. See critiques by Vigen (2006) and Cahill (2005).

Where Treatment Is Abundant: Is More Always Better?

END OF LIFE CARE

To illustrate the plethora of treatment options available to some in the United States, consider end-of-life care. CBS correspondent Steve Kroft reports that in 2008, "Medicare paid $50 billion just for doctor and hospital bills during the last two months of patients' lives—that's more than the budget of the Department of Homeland Security or the Department of Education" (CBS *60 Minutes* 2009). If public education is an integral part of primary prevention, ponder the fact that more public financial resources are being allocated for *one segment* of the Medicare population than for the *entire* school aged population that relies on Department of Education funding.[19]

To put such statistics into context, Kroft interviews the daughter of Dorothy Glas. Glas, a former nurse, had advanced liver and heart disease. She died at 85 after spending the last 2 months of her life in hospitals and nursing homes, despite having a living will "expressing her wishes that no extraordinary measures be taken to keep her alive." Yet 25 specialists attended her and ordered countless tests and medical procedures, including a Pap smear (CBS *60 Minutes* 2009).

Does such treatment make sense—financially, ethically, or from a faith perspective? What hopes, values, and goals does it represent? Christians have an obligation to wrestle with such questions. If we can put aside the unfounded paranoia of "death panels," the Christian theological and ethical insights highlighted above can help us search our hearts and minds for the deeper values by which we hope to live and, eventually, die.

To explore these questions, I will share a bit about a woman whom I will call "Iris." Iris was a friend of my mother's who loved choral music, languages, tennis, and art, and who had a sharp wit. She was physically active and had the appearance of a woman in her late fifties. Her father had been a Missouri Synod Lutheran pastor and she was a life-long Christian. Iris worked up until she had emergency surgery to repair a ruptured colon. She developed sepsis and was in the ICU for several weeks, often unconscious, and on periodic dialysis. As they tried to stabilize Iris, doctors discovered colon cancer.

We visited Iris in the ICU. She had just turned 76 years old. Her first words were: "They won't let me die. I just think it's unethical." The hospital had a copy of her Advanced Directives in which Iris was clear about her wishes. Yet it was

---

19. One problem is that doctors and hospitals are paid according to the number of patients they see and admit, and the procedures they administer, with no financial incentives to keep people healthy (CBS *60 Minutes* 2009; Fischer 2009).

difficult for her family to act upon them because it was not always certain how much Iris might recover or what kind of quality of life she might have. How fast-moving was the cancer? Would the kidneys begin functioning? Would Iris remain bedridden? No one wanted to give up prematurely.

Still, Iris consistently stated that she did not have any hope for recovery and that she did not want aggressive interventions. She was transferred to a rehabilitation center where some therapeutic efforts continued, but she grew increasingly despondent. A doctor conferred with her and concluded she was competent and could discontinue treatment. In hospice, Iris sat up in bed and conversed with many visitors; she expressed peace with her situation. After approximately 14 weeks of medical care, Iris died in her sleep surrounded by loved ones.

Iris was on Medicare and my guess is that she had supplemental insurance. Not all of her care was covered by insurance, but she probably had sufficient savings. She was also white, well-educated, independent, and accustomed to exercising her autonomy. In her last months, Iris received the most advanced medical technologies available in the United States or anywhere. Yet she did not want them. Her story speaks to how a person's existential and/or spiritual grappling with his or her finitude can collide with a medical culture that is often driven by a compulsion to treat.

OTHER AREAS OF HEALTH CARE CONSUMPTION

The tendency to err on the side of medical intervention rather than accept human limits can be seen in other sectors of U.S. health care as well. Over one million U.S. inhabitants had some kind of fertility treatment in 2004, "participating in what had become a nearly $3 billion industry" (Spar 2006, 3). Ubiquitous ads promise pharmaceutical remedies for erectile dysfunction, sleep problems, depression, restless legs, high blood pressure, high cholesterol, and menstrual cycles. Ezekiel Emanuel and Victor Fuchs report that the United States has the "fourth highest per capita consumption of pharmaceuticals" in the world (Emanuel and Fuchs 2008, 2789). Yet there is comparatively less investment in televised public education campaigns promoting lifestyle choices that improve our health and lower stress, or in addressing the fact that many public schools are slashing physical education and nutrition programs.

As a perplexing aside, elective cosmetic surgery is increasingly popular among teenage girls who get plastic surgery as Christmas, birthday, or graduation gifts (Singer 2005) and bridesmaids who get Botox (Ellin 2008). In 2004 alone, people ages 19–34 had "427,368 Botox procedures, 100,793 laser resurfacing treatments ... and 1,094 face-lifts" (Tannen 2005). Are such elective treatments the best use of medical equipment, resources, and expertise? U.S. inhabitants often prioritize health care consumption over need.

Indeed, plastic surgery and dermatology specializations increasingly draw the best and brightest medical students, although the United States suffers from a dearth of internists and family practitioners who could serve on the front lines of effective public health (Singer 2008). Only about 10% of all medical school graduates go into primary care (Lohr 2010). Physicians specializing in select treatment (e.g., infertility, plastic surgery, and dermatology) earn more (often twice as much) than primary care physicians. They also have more control over their schedules and can often limit on-call duties. Yet primary care physicians are the gateway to *both* effective prevention and treatment.

As I reflect on these complicated realities, I observe how accustomed to care some in the United States have become, perhaps to the point of feeling "entitled" to whatever treatment is available. Many with generous insurance programs and ample, personal resources benefit from the luxury of being able to turn to a pill, surgery, or other treatment to address whatever irritates—stress, weight, appearance, libido. Others use credit cards to access these medical services and products.

In dramatic contrast, people—neighbors in the United States and around the world—struggle daily to survive due to a complete lack of prevention, treatment, or both. Ironically, Dorothy Glas and Iris got more of what neither wanted—a burdensome (and expensive) use of medical technologies and expertise, whereas Trina Bachtel (along with thousands of others in the United States and millions worldwide) could have lived longer with earlier and more consistent preventive and treatment interventions if they had been available to her.

Holding these paradoxical realities in tension, I resonate with Catholic ethicist Lisa Sowle Cahill's pointed questions to a privileged world:

> While Americans and Europeans seek answers to cancer and other enigmatic diseases, millions die around the world from treatable causes such as malaria, anemia, and tuberculosis. Does it serve the common good, even in the United States, to provide new genetic treatments for the privileged, while so many go uninsured? Does it serve the global common good to devote billions to new genetic interventions while more basic health needs are so dire and while great gaps in other basic needs such as food, housing, education, and clean water bring early death to so many? (Cahill, 2005, 215)

Whether, or to what extent, to pursue things such as artificial reproductive technologies, genetic research, or embryonic stem cell research are questions, for the most part, particular to contexts of wealth and abundance. With specific respect to prevention and treatment, the point is this: in certain sectors of the affluent, industrialized world, we spend a great deal on the treatment side of the equation, often to the detriment of prevention. However, with respect to other U.S. and international contexts, too little attention is given to *both* pressing prevention and treatment needs. In many impoverished and hurting places, thousands of lives could be, and sometimes are, saved by sustained investments in strategic, *integrated* preventive and treatment efforts.

IMPLICATIONS FOR TWENTY-FIRST-CENTURY PRIORITIES: PROTESTANT BENCHMARKS

Before highlighting three Protestant benchmarks for assessing the merits of any proposed allocation of prevention and treatment resources, a caveat is needed: Protestantism is not a monolith. Starting notably with the Reformation, we cannot speak of a single Christianity, and we also cannot speak of "*the* Reformed tradition." Lutherans, Calvinists, Anabaptists, and Anglicans represent the earliest outgrowths, but they are certainly not the only ones. For many, lines blur between "mainline" Protestant denominations and Evangelicals.[20] Increasingly, people grow up in one tradition but gravitate to another, often sampling various denominations. Moreover, the traditions themselves are not stagnant.

In terms of medical care, some Protestants believe more in miracles (via prayer and/or modern medicine) than others. Some focus on individual notions of care, entitlement, and access while others have a more robust social ethic. Consequently, I will not claim to speak for all U.S. Protestants even as I elucidate three primary features of "*a* Protestant ethic" that may assist in assessing proposals for the allocation of prevention and treatment. They are an integrative vision of health and healing, an honest acknowledgment of limits (human, medical, technological, biological, financial), and a keen focus on the common good (with special concern for the plight of the poor, vulnerable, and sick). They extend the earlier theological discussion and Allen Verhey is a central dialogue partner. These qualities, although they may resonate with some contemporary Protestants more than others, are nonetheless integral to the history, theology, and ethics of Protestant thought. Together, they give clues for holding prevention and treatment in dynamic tension, prioritizing them in differing ways, depending on particular contexts.

---

20. Six denominations are generally considered to constitute mainline U.S. Protestantism: The American Baptist Churches U.S.A., the Episcopal Church, the Evangelical Lutheran Church in America (ELCA), the Presbyterian Church U.S.A., The United Church of Christ, and The United Methodist Church.

Integrative Vision of Health and Healing

Expressed as a benchmark, this theological theme bridges to public policy. It asks whether a given policy proposal has a sufficiently broad and deep understanding of health and healing behind it. Does the allocation proposal recognize the socioeconomic and psychological dimensions to both preventive care and treatments? Does it define health in biological terms and also in social ones? As Blacksher emphasizes, "[R]eal gains [in improving prevention] depend on embracing serious primary prevention. In the absence of efforts that address the social and environmental determinants of health, those who are at risk or sick are very unlikely to improve their health outcomes" (Blacksher 2009).

Thus, a comprehensive prevention strategy for diabetes and/or obesity goes beyond increasing early screenings and detection programs to explore the infrastructures needed to create healthy and affordable neighborhoods, grocery stores, school meals, and lifestyles. Similarly, adequate prenatal health only begins with clinic access; it continues with ensuring access to social, educational, nutritional, and economic supports for pregnant women in need.

A holistic sense is needed not only for prevention, but for treatment as well. As noted above, for Christians and many people of various faith traditions, healing is not limited to the preservation or restoration of physical health. So much healing can happen—socially, psychologically, interpersonally, and spiritually—whether medical treatments *succeed or fail* in curing the pathology.

Historically, there has arguably been relatively little public support in the United States for the funding and implementation of preventive and public health programs compared to acute treatments. Why? To other contributors' observations, I add two musings on the values implicit in such an orientation. First, some health providers and researchers find the cutting edges of therapeutic and high-tech medicine more interesting (and more lucrative) than community health. Some U.S. health care consumers and providers alike value the technological and heroic more than the day-to-day trenches of maximizing a community or person's well-being. This observation gets at the larger questions noted above of how we value life, what we perceive as ultimately important, and what we hope for in terms of our life trajectories. What kind of health and beauty improvements do we expect to see—for ourselves or our children? Pragmatic allocation debates are *also* about questions of these kinds of existential values and hopes. The theological themes presented here (e.g., encountering divine grace and human limits) suggest distinct answers to such questions that might shift predominant priorities in significant ways.

Second, it seems many in the United States worry about excessive "government handouts" to the undeserving. They see health and health care, *particularly health promotion and disease prevention*, as goods that are up to individual persons to secure—through employment, private resources, education, and personal initiative/responsibility. Again, questions of values are integral to the perceptions. Do we conceive of—and value—good health and access to quality health care as a privilege, a human right, or a consumer product available for purchase? How *ought* we? How might "neighbor-love" inform an answer?

Allen Verhey contends that even as it is ethically justifiable to distribute some goods relative to the ability to pay, others ought to be understood less as commodities and more as public goods: "Like police protection, medical care responds to threats against our basic well-being ... Like education, medical care provides and protects a certain range of opportunities" (Verhey 2003, 383). Seeking justice in access and quality of *both* prevention and treatment is the foundation upon which *any* allocation policy must be built. Without it, the prospects for enjoying other social goods—education, vocation, and relationships—are significantly diminished during a person or community's life. An integrative vision of health and healing helps discern an appropriate balance.

Advocating for a holistic social and medical safety net does not mean that "everyone gets anything and everything" that medicine has to offer. Limits are undeniable and compassion means more than simply attending to the person who needs immediate treatment. To illustrate, Verhey notes that the parable of the Good Samaritan presents a moral dilemma for contemporary Christians:

> Suppose the oil and wine and the stay at the inn left the wounded man in the story only half alive. Would the Samaritan continue to pay for his care? Or suppose he encountered another neighbor on the side of the road when he returned to pay the bills for the first wounded traveler. Would he do the same for this second neighbor? Suppose he encountered not just one other but more than his donkey could bear, more than his purse could afford, more than even the most hospitable innkeeper could receive ... Can we live this story we love to tell—as citizens, as physicians, as churches—*and* recognize scarcity? (Verhey 2003, 361)

A dual focus on compassion and justice means that, in the United States especially, primordial prevention *along with* access to basic, highly effective treatments for all (rather than advanced and costly treatments for fewer people) assumes a higher priority in allocation than it currently receives. Taking justice seriously means that our policy proposals will take scarcity seriously.

Honest Acknowledgment of Limits—Human, Medical, Technological, Financial

Few people embrace limits. Perhaps part of human nature is to press against them. And in our restless quests, we witnessed astounding achievements in the twentieth century—from telephone wires to wireless communications; from realizing how to harness fossil fuels to building alternate power systems to mitigate overdependence on them; from antibiotics and vaccines to space travel. Indeed, various societies would have seen far fewer innovations, which have greatly improved the quality and length of lives of millions, if persistent, resilient human beings had not doggedly striven to break through the bounds of "impossibility." Many religious ethicists and theologians (e.g., Ronald Green, Ted Peters) celebrate the human capacity to "co-create" with God—to innovate and modify aspects of nature to continue to improve our lives and diminish human suffering.

Yet no one gets unlimited life, happiness, or health. Ultimately, everyone's mortality makes itself apparent. We live in a society in which "40 percent of Americans believe that medical technology can always save their lives" (Callahan 2008). In light of such unfounded "faith," responsible public policy will attend both the possibilities *and* limits of all medical strategies and interventions. It will avoid promoting a false "gospel" of infinite medical possibilities, control, and resources.

As much as some in affluent, technologically-driven cultures celebrate increased autonomy, the harsh, but no less true, mirror held up by Christianity (and other religious traditions) reveals that, ultimately, human beings are *not* in control. We cannot become immortals on earth. We can, however, embrace mortality *even as* we make the case that we have a moral obligation to prevent premature, untimely, and reasonably avoidable deaths. Responsible public policy will find ways to live and work dynamically in the tension between human capabilities and limits—both of which for Christians are God given.

However we choose from among competing goods (preventive care, therapeutic care, heroic technologies, medical research, and public health infrastructures), there will be an element of tragedy in how we prioritize.[21] There will always be casualties. Given this fact, what clues to policy might guide us? For Verhey, two options—both commonly utilized in public debate—are equally untenable: denying scarcity (and mortality) *and* denying sanctity (Verhey 2003, 367). First, putting unqualified hope and resources in medical progress and therapies to increase longevity (for some, but not all, human sectors) is ethically unsound. Such an approach constitutes a kind of idolatry and leads primarily to

21. Verhey (2003, 365).

increased debts (personal, professional, institutional, social, and governmental) and bitter disillusionment and despair when even the best medical efforts fail.

On the other hand, a Christian ethos will oppose public policy that reduces human lives to dollar signs. Christians profess that human beings are made in the image of God (*imago dei*). If we take dignity and justice seriously, then we will do more *both* to prevent ill health *and* to treat those already afflicted who subsist on the margins of health and medical care. Indeed, the arc of the Christian witness continually focuses our collective attention squarely on the plights of those who are poor, sick, dispossessed, invisible, and vulnerable.

Strong Attention to the Common Good

This last benchmark concretizes the analysis above, namely that attending to both the preventive and treatment needs of those most often disregarded is the appropriate starting place for ethical analysis. To arrive at ethical policies, we must first explore specific contexts. One particular place may require more robust prevention, but another may require the reverse, whereas still another calls for equal parts.

The notion of the common good runs throughout the historical ethos and theologies of many Christian denominations. It has incredible relevance for thinking about prevention and treatment because it is connected to aspects of human life that are universally shared. To survive, all people (all living things) need food, water, air, a protective habitat, and a web of interdependent relationships with other living beings. Creation itself embodies a relational matrix— whether envisioned as a mutually beneficial cooperation of flowers, bees, and the production of oxygen and nitrogen or as the food chain. Simply put, biologically and ecologically speaking, no living thing exists completely insulated from the well-being and functioning of others. This simply *is* Creation.

Thus, human beings are intrinsically social beings. Yet at least in the United States, many people have fallen in love with the image of rugged, independent, free individuals. Certainly, a prominent ethical theme for many Christians is that sense that each individual person must be respected as an end in himself or herself (borrowed from Kant). This is one side of the common good: individuals have intrinsic worth/dignity in and of themselves. The other side of the common good, however, is not as fully embraced, namely that humanity's flourishing is bound up with that of others and that we need to seek the well-being of all.

Bluntly put, all of us will die and most will get sick before we die and need health care. Similarly, many people, especially (but not exclusively) in affluent countries, will develop chronic conditions that, over time, require medical care that is technologically complex, sustained, and so expensive that it exceeds what most of us in the world could ever pay alone. Thus, a pivotal Christian task in this era of increasing inequalities is not only to be compassionate, but fair. "A Fair Samaritan will attempt to assure that people—young people, elderly people, disabled people, dying people—have a range of opportunities appropriate to their age and condition" (Verhey 2003, 383).[22]

And to approximate fairness, we—as individuals and as a society—need to move beyond focusing on the requirements of charity to those of justice. Verhey describes the distinctive Christian sense of justice in this way:

> The test for justice in the story of Scripture is not the impartial and rational standard ... that simply identifies justice with "maximum freedom." When the contemporary Good Samaritan invokes the standard of justice ... she encourages people to test policy recommendations not just against a standard of impartial rationality but against the plumb line of "good news for the poor," including especially the sick poor. (Verhey 2003, 371–72)

Interestingly, the Christian vision is not rooted in an "objective" nature of justice or in individualistic notions of liberty and rights. Numerous biblical scholars and theologians come to the same conclusion and social and statements from various Protestant denominations emphasize these same qualities.[23]

Moreover, Verhey cautions against a Christian ethic that focuses solely on the virtues of individual heroism or benevolence. He explains that the Good Samaritan "is the story of living in a community that shares in the human vulnerability to suffering—and communally supports care for the members of the community ... To love God and the neighbor is not an invitation to the conceit of philanthropy; it is an invitation to be part of a community that includes the sick and the poor" (Verhey 2003, 376–77). Thus, a just adjudication of prevention vs. treatment will not be one that boasts of generosity or charity (of government, individuals, institutions, or other providers of medical care). Instead, it will ground itself in the sense that we are our brother's and sister's keepers—that we are all part of interdependent communities and we all have real needs. It will strive to enact and embody (even if imperfectly) justice and fairness.

---

22. The Consortium of Jesuit Bioethics Programs issued this statement on U.S. Healthcare Reform: "A just and compassionate society is obligated to try to meet the basic needs of all members of the community—not every imaginable desire, but our most basic needs such as food, a foundational education, and basic health care" (Consortium of Jesuit Bioethics Programs 2009).

23. Brueggemann (1997, 2001, 2009, 2010), Birch and Rasmussen (1988), Long (1997), (Wheeler 1995), and Evangelical Lutheran Church in America (2003).

This insight is not novel. For Luther, one of the most profound meanings of freedom was not *from* responsibility/obligation/relationships, but rather *freedom for*—the neighbor, *for* service in the world.[24] As highlighted above, one of his largest concerns was to free human beings from the anxious desperation that comes when people try to justify themselves before God. Luther concluded that only God can save—and has already done so. The believer's task and vocation is to accept the unmerited gift of God's love and grace *and to then embody it for others*. Once we accept that God has accepted us, we are finally free *for* love and free *to* serve neighbors in need (even if they are also strangers).

The common denominator of mortality means that we are profoundly connected—and accountable—to one another:

> The ordinary human events of giving birth, suffering, and dying are extraordinarily significant as points at which we express and gesture our *inter*dependence. As in providing police protection, members of a society say to one another, "We will protect you and your goods against violence," and as in providing an education members of a society say to one another, "We will nurture your children," so in providing medical care members of a society can say to one another, "We will care for you; we will not pass by your suffering" (Verhey 2003, 383–4).

Providing a safety net of medical treatment and preventive programs builds up the social bonds within a society. It helps us know we are not ultimately strangers to one another. It is a visceral way to embody responsible, just, and caring love—for self and for others.

These observations indicate my sense that primordial prevention merits more investment in the United States. Yet when I contemplate the global poor, the equation shifts and I conclude that in order to attend fully to the common good, more investments in both prevention and treatment are desperately needed. Within the United States, we hotly debate the nature and limits of our social obligations to one another. So, it may seem even more unwieldy to ask whether such obligations extend beyond national borders. Yet I am convinced—for the sake of our moral integrity—we must do so.

Consider again the situation of pregnant women in Malawi. One of the two obstetricians on staff showed Paul Farmer that his hospital was in dire need of blood, equipment, skilled professionals, and facilities:

> Outside the doors of the single OR was a gurney piled high with surgical drapes in tatters. [Dr. Meguid] referred to the hallway as "post op." ...

---

24. Vigen (2006, Chap. 3).

"This is an abuse of human rights," he said, lifting up one of the rags. "It would never happen if people considered the women we serve as human beings." The doctor felt sick, he said that maternal mortality within the hospital was 300 per 100,000 live births, even though one might note ... that this was a six-fold reduction in the national rate. (Farmer 2008, 9).

In light of pernicious shortages that Dr. Meguid and untold others stubbornly face every day, Farmer asks a provocative question: "Should there be a right to sutures? To sterile drapes? To anesthesia?" (Farmer 2008, 9). Both doctors define these issues, not merely as public health challenges, but as a moral indictment. The humanity of the relatively affluent depends upon our resolve to confront honestly and tenaciously these fundamental needs of other human beings.

Some fall back on the rationale that substantial change is not feasible; that too many structural obstacles exist (e.g., cultural taboos, ineffectual or corrupt governments, the severity and complexity of health problems; steep costs, and limited resources). Farmer's retort underscores a troubling irony: "Humanitarian and health professionals have spent a generation now shaking our heads at the fact that, in many of the settings where we are unable to provide food, health care, and primary education with any reliability, global corporations consistently deliver chilled soft drinks, and arms traders have no trouble at all delivering weapons" (Farmer 2008, 14). Moreover, the collaborative efforts of Partners in Health, The Bill and Melinda Gates Foundation, Doctors without Borders, The World Health Organization, The United Nations Population Fund, and countless indigenous organizations have achieved significant preventive and treatment results in some of the poorest and underserved regions.

Credit must also be given to faith-based organizations, such as Catholic Relief Services, *Caritas*, and Lutheran World Relief. Protestant Evangelicals also play a key role. Nicholas Kristof illustrates that it is not only "social justice" progressive Christians who address global health inequalities and injustice, but that significant numbers of Evangelicals do as well.

As just one example, Kristof may surprise some with the fact that the largest U.S.-based international relief and development organization is not secular (i.e., Save the Children or CARE) but rather the Christian Evangelical organization, World Vision, which has "40,000 staff members in nearly 100 countries" (Kristof 2010).[25] Kristof quotes Richard Sterns, the head of the World

25. "That's more staff members than CARE, Save the Children and the worldwide operations of the United States Agency for International Development—combined" (Kristof 2010). See also Kristof and WuDunn (2010) and Sterns (2009).

Vision in the United States, who reflects on his life-changing encounter with a 13-year-old AIDS orphan who was the only surviving head of his household and who cared for his younger brothers:

> What sickened me most was this question: where was the Church? ... Where were the followers of Jesus Christ in the midst of perhaps the greatest humanitarian crisis of our time? Surely the Church should have been caring for these "orphans and widows in their distress." (James 1:27) ... "How have we missed it so tragically, when even rock stars and Hollywood actors seem to understand?" ... In one striking passage, Mr. Stearns quotes the prophet Ezekiel as saying that the great sin of the people of Sodom wasn't so much that they were promiscuous or gay as that they were "arrogant, overfed and unconcerned; they did not help the poor and needy (Ezekiel 16:49)." (Kristof 2010)

Even as prominent ethical and theological divisions exist among varying Protestant faith communities, it is important to highlight common bonds and commitments that can transcend at least some of the differences and disagreements.

CONCLUDING QUESTIONS

Rather than offer definitive or absolute answers, this chapter concludes with questions. Christians who wish to contribute to a broader social and public ethic regarding the appropriate balancing of prevention and curative therapies might pose these queries to the dialogue:

- What ought we hope for/expect from preventive and curative efforts?
- Are we in danger of asking/expecting too much or too little of either?
- In what ways will a particular proposal for the use of preventive care and/or medical treatments serve and/or neglect justice concerns?

This chapter's purpose has been to reflect on how to frame questions related to prevention and treatment in light of Protestant thought. Such a framework will hopefully assist nuanced moral discernment within specific contexts. Dynamic and particular allocations between prevention and treatment will be continually needed.

In their introduction, Faust and Menzel invite contributors to engage a mental exercise that exemplifies the tensions and tragic choices that can arise between preventive and curative efforts. It is an interesting one and I find the

various responses to it thought provoking. However, I wish to respond by inter-
rupting it with two questions.

First, as a Lutheran and liberationist ethicist, I hesitate to answer hypothetical questions both because of their implicit assumptions and because, in my
methodological approach, more context is needed to do sufficient ethical analysis. Consequently in contemplating the scenario, I wonder if we (bioethicists,
policy analysts, health care providers, etc.) attend sufficiently to the structural
dynamics that have given rise to the individual levels of provider dilemmas
such as this one. Do we need to focus our analysis on "what the provider should
do" or rather on how to change the structures that created the crisis in the first
place?

Second, how can we imagine and develop descriptions and analyses of prevention and treatment in ways that show not only how they compete, but how
they may work together? The task of relating prevention to treatment in creative
and thoughtful ways is acutely relevant in global contexts. Farmer compellingly
argues:

> Prevention is, of course, always preferable to treatment. But epidemics of
> treatable infectious diseases should remind us that although science has
> revolutionized medicine, we still need a plan for ensuring equal access to
> care. As study after study shows the power of effective therapies to alter the
> course of infectious diseases, we should be increasingly reluctant to reserve
> these therapies for the affluent, low-incidence regions of the world where
> most medical resources are concentrated. Excellence without equity looms
> as the chief human rights dilemma of health care in the 21st century.
> (Farmer 2001, 210)

State of the art care for a minority of the world's population while making
available only the most rudimentary medications and treatments for the
majority is a shameful trade-off. Offering people free condoms or an HIV/AIDS
test, but no treatment options if they test positive, is ethically tenuous. Besides,
the courage to get tested often diminishes drastically if there is no hope for
treatment.

Even more, if relatively affluent citizens and Christians truly believe that all
people have inherent dignity, then how can we turn into our shining medical
centers and simultaneously turn away from the human suffering bleeding
out from the streets, huts, apartments, and hillsides of the impoverished, at
risk, or sick? Nuanced and fair combinations of advanced treatments and
front-line prevention are absolutely possible. Such agile balancing requires
moral fiber even more than mathematical and economic gymnastics. My
fervent hope is that Christians may collaborate constructively with others in

addressing both human limits and needs in powerful, just, imaginative, and grace-filled ways.

REFERENCES

Althaus, P. 1972. *The Ethics of Martin Luther.* Minneapolis, MN: Fortress Press.

Amundsen, D.W., and Ferngren, G. 1982. Medicine and Religion: Pre Christian Antiquity. In M. Marty and K. Vaux, Eds., *Health Medicine and the Faith Traditions.* Minneapolis, MN: Augsburg Fortress: 53–92.

Birch, B., and Rasmussen, L. 1988. *Bible and Ethics in the Christian Life.* Minneapolis, MN: Augsburg Books.

Blacksher, E. 2009. Health Reform: What's Prevention Got to Do with It? *Hastings Center Report* 39 (6):inside back.

Brueggemann, W. 1997. *Theology of The Old Testament.* Minneapolis, MN: Fortress.

———. 2001. *The Prophetic Imagination,* 2nd ed. Minneapolis, MN: Fortress.

———. 2009. *An Unsettling God.* Minneapolis, MN: Fortress.

———. 2010. *Journey to the Common Good.* Louisville, KY: Westminster John Knox.

Cahill, L.S. 2005. *Theological Bioethics.* Washington, DC: Georgetown University Press.

Callahan, D. 2008. Curbing Medical Costs: The "Unpopular" Problem. *America* 193 (8):9–12.

CBS 60 Minutes. 2009. *The Cost of Dying: Patients' Last Two Months of Life Cost Medicare $50 Billion Last Year; Is There a Better Way?* November 22. Available at http://www. cbsnews.com/stories/2009/11/19/60minutes/main5711689.shtml?tag=contentMain; contentBody, accessed January 2, 2011.

The Commonwealth Fund. 2008. *Racial and Ethnic Disparities in U.S. Health Care.* March. Available at http://www.commonwealthfund.org/Content/Publications/ Chartbooks/2008/Mar/Racial-and-Ethnic-Disparities-in-U-S—Health-Care— A-Chartbook.aspx, accessed May 8, 2011.

The Consortium of Jesuit Bioethics Programs. 2009. *The Moral Case for Insuring the Uninsured.* Available at http://www.jesuitbioethics.net/files/Moral_uninsured2009. pdf, accessed May 10, 2011.

Ellin, A. 2008. It's Botox for You, Dear Bridesmaids. *The New York Times,* July 24.

Emanuel, E., and Fuchs, V. 2008. The Perfect Storm of Overutilization. *JAMA* 299 (23):2789.

Evangelical Lutheran Church in America (ELCA). 2003. *Caring for Health: Our Shared Endeavor. Available at* http://www.elca.org/What-We-Believe/Social-Issues/Social-Statements/Health-and-Healthcare.aspx, accessed May 10, 2011.

Farmer, P. 2001. The Major Infectious Diseases in the World—To Treat or Not to Treat? *New England Journal of Medicine* 345(3): 208–210.

———. 2005. *Pathologies of Power.* Berkeley, CA: University of California Press.

———. 2008. Challenging Orthodoxies: The Road Ahead for Health and Human Rights. *Health and Human Rights* 10 (1):5–19.

Farmer, P., and Kim, J. 2008. Surgery and Global Health: A View from Beyond the OR. *World Journal of Surgery* 32:533–36.

Fischer, E. 2009. Getting Past Denial: The High Cost of Health Care in the United States. *New England Journal of Medicine* 361 (13):1227–30.

Hauerwas, S. 1986. *Suffering Presence.* Notre Dame, IN: University of Notre Dame Press.

———. 1994. *God, Medicine, and Suffering.* Grand Rapids, MI: Eerdmans.

———. 2001. *The Hauerwas Reader.* Durham, NC: Duke University Press.

Hicks, L.S., Tovar, D.A., Orav, E.J., and Johnson, P.A. 2008. Experiences with Hospital Care: Perspectives of Black and Hispanic Patients. *Journal of General Internal Medicine* 23 (8):1234–40.

Ivers, L.C., Garfein, E.S., Augustin, J., Raymonville, M., Yang, A.T., Sugarbaker, D.S., and Farmer, P.E. 2008. Increasing Access to Surgical Services for the Poor in Rural Haiti: Surgery as a Public Good for Public Health. *World Journal of Surgery* 32:537–42.

The Kaiser Family Foundation. 2007. *Key Facts: Race, Ethnicity, and Medical Care, 2007 Update.* Available at http://www.kff.org/minorityhealth/upload/6069-02.pdf, accessed May 8, 2011.

———. 2009a. *Black Women Develop Breast Cancer at Earlier Ages, Have Higher Mortality Rates Than Other Women, Study Finds.* May 13. Available at http://dailyreports.kff.org/Daily-Reports/2009/May/13/dr00058433.aspx, accessed May 20, 2011.

———. 2009b. *Putting Women's Health Care Disparities on the Map.* Available at http://www.kff.org/minorityhealth/7886.cfm, accessed May 8, 2011.

Kidder, T. 2003. *Mountains Beyond Mountains.* New York: Random House.

———. 2009. *Strength in What Remains.* New York: Random House.

Kim, J., and Farmer, P. 2006. AIDS in 2006—Moving Toward One World, One Hope? *New England Journal of Medicine* 355(7): 645–647.

Kristof, N. 2009. The Body Count at Home. *The New York Times,* September 12. Available at http://www.nytimes.com/2009/09/13/opinion/13kristof.html, accessed May 5, 2011.

———. 2010. Learning from the Sin of Sodom. *The New York Times,* February 27. Available at http://www.nytimes.com/2010/02/28/opinion/28kristof.html, accessed May 20, 2011.

Kristof, N., and WuDunn, S. 2010. *Half the Sky.* New York: Vintage.

Krugman, P. 2008. Health Care Horror Stories. *The New York Times,* April 11. Available at http://www.nytimes.com/2008/04/11/opinion/11krugman.html, accessed May 5, 2011.

Lammers, S., and Verhey, A., eds. 1998. *On Moral Medicine,* 2nd ed. Grand Rapids, MI: Eerdmans.

Lazareth, W. 2001. *Christians in Society.* Minneapolis, MN: Augsburg Fortress.

Lindberg, C. 1993. *Beyond Charity.* Minneapolis, MN: Augsburg Fortress.

Lohr, S. 2010. Study Shows "Invisible" Burden of Family Doctors. *The New York Times,* April 28. Available at http://www.nytimes.com/2010/04/29/business/29doctor.html?ref=health.

Long, E. 1997. *To Liberate and Redeem.* Cleveland, OH: The Pilgrim Press.

Luther, M. 1529. Large Catechism. In T. Tappert, Ed., and trans., *The Book of Concord.* Minneapolis, MN: Fortress.

Marty, M., and Vaux, K., Eds. 1982. *Health Medicine and the Faith Traditions.* Minneapolis, MN: Augsburg Fortress.

McNeil, D. 2010. At Front Lines, AIDS War Is Falling Apart. *The New York Times,* May 9. Available at http://www.nytimes.com/2010/05/10/world/africa/10aids.html?ref=africa, accessed May 20, 2011.

Moe-Lobeda, C. 2002. *Healing a Broken World.* Minneapolis, MN: Augsburg Fortress.

———. 2004. *Public Church.* Minneapolis, MN: Augsburg Fortress.

Ramsey, P. 1970a. *The Patient as Person.* New Haven, CT: Yale University Press.

———. 1970b. *Fabricated Man.* New Haven, CT: Yale University Press.

Ramsey, P., Farley, M., Jonsen, A.R., and Wood, M.R. 2002. *The Patient as Person, 2nd Edition: Exploration in Medical Ethics.* New Haven, CT: Yale University Press.

Rodriguez, M., Bustamante, A.V., and Ang, A. 2009. Perceived Quality of Care, Receipt of Preventive Care, and Usual Source of Health Care among Undocumented and Other Latinos. *Journal of General Internal Medicine* 24 (suppl 3):508–13.

Sansom, D. 1998. Why Do We Want To Be Healthy? Medicine, Autonomous Individualism, and the Community of Faith. In S. Lammers, and A. Verhey, Eds., *On Moral Medicine* (2nd ed., pp. 262–66). Grand Rapids, MI: Eerdmans.

Scharen, C. 2000. *Married in the Sight of God.* Lanham, MD: University Press of America.

Siegel, B. 2009. Leveling the Field—Ensuring Equity through National Health Care Reform. *New England Journal of Medicine* 362 (25):2401.

Singer, N. 2005. Skin Deep; For You, My Lovely, A Face-Lift. *The New York Times,* December 29.

———. 2008. For Top Medical Students, an Attractive Field. *The New York Times,* March 19.

Smedley, B., Stith, A., and Nelson, A., Eds. 2003. *Unequal Treatment.* Washington, DC: National Academies Press.

Spar, D. 2006. *The Baby Business.* Cambridge, MA: Harvard Business School Press.

Sterns, R. 2009. *The Hole in Our Gospel.* Nashville, TN: Thomas Nelson.

Tannen, M. 2005. Botox Babies. *The New York Times,* August 28.

Townes, E. 1998. *Breaking the Fine Rain of Death.* New York: Continuum.

Verhey, A. 2003. *Reading the Bible in the Strange World of Medicine.* Grand Rapids, MI: Eerdmans.

Vigen, A. 2006 (paperback edition with new material 2011). *Women, Ethics, and Inequality in U.S. Healthcare.* New York: Palgrave Macmillan.

Walton, D.A., Farmer, P.E., Lambert, W., Leandre, F., Koenig, S.P., and Mukherjee, J.S. 2004. Integrated HIV Prevention and Care Strengthens Primary Health Care: Lessons from Rural Haiti. *Journal of Public Health Policy* 25 (2):137–58.

Wheeler, S. 1995. *Wealth as Peril and Obligation.* Grand Rapids, MI: Eerdmans.

World Health Organization (WHO). 2009a. *Children: Reducing Mortality Factsheet.* Available at http://www.who.int/mediacentre/factsheets/fs178/en/.

———. 2009b. *Women and Health.* November. Available at http://www.who.int/gender/women_health_report/en/index.html.

———. 2009c. *World Malaria Report 2009.* Available at http://www.who.int/malaria/world_malaria_report_2009/en/.

———. 2010. 2001–2010 *United Nations Decade to Roll Back Malaria, Children and Malaria Fact Sheet.* Available at http://www.rollbackmalaria.org/cmc_upload/0/000/015/367/RBMInfosheet_6.htm, accessed May 8, 2011.

Yang, R., Cheung, M.C., Franceschi, D., Hurley, J., Huang, Y., Livingstone, A.S., and Koniaris, L.G. 2009. African American and Low-Socioeconomic Status Patients Have a Worse Prognosis for Invasive Ductal and Lobular Breast Carcinoma: Do Screening Criteria Need to Change? *The Journal of American College of Surgeons* 208 (5): 853–68.

15

Apocalypse and Health

Treatment and Prevention in the Seventh-day Adventist Tradition

ROY BRANSON, PhD ■

Seldom while expecting a Kingdom of God from heaven has a group worked so diligently for one on earth.
—Edwin Gaustad, *A Religious History of America*

Adventists are perhaps the longest-lived population that has yet been formally described. ... For the common causes of death, low-risk Adventist men die at ages about 13 years older and women about nine years older than other Californians.
—Gary E. Fraser, *Diet, Life Expectancy, and Chronic Disease*

The largest Adventist Christian denomination—over 16 million adult Seventh-day Adventist members worldwide—also runs the largest number of acute-care medical institutions of any Protestant denomination: 179 throughout the globe (Office of Archives and Statistics SDA). In places such as Orlando, Florida and in the Inland Empire of Southern California (Riverside and San Bernardino counties east of Los Angeles), Seventh-day Adventist (SDA) hospitals and health care corporations are the second-largest employers.

News media have widely reported novel acute-care procedures performed in Adventist hospitals: in early 1984, infant heart transplantations, and in 1991, the first radiation treatments using a hospital-operated proton accelerator. Both were done at the Loma Linda University Medical Center. Not as widely reported is the commitment of the SDA community, from its beginnings, to prevention.

I will discuss how Seventh-day Adventism's history, understanding of scripture, and fundamental beliefs undergird its commitment to prevention.

FROM THE GREAT DISAPPOINTMENT TO PREVENTION

The SDA denomination is the largest to emerge out of the 1840s revivals in the United States led by William Miller. A licensed Baptist minister, Miller preached that Christ's Second Coming was imminent, predicting it would take place on October 22, 1844. After the nonappearance of Christ, what came to be known as The Great Disappointment, one group of former "Millerites" concluded that the time had been correct, but the activity had been misidentified. Rather than returning to earth, Christ had entered the "most holy" place of a "heavenly sanctuary."

Prevention was embedded early in the life and thinking of the SDA community. Joseph Bates is often regarded as having cofounded, along with James and Ellen White, the SDA denomination. A prosperous sea captain roaming the Mediterranean, Atlantic, and Pacific, Bates retired to become a social reformer, advocating total abstinence from tobacco, alcohol, and meat, abolition of slavery, educational innovation, and apocalyptic revivalism. Soon, in 1827, Bates joined through baptism the Christian Connection, an early nineteenth-century movement that took the Bible as the only rule of faith and practice. He also fought for radical religious, social, and health reform. In the 1830s, Bates helped found the Fairhaven Antislavery Society near New Bedford, Maine. By 1843, he had adopted a vegetarian diet, and along with many Christian Connection ministers, such as James White, became deeply involved in what he understood as another reform movement—the Millerite revival (Bates 1878; Knight 2004, 28).

Bates and the Whites led a small group through crucial early steps that contributed to the forming of an enduring American-founded denomination. After 1844, sooner than the majority of Adventists, they stopped setting dates for Christ's return and adopted the celebration of the weekly seventh-day Sabbath. By the early 1850s the former Millerites stopped making accounts of miraculous healings a staple in their publications and decided to establish enduring institutions (White 1860).[1] The first, in 1860, was a publishing corporation to operate the weekly *Review and Herald*. Sixteen years after the Great Disappointment, these Millerites had become Seventh-day Adventists planning a future that included advocating health reform (Branson 1976).

1. For further discussion see Land (1986).

In February 1863, the year that the Seventh-day Adventists formally established themselves as a denomination, James White started publishing articles on health reform in the *Review and Herald*. In June, in the home of some fellow Seventh-day Adventists, Ellen White experienced a vision that she shared in print 18 months later. The vision coincided with the views of contemporary health reformers: healthful living could be achieved through use of "pure soft water," liberal exposure to sunshine, and a simple vegetarian diet that excluded tobacco, tea, and coffee. Water treatments were acceptable;drugs such as opium, mercury, calomel, quinine, and strychnine were not (White 1864, 1867).[2]

By now, SDA leaders were exhausted by 20 years of theological, social, and institutional drama. In 1864–1865 several checked into "Our Home on the Hillside" in Dansville, New York, an institution run by James Caleb Jackson, an all-purpose reformer: antislavery, pro-temperance, pro-vegetarian. At Our Home on the Hillside, some of the leaders of the new denomination—including James White, who was recovering from a stroke—became increasingly steeped in the combination of religious, social, and health reform that Joseph Bates had advocated decades earlier.

Several of the early Adventists had come to the Millerite revival from Methodism, whose founder, John Wesley, had stressed the connection between religion and healthful living in his well-known work, *Primitive Physic: An Easy and Natural Way of Curing Most Disease*. Larkin B. Coles, preacher, physician, and leading hydropathic (emphasizing baths and "water-cures") health reformer, became a part of the Millerite movement. His best-selling book, *Philosophy of Health* (Coles 1855), sold a hefty 35,000 copies.

However, it was a minister from the Calvinist tradition, the Presbyterian Sylvester Graham, who most prominently made healthful living a part of both religious revival and social reform. His teachings dominated life at Our Home on the Hillside: plenty of fresh air and exercise, cold water (not tea, coffee, or alcohol), and a diet of vegetables (not meat, particularly pork), fruits, nuts, and wheat bread, including his famous Graham crackers. Tobacco was totally proscribed. This approach became a hallmark of the facility founded by Seventh-day Adventists in 1866, the "Western Health Reform Institute." The institute was initially headed by Horatio S. Lay, a physician who had also served as vice-president of the National Health Reform Association. The experience of SDA leaders at Danville guaranteed that the newly organized Adventist denomination would permanently include in its belief and practice a commitment to health reform and prevention (Blake 1974; Reid 1982).

---

2. On Ellen G. White's visionary experience and the reception of this particular vision see Numbers (1976).

In the 1870s, James and Ellen White financially supported young protégés, such as John Harvey Kellogg and E.J. Waggoner, to obtain medical training at both health reform and orthodox medical institutions.

In 1875, Kellogg became director of what was by now known as the Battle Creek Sanitarium. He and other physicians on the staff combined orthodox medicine, including surgery, with hydrotherapy, vegetarian diet, and the full panoply of health reform practices. The combination allowed Battle Creek Sanitarium to become one of the largest medical institutions in the United States.

THE BODY AS A TEMPLE

Early Adventists made prevention an intrinsic part of both their practice and their thinking. Their theology of health was shaped by at least three biblical motifs: temple, law, and cosmic conflict. In their minds, all three were connected to health and prevention of disease. All took on special urgency within the Adventists' understanding of the biblical apocalyptic vision.

The *locus classicus* for connecting the biblical motif of the temple with health is in Paul's letter to the Corinthians. "Do you not know that your body is the temple of the Holy Spirit within you, which you have from God?" (I Corinthians 6:19 NRSV). It is one thing to oppose practices as unhealthful; it is another to do what nineteenth-century Protestants did: fight tobacco as a barrier to holiness. But Adventists upped the ante even further. Using tobacco, they said, prevented a person from stepping immediately into heaven, pure and undefiled. Following the Great Disappointment of 1844, the earliest Adventists, including those who were to become Seventh-day Adventists, continued to regard abstaining from smoking and drinking as rituals of purification, preparing one for entry at any moment into the presence of Holiness itself. Four years later, in 1848, Ellen White reported that she had seen in a vision that (White 1851) "tobacco was a filthy weed, and that it must be laid aside or given up…and unless it is given up the frown of God will be upon the one that uses it, and he cannot be sealed with the seal of the living God." In 1854, Ellen White told Adventists still expecting to be translated to heaven before death that "unless we are clean in person, and pure, we cannot be presented blameless to God" (White 1854).

By the time Seventh-day Adventists officially organized in 1863, Ellen White was not as focused on tobacco use as a bar to immediate entry into heaven. But she did emphasize how use of tobacco violates biblical scenes of worship.

The priests, who ministered in sacred things, were commanded to wash their feet and their hands before entering the tabernacle in the presence of

God... Yet professed Christians bow before God in their families to pray with their mouths defiled with the filth of tobacco... Instead of the cloud of fragrant incense filling the house as in the case of the ancient tabernacle, it is filled with the sickening, polluted odor of ejected tobacco spittle and quids, and the air breathed by the congregation is poisoned. (White 1944, 2:127)

From then to now, total abstinence from tobacco and alcoholic beverages has been required of SDA church members, "because our bodies are the temples of the Holy Spirit" (Christian Behaviour 2010). A person must give up smoking before joining the church; the disciplining or "disfellowshipping" of a person who subsequently lapses is a responsibility of local congregations.

Adventists, born out of the same Methodism that gave rise to the holiness movements of late nineteenth-century and early twentieth-century America, wrestled with just how to relate health to holiness. At the 1901 meeting of the General Conference, the highest jurisdiction of the church, Ellen White successfully put a stop to what had become known as the "holy flesh movement," an extension of the biblical motif of the body as a temple into a guarantee of perfect health (Haloviak 1983). She denounced any teaching that claimed sanctified believers would be able to avoid aging and death. Within this contentious environment, Kellogg's 1902 book, *The Living Temple,* stressed that God "filled all space, and every living thing," that "there is a tree-maker in the tree, a flower-maker in the flower," and "God himself enters into our bodies in the taking of food" (Schwarz 1964, 1979, 290, 1986, 106). Kellogg was warned by the President of the General Conference that he was coming close to being a pantheist (Schwarz 1979, 289). Adventist theology has, ever since, strictly avoided worshipping health or the human body.

However, the body has remained important in Adventist theology. That has been particularly true in the denomination's health care university, Loma Linda University. In the late 1950s it adopted a motto that has come to be understood as expressing its central purpose: "to make man whole" (Loma Linda University 2008). From the 1950s through the 1970s, Jack Provonsha, an MD and a PhD in ethics who taught religion classes to medical and nursing students, emphasized that wholeness flowed from a view of human nature as a "multidimensional unity" (Provonsha, no date). As the statement of *Fundamental Beliefs of the Seventh-day Adventist Church,* officially adopted in 1980, states, each human being "is an indivisible unity of body, mind, and soul, dependent upon God for life and breath and all else" (General Conference of Seventh-day Adventists 1984). The body is not separate from any part of a person, and does not take second or third place to any other aspect. Cure of the body is inextricably bound up with care of the whole person.

What has remained a constant in the Adventist tradition, from the time that its founders believed that they would momentarily enter into God's presence to now, is the sense that the human person, including the body, can be a dwelling place of God's Spirit. Proscriptions, such as abstaining from tobacco and alcohol, rise from scientific evidence, but they point beyond themselves. The biblical motif of the body as the temple of God hints at something further: keeping the body healthy and preventing its premature demise can be regarded as a sacramental act. For Adventists steeped in apocalyptic expectations of a future culminating in resurrection of bodies made whole, healthful practices are harbingers of the holy.

HEALTH THROUGH OBEDIENCE TO LAW

As the reality of the 1844 Disappointment sank in, many Millerites realized that their present might not be filled by God's Second Advent, i.e., that His coming might be delayed. For the disappointed, the longed-for "translation," or transformation of the body at the second Coming of Christ, receded day by day. Still they affirmed the concreteness of a future resurrection of the body at the general resurrection of humanity at the Last Day. The affirmation endures among many Christians, certainly among Seventh-day Adventists. We believe that the human body stretches across the chasm between the present and the future.

D.P. Hall wrote the first systematic statement of Sabbatarian Adventist beliefs concerning the nature of humanity, death, and resurrection (Bull and Lockhart 2007, 89). He insisted that the present body does not dissolve at death but rises again at the final resurrection. There is "no mixing up or mingling of mortality with immortality." Rather, *man is a unit, composed of dust, his mental and moral nature inhering in the organized man*" (original text in italics) (Hall 1854). Hall explicitly rejected the immortality of the soul, with its implied denigration of the body. When humans die, the whole person remains in the grave. At the resurrection at the Second Advent the whole person rises. The present body, mind, and character, albeit transformed, persist via a future resurrection into a restored creation.

The continuing Adventist commitment to the biblical future scenario of a resurrection of the whole person, with the physical, intellectual, and even moral character of the individual persisting in some form into a new earth, is a crucial theological foundation for valuing the whole person in the present. Ellen White consistently taught that "Jesus does not change the character at His coming. The work of transformation must be done now" (White 1953). Seventh-day Adventists created educational and health institutions not as a betrayal, but as a confirmation of their commitment to the biblical picture of a future resurrection.

As the years went on, Adventists developed their life and thinking in directions similar to those of their fellow Protestants. Ellen White was inspired in her childhood Methodist home by John Wesley's teaching that sanctification entailed conformity to law, including the "law of our physical being" (Holifield 1986). Adventists also imbibed deeply from the Calvinist tradition that emphasized law. For example, the Kelloggs sent three sons to Oberlin College where they met the Presbyterian lawyer-turned-evangelist and theologian, Charles Finney. He urged "perfect obedience to the law of God," including learning to eat and drink and sleep according to God's laws of health (Finney 1878, 1986). By the time the Kellogg boys arrived in the mid-1850s, most of the Oberlin College faculty and students had adopted Sylvester Graham's proscription of meat, pastries, and condiments, including pepper, mustard, and vinegar (Numbers 1976, 79).[3] This program was justified by the American Physiological Society because "the millennium, the near approach of which is by many confidently predicted, can never reasonably be expected to arrive, until those laws which God has implanted in the *physical* nature of man are, equally with his moral laws, universally known and obeyed" (original in italics) (Third Annual Report of the American Physiological Society, 1837, quoted in Blake 1974, p. 43).

In 1876 the 24-year-old John Harvey Kellogg returned from his training in orthodox medicine to head up the freshly named Battle Creek Medical and Surgical Sanitarium (a word Kellogg popularized). Kellogg realized that Adventists, understanding themselves as a part of America's mix of religious, social, and health reform, were emerging on the scene just as medicine was studying the laws of nature and becoming a part of science. Kellogg self-consciously set out to develop his own skills in both acute care and prevention by visiting medical centers in New York, London, and Vienna. At the same time, he did not abandon his hydropathic health reform roots; his institution became famous for its heavy reliance on water treatments. Kellogg even produced a book that became the accepted text in the field, *Rational Hydrotherapy* (Schwarz 1964).

He knew that what the evangelists of health reform and orthodox physicians had in common was commitment to law—divine, moral, natural, and scientific. Kellogg further realized that the turn-of-the-century American public would respond to a Battle Creek institution that combined education in health reform and prevention with scientific medicine, increasingly focused on cure. Before the onslaught of the Great Depression, Kellogg was supervising an institution of 1,300 beds, which in 1926 admitted 7,462 patients (Schwartz 1964, 73).

---

3. The single most important work on health in the Adventist tradition has been published in a revised edition, with an introduction by Jonathan M. Butler (1992).

Eventually, Kellogg and the Adventist denomination came to a painful part-ing of the ways. By 1905, when it became clear that Kellogg would retain com-plete control of the Battle Creek Sanitarium, a 78-year-old Ellen White had already sprung into action, cajoling, promoting, and demanding that Adventists in Southern California purchase and open health care institutions. In 1904–1905, three new sanitaria opened: one in San Diego, one in Glendale, and a third in Loma Linda. The next year she convinced church leaders to start a school, the Loma Linda College of Evangelists, to train nurses and "gospel med-ical missionaries" committed to law.

But would the school adopt a curriculum that provided students with a knowledge of the laws of science, a curriculum that prepared graduates to obtain legal certification as practitioners of orthodox scientific medicine? After a 4-year debate, Ellen White settled the matter by proclamation that the SDA medical school would prepare students "to pass the examinations required by law of all who practice as regularly qualified physicians" (Neff 1964). Adventists' rough and ready appreciation for what they have indiscriminately called divine law, laws of nature and laws of health, meant that Adventists were not threat-ened by the rise of scientific medicine.

For many years SDA medical institutions determined for themselves how to relate medical science and technologies to the beginnings of life. It was not until the 1990s that the General Conference of Seventh-day Adventists, the world church's highest governing body, began adopting advisory guidelines concern-ing medical practices. A statement on abortion (1992) was followed by guide-lines in 1994 on birth control and human reproduction technologies (including IUDs, hormonal methods of birth control, RU486, and in vitro fertilization) and in 1995 on genetic interventions. The general approach of the guidelines toward all these topics assumes a respect for the scientific study of God's nature. The statements typically start with a review of the current state of scientific knowledge, proceed to articulate general biblical and moral principles, and finally urge institutions and individuals to decide for themselves how to apply the guidelines.

Commitment to law is also a major reason why Seventh-day Adventists believe in prevention as well as acute care and why they follow a lifestyle that has come to be studied as a way individuals can lead longer, healthier lives. At the same time that Adventist hospitals through the twentieth century increas-ingly became acute-care facilities, Adventist members continued to demon-strate in their daily lives how obeying the laws of health helped prevent disease.

In 1958, the lifestyle of Adventists drew the attention of the American public health community. The American Cancer Society funded the first of a series of studies of the relationship between SDA behavior and health. Studies of

Adventist members from 1958 through 2010 have resulted in well over 320 articles in peer-reviewed journals. They focused on how key aspects of Adventist behavior—particularly diet and exercise—correlate with extension of longevity and prevention of disease (Fraser 2003).[4]

The studies are ongoing, but more than 50 years of research reveals some clear results. California Adventists as a whole live longer than other Californians—over 4 years for Adventist women and over 7 years for Adventist men. Even more dramatically, low-risk Adventists carefully following their laws of health (vegetarian, physically active, and slender) live longer than other Californians by an amazing 9 years (women) and 13 years (men).

In addition to exercise and abstention from tobacco, diet appears to be a crucial reason common diseases appear less often among Adventists. Incidences of cancer are lower among Adventists as a whole, but meat-eating Adventists are significantly more likely to develop colon, bladder, and ovarian cancers than vegetarian Adventists. Eating vegetables and fruits reduces the likelihood of developing many types of cancer; for instance, frequent consumption of legumes is associated with lower rates of pancreatic and colon cancer, and eating more fruit correlates with lower rates of pancreatic and prostate cancer. Men drinking soymilk more than once per day have a much-reduced risk of prostate cancer (Fraser 2003).

Heart disease rates are lower among Adventists, particularly those who are vegetarian. A daily, small quantity of nuts protects against heart attacks, as does the consumption of whole grain bread and fatty fish. Also, vegetarian Adventists have lower rates of diabetes and rheumatoid arthritis than meat-eating Adventists (Fraser 2003).

We know there is a significant disparity of dietary and exercise patterns among Adventists. For example, half of Adventists surveyed did not follow the (nonmandatory) meatless diet the church recommends (Fraser 2003). Most of the Adventists in these studies have lived in the United States. If future studies examine Adventist lifestyles outside the United States, where over 90% of Adventists live, an even greater diversity of lifestyles might manifest itself. Would they show different correlations between lifestyles and health and longevity from the studies conducted on Adventists in California? How does the Adventist community affect the non-Adventists in their midst? Will information provided to Adventist communities predisposed to observe the laws of health actually result in healthier behavior?

---

4. For the most thorough overview of these studies see Fraser (2003). The total of 320 peer-reviewed articles comes from Fraser's 2003 edition, viii. Longevity is the focus of Chapter 4, summary of statistics, 58.

In 1967, 9 years after American health leaders started funding studies of Adventist lifestyle behavior, the SDA church acknowledged the importance of studying preventive adherence to the laws of health by establishing a School of Public Health at Loma Linda University.

PREVENTION AS COSMIC CONFLICT

Opening the School of Public Health at Loma Linda University had a firm footing in the biblical metaphors emphasized in the Adventist tradition. The biblical motif of the body as a temple sacralizes abstention from unhealthful practices. The motif of law, understood as including laws of health, produces regimens human beings can follow to extend the quality and length of their bodily lives. Both motifs appear in parts of the Bible that colorfully and vividly portray divine activity through history and the cosmos—the apocalyptic books. But those books, particularly the book of *Revelation* so important to Seventh-day Adventists, also include the more encompassing motif of cosmic conflict— the battle in the past and in the present between good and evil and between life and death.

Apocalypse, apocalyptic, and apocalyptic consciousness do not mean, in this chapter, disaster, destruction, and a sense of doom. Apocalyptic means uncovering and revelation; an apocalyptic consciousness is the awareness that our present existence dwells within a transcendence extending throughout the cosmos, throughout the future, and throughout time. That transcendence brings the cosmos and the future into confrontation with the here and now. The result is the clash of the ideal and the imperfect, of justice and oppression, of health and disease, and of life and death (Collins 1986).[5]

This sense of cosmic conflict was emphasized much more for the church's founders in the second half of the nineteenth century than more recently. Joseph Bates' commitment to reform was a part of his apocalyptic consciousness. Bates, who had been involved in the manual-labor school movement, who had been a founder of the abolitionist Fairhaven Anti-slavery Society, and who had seen his local Fairhaven Temperance Society spread nationwide, was certain that these reforms were a part of God's cosmic reform. Just after a shower of stars in New England, interpreted by Millerites as a sign of the impending climax to history, Bates (1878, 241) reported triumphantly, "in connection with these

---

5. Apocalyptic writings were "intended," according to Adela Yarbro Collins (1986), "to interpret present, earthly circumstances in light of the supernatural world and of the future, and to influence both the understanding and behavior of the audience by means of divine authority."

portentous signs in the heavens, moral reform was working its way like leaven throughout the United States...moral-reform societies were multiplied in various places, as were also peace societies." Bates insisted that social reform and the Second Coming were intertwined. "All who embraced this doctrine would and must necessarily be advocates of temperance and the abolition of slavery, and those who opposed the doctrine of the second advent would not be very effective laborers in moral reform" (Bates 1878, 262).

Bates and his community of Adventists were not alone. R. Laurence Moore, in his book *Religious Outsiders and the Making of Americans* (1986, 132), insists that "the evidence from antebellum America is overwhelmingly on the side of proving a connection between a belief in Christ's imminent return and energetic efforts to perfect this world."[6]

In 1894 Ellen White's eldest son, Edson, acted in response to his mother's words, chastising the U.S. government and "the Christian churches" for not establishing sanitaria, constructing schools, and introducing crops other than cotton (White 1948, 7:227–228). He sailed a small steamer, the *Morning Star*, down the Mississippi river, stopping at St. Louis, Cairo, Memphis, and Vicksburg on the way to Yazoo City, the gateway to the Mississippi Delta. Edson was determined to improve not only the spiritual but the physical health of Mississippi's "colored people." He assumed that entailed changing society. Despite the threats of violence from ruffians in the employ of cotton plantation owners, Edson and his crew of blacks and whites preached temperance and the gospel of crop diversification. They worked with black sharecroppers to vary their diet and improve their income by raising chickens, caring for bees, and planting a greater variety of crops on their own small plots (Graybill 1971).

Along with other social reformers in America, the new SDA community easily moved from abolition of slavery to confrontation with liquor interests. In 1865, only 2 years after the denomination had officially come into existence, the General Conference adopted a statement that linked apocalyptic concerns with social reforms. "The casting of any vote that shall strengthen the cause of such crimes as intemperance, insurrection, and slavery, we regard as highly criminal in the sight of heaven" (Morgan 2001).[7]

Adventists considered temperance as more than individuals keeping their bodies pure, or following the laws of nature. Ellen White considered this battle against liquor interests key to reforming the American nation. "Society is corrupted, work-houses and prisons are crowded with paupers and criminals, and the gallows are supplied with victims... The burden of taxation is increased, the

6. See the chapter entitled "Health as Cosmic Struggle."

7. Morgan's (2001) volume is the essential work on the history of Adventist involvement in the public square.

morals of the young are imperiled, the property and even the life of every member of society is endangered" (White 1882). Adventists' confidence in the Lord's return coincided with their energetic joining His cosmic battles against evils, including those threatening the public's health. In 1882 Ellen White passionately summoned fellow believers to man the front lines: "We need not expect that God will work a miracle to bring about this reform, and thus remove the necessity for our exertion." From the perspective of the apocalyptic, biblical motif of cosmic battle—what Ellen White called the Great Controversy— political, social, and health reform could be seen as an appropriate part of worship. She might shock some, Ellen White wrote to Seventh-day Adventists in Iowa, but if it proved to be necessary, she firmly believed that they should go to the polls on the Sabbath day to vote for temperance legislation (White 1964).

Saturated with biblical apocalyptic images of *divine* action bringing sudden and *pervasive human* action, Adventists were drawn into participating in another ambitious reform movement: improving the physical and social health of turn-of-the-century American cities (Bull and Lockhart 2007, 13–14).[8] Kellogg visited the Bowery Mission started by idealistic church people in New York City, and the even more renowned Hull Settlement House, founded by Jane Addams in downtown Chicago. In 1893, Kellogg received $40,000 from the Wessel brothers of South Africa, whose family held part of the Kimberly diamond mine.

Kellogg moved quickly. Shortly after receiving the Wessel donation he purchased property for the Chicago Branch of the Battle Creek Sanitarium, which could admit 70 paying patients. A month later, Kellogg opened the Chicago Medical Mission, which operated with a broad understanding of "medical," including free baths, a laundry, a kindergarten, a medical dispensary, a visiting nurse service, and an evening school. Within 3 years, he was operating seven institutions in downtown Chicago, including a five-story College Settlement Building manned by student physicians and nurses operating a day nursery, a school of health, classes in home hygiene, a free employment agency, a placement service for orphans, and at one point 75 clubs among the city's newsboys and bootblacks.

Growing out of its involvement in Chicago, the Seventh-day Adventists also started a journal, the *Life Boat*, which published articles on juvenile delinquency, child-labor problems, and prison reform. The journal quickly grew to a surprising circulation of 200,000 (Butler 1974). Because the curriculum at the Adventist medical school at Battle Creek pressed students on to the front lines

---

8. Bull and Lockhart (2007) provide a fascinating account of Seventh-day Adventists and the progressive Upton Sinclair, whose muckraking writings led to the Pure Food and Drug Meat Inspection Acts of 1906.

of social reform in America, they gained an understanding that health includes public health and health care begins with prevention (Rice 1970).[9]

But it was in the area of nutrition and diet that the SDA expansive apocalyptic consciousness heightened the social and health reforming zeal of their time most dramatically. Out of the Adventist health care institution at Battle Creek came one innovation after another. Kellogg developed a coffee substitute that one of his former patients, Charles W. Post, turned into *Postum*. Kellogg was one of those who turned healthful nuts into the enormously popular peanut butter. He took one of Sylvester Graham's wheat dishes, "granula," added cornmeal and oatmeal, and called the result "granola." Most famously, John Harvey Kellogg and his brother W.K. Kellogg experimented long enough in the Sanitarium kitchens, and on its patients, to produce corn flakes. Although it was only W.K. Kellogg who made corn flakes into an industry, the Kellogg brothers together transformed America's breakfasts into lighter, more nutritious fare.

Part of the complex dispute between John Harvey Kellogg and the Seventh-day denomination at the beginning of the twentieth century was whether SDA should stay focused on their social and health reform efforts in Chicago or expand globally. One of Kellogg's prize students, Harry Miller, exemplified the global option. Harry and his wife Maude entered the American Medical College in 1898, spent their junior and senior years at Rush Medical College in Chicago, passed the Illinois state medical examinations, and, against Kellogg's advice, went to central China, where tragically Maude died.

Harry Miller carried on from 1903 into the 1960s, establishing hospitals throughout China and Southeast Asia. Like Kellogg, Miller's imagination expanded beyond providing acute care to developing global-wide advances in prevention through changes in diet. The greatest passion of his life was experimenting with vegetables he discovered in one part of the world in order to develop inexpensive, healthful foods available to all. Throughout his life, Miller conducted experiments on soybeans. During his periodic assignments by the Adventist church to the United States, Miller worked with J.A. La Clerc, the chief chemist of the United States Department of Agriculture, to study how the soybean Miller had encountered in China could be made into both nutritious and tasty products. The result was an increasing number of soy foods and drinks. One example is Vitasoy (http://www.vitasoy-usa.com/). By 1974, it had surpassed Coca Cola as Hong Kong's favorite beverage. According to La Clerc, Miller's soy drinks and dishes helped preserve many thousands more lives than

---

9. That may be the reason that Dr. Stephen Smith, founder of the American Public Health Association, at one point called the American Medical Missionary College "the most important educational institution in the world."

did the 15 hospitals he had built. Miller's work drew the admiring attention of UNICEF and the World Health Organization. Miller was said to have improved the health of a quarter of the world's population (Shurtleff 1981; Moore 1961).

Whereas individuals such as Harry Miller in Asia and others in Australia and South America understood health as prevention within the encompassing apocalyptic motif, most SDA denominational leaders in the twentieth century connected health with the observance of divinely ordained laws of science and health, not social and public health crusades. However, when such crusades did come knocking at their doors, Adventists, because of their lifestyle committed to prevention, were girded for battle.

Part of their recent contribution to the larger health of the United States and other societies has come through the specific interest in Adventists for epidemiological studies. Dr. Ernest Wynder, of the Sloan-Kettering Memorial Cancer Institute of New York, and a central figure in developing scientific data to confront the tobacco industry, contacted Loma Linda. The result was the Adventist Mortality Study, the first of a series of such epidemiological studies. The study, begun in 1958, compared rates of death from cancer among 27,530 nonsmoking Adventists to a million persons from the general population. The significantly higher incidence of cancer and heart-related deaths found among the general population was used to bolster the landmark 1964 Surgeon General's Report on smoking and health (U.S. Department of Health, Education and Welfare 1964).

In 1995, I directed the Adventist Center for Law and Public Policy and organized the first Interreligious Coalition on Smoking or Health, representing tens of millions of members in Protestant, Catholic, Jewish, and Muslim denominations and organizations in the United States. Working closely with the Cancer, Heart, and Lung Associations, the Interreligious Coalition and its member denominations testified before Congress, encouraged the Food and Drug Administration (FDA), heads of departments in the executive branch, the President, and the Vice-president to take action, and lobbied at the state, national, and international levels for tobacco-control legislation. As a result of the Coalition's pioneering efforts, for the first time faith-based organizations became an integral part of the country's tobacco-control advocacy groups, successfully convincing state governments to raise taxes on tobacco products, and eventually convincing the U.S. Congress to authorize the FDA regulation of tobacco.

The Adventist Mortality Study and the subsequent Adventist Health Studies conducted by the Loma Linda School of Public Health have also led Adventists to address issues of diet being debated in the public square. These studies have compared the diets and disease rates between Adventists and non-Adventists, and have carried out prospective cohort studies among successively larger populations of Adventists (Fraser 2003). Walter Willet, chair of the department of nutrition in the Harvard School of Public Health, has praised these studies for contributing greatly to understanding the close relationship between nutrition and health, pointing to two areas in particular. First, the studies show the importance of maintaining lean body weight throughout life. Second, they demonstrate the importance of eating abundant amounts of fruits, vegetables, nuts, and grains in order to prevent heart disease and cancer (International Congress on Vegetarian Nutrition 2002).

The founders of Adventism would have been delighted both with Dr. Willet's conclusions and also by the fact that the Fifth International Congress on Vegetarian Nutrition, held on the Loma Linda University campus in 2008, explored the relevance of vegetarian diet to the encompassing, contentious issues of global warming and climate change. For Adventist founders, participating in the sweeping drama of biblical apocalyptic meant that health reform was much more than concern that individuals attain purity or observe the laws of health in their lifestyles; it meant participating in God's healing of the nations.

HEALTH IN AN APOCALYPTIC TRADITION—SOME PORTENTS

The Adventist tradition will continue to commit itself to both acute care of individuals and also prevention of disease and promotion of health of communities—local and national. Seventh-day Adventists will continue to operate and expand its international system of acute-care hospitals. The Adventist community will remain committed to employing treatments and procedures—some innovative and ambitious—as long as they are developed by scientific medicine that conforms to laws operating in a divinely sustained creation. Adventists will continue to encourage their ethicists to reflect on the application of moral laws to quandaries arising from the practice of clinical care in its hospitals.

Confronted with the thought experiment presented in the introductory chapter to this volume, and despite the religious community's long history of emphasis on prevention, including diet, exercise and healthy lifestyle practices, I believe that individual Adventist physicians, like most of their medical colleagues, would think that their primary duty in the clinical setting assumed in the case is to Bill or John, not to the public health department. The physician's professional, even contractual, obligations have been strengthened through a long-established doctor–patient relationship with both patients (see Faust in Chapter 7 of this volume). The doctor's duties to Bill and John are thick with explicit and implicit promises, commitments, and obligations. Sometimes the relationship between a physician and patients of the sort described in the case has been characterized as a friendship (Fried 1974). If not that close, a physician does have a special relationship (accompanied by obligations) with his or her patients, particularly those that are long established—a special relationship and obligations that the physician does not have with some unknown individual in the community (Jeske 2008).

Should the physician in the book's hypothetical case treat Bill or John? Again, like many primary care physicians, most Adventist physicians would treat Bill. The physician has read test results that establish that Bill's epigastric discomfort, according to the wording of the case, "is really ischemic heart disease." The physician has not yet assessed John's risk factors for heart disease, but knows that Bill needs immediate physical treatment and that available treatments are very likely to improve Bill's condition. Bill is the "burden" in the hand.

In the center of the Loma Linda University, near both the SDA University Church and the medical school, stands a group of oversized statues depicting the Gospels' story of the Good Samaritan. This visual center of the campus evokes the biblical account that has become paradigmatic of extravagant care given to the specific needs of a specific individual. The act of care in the story established a "special relationship," akin to the relationship of the mother's care of a child, or a physician's caring for an acutely ill, dependent patient, a relationship that can take precedence over other relationships (Dunbar 2008).

Early nineteenth-century Adventists were drawn to caring for individuals suffering acute physical disability and pain. One year after the Great Disappointment of 1844, Ellen White and her husband James toured groups of believers in Maine and reported that prayer had resulted in healings. By 1854, she was saying that those who were ill should not be treated solely by prayer, but by physicians (White 1860). But Adventists, steeped in biblical accounts of sudden healings achieved in the midst of the cosmic battle for life over death, have continued to be drawn to the idea that physicians can achieve dramatic results in overcoming the power of disease in the lives of individuals. That may be a contributing factor to the Adventist Medical Center at Loma Linda feeling no hesitation, when immunosuppressant agents became available, to use them for the first-ever infant heart transplants. Similarly, Adventist ministers on the center's Board of Trustees readily voted special appropriations to purchase the first proton accelerator to be housed in a medical center, an accelerator which brought decisive relief to individuals suffering from cancer.

The story of the Good Samaritan also pointedly expresses the need to extend the scope of care, whether or not the person who needs help is a member of your own tribe. The villains of the story refrain from providing emergency care to the injured. The hero, marginalized as a Samaritan, understands that care must be expanded to include not only binding up wounds, but providing housing and food, that the neighborhood should be inclusive. Through the first half of the twentieth century, Adventists became more and more focused on one aspect of the Good Samaritan story—the care of the individual. They sometimes overlooked the other side of the account—the emphasis on enlarging the sphere of our good works. Adventists largely forgot the connection between the biblical motif of cosmic conflict and social reform within which the Adventist founders lived and breathed.

In the 1960s, however, black Adventist leaders defended their participation in civil rights marches, and Adventist historians began to rediscover their church founders' involvement in reform movements. Beginning in 1985, statements from the president of the church were released at General Conference Sessions on peace, arms, and the environment. Neal Wilson described the arms race as a "colossal waste of human funds and resources," and "one of the most obvious obscenities of our day." Ecological responsibility, he said, and "belief in the imminent Advent" were "not mutually exclusive" (Morgan 2001).

In the same decades Loma Linda University, whose self-understanding has often had an impact on that of the church as a whole, increasingly expanded its identity to include societal reform. The University's motto is "To Make Man Whole." Although this formulation can be seen as focusing on the comprehensive care of individuals, its meaning has expandede in the 50 years since it was adopted. Perhaps most importantly, the School of Public Health has involved professors and students in advocating the health interests of the poor in developing nations, and the need for greater protection of the environment. The School of Medicine in 1995 asked their graduating medical students to commit themselves publicly to a "Physician's Oath" that included new wording: "Acting as a good steward of the resources of society, I will endeavor to reflect God's mercy and compassion by caring for the lonely, the poor, the suffering, and those who are dying" (The LLUSM Physician's Oath—Our Own 1996).[10] The School of Religion in 2009 formally adopted five goals for the religion courses it teaches to all of Loma Linda University's 4,000 university students. One of these is to describe in every School of Religion course "ways in which moral advocacy can shape society" (Branson 2009). The following year the Center for Spiritual Life and Wholeness, directed by Carla Gober, Ph.D, led the university in revising and adopting a more encompassing definition of wholeness. The definition now includes phrases such as "caring for creation," and the book of *Revelation's* (22:2) "healing of the nations" (Gober 2009).

Other signs point to the renewal within the Adventist community of the concern for social justice characteristic of biblical apocalyptic. The Adventist Development and Relief Agency (ADRA), growing out of the church's efforts to

10. See reflections on the oath (1996, 32).

aid victims of disaster, self-consciously expanded its mission in 2007 to lead the Adventist community into the intersection of prevention and social justice. ADRA involves Adventists in struggles to protect the vulnerable, including fighting organized violence against women and multinational tobacco companies targeting children and women in third-world countries.

A 2010 General Conference *Statement on Global Poverty* dramatically demonstrates Adventism's increasing reappropriation of its historic commitment to reform—religious, social, political, and health. The statement opens by decrying poverty's undermining of human rights, including health. "It keeps people hungry; it deprives them of medical care, clean water and education, the opportunity to work." The second paragraph begins with the assertion that "Seventh-day Adventists believe that actions to reduce poverty and its attendant injustices are an important part of Christian social responsibility." The paragraph ends by declaring that "as a spiritual community Seventh-day Adventists advocate justice for the poor and 'speak up for those who cannot speak for themselves' (Proverbs 31:8 NIV) and against those who 'deprive the poor of their rights' (Isaiah 10:2 NIV). We participate with God who 'secures justice for the poor' (Psalm 140:12 NIV)."

The third paragraph would have made Joseph Bates, Ellen White, and the early founders of the Seventh-day Adventist community proud. "Working to reduce poverty and hunger means more than showing sympathy for the poor. It means advocating for public policy that offers justice and fairness to the poor, for their empowerment and human rights." The statement goes on to support the United Nations' Millennium Development Goals for reducing poverty by at least 50% by 2015 and pledging that "Seventh-day Adventists partner with civil society, governments and others, working together locally and globally to participate in God's work of establishing enduring justice in a broken world."

Appropriately, the statement ends by invoking the apocalyptic vision of the good earth, the New Jerusalem:

> As followers of Christ we engage this task with determined hope, energized by God's visionary promise of a new heaven and a new earth where there is no poverty or injustice. Seventh-day Adventists are called to live imaginatively and faithfully inside that vision of God's Kingdom by acting to end poverty now.

Adventist thinking and tradition certainly endorse prevention. Adventists will no doubt continue to value dramatic treatments of individuals. Even heroes of prevention in the Adventist tradition—such as Kellogg and Miller—developed surgical skills. However, recent official statements by the church and its institutions recognize social reform as part of the historic mission of the

Adventist community. The degree to which Adventists increasingly place a priority on prevention and social reform depends on how vividly they remember their apocalyptic tradition, not in the sense of how accurately they can predict the Second Advent, but how sweeping their vision of good and evil is and how passionately they confront the powers that take away the health and lives of the vulnerable.

Apocalyptic thrusts treatment of individuals onto a vast panorama, where powerful institutions clash, where whole populations are affected, and where change comes not only dramatically but pervasively. The apocalyptic consciousness propels entire communities into advocacy of practices they believe prevent harm and improve the health of both individuals and entire societies, indeed of the world. Seventh-day Adventists involve themselves in prevention and social reforms not in spite of apocalyptic, but because of it.

REFERENCES

Bates, J. 1878. *The Autobiography of Elder Joseph Bates; Embracing a Long Life on Shipboard, With Sketches of Voyagers on the Atlantic and Pacific Oceans, the Baltic and Mediterranean Seas; Also Impressment and Service on Board British War Ships, Long Confinement in Dartmoor Prison, Early Experience in Reformatory Movements; Travels in Various Parts of the World; and a Brief Account of the Great Advent Movement of 1840–44.* Battle Creek, MI: *Seventh-day Adventist Publishing Association.* Reprint 2004. Berrien Springs, MI: Andrews University Press.

Blake, J.B. 1974. Health Reform. In E. Gaustad, Ed., *The Rise of Adventism* (pp. 30–49). San Francisco, CA: Harper & Row.

Branson, R. 1976. Adventists Between the Times: The Shift in the Church's Eschatology. *Spectrum* 8 (1):15–26.

———. 2009. *The Five Goals of the School of Religion Curriculum, School of Religion,* Loma Linda University. A Case Study Prepared for Loma Linda University's Accreditation Report to the Western Association of Schools and Colleges.

Bull, M., and Lockhart, K. 2007. *Seeking a Sanctuary: Seventh-day Adventism and the American Dream,* 2nd ed. Bloomington, IN: Indiana University Press.

Butler, J. 1974. Adventism and the American Experience. In E.S. Gaustad, Ed., *The Rise of Adventism* (p. 199). New York: Harper & Row.

Butler, J.M. 1992. *Prophetess of Health: Ellen G. White and the Origins of Seventh-day Adventist Health Reform.* Knoxville, TN: University of Tennessee Press.

Carlson, D. 1996. The LLUSM Physician's Oath, Loma Linda University School of Medicine. *Alumni Journal* (Jul.-Aug.): 32.

Christian Behaviour. 2010. Article 21. *Seventh-day Adventist Yearbook.* Hagerstown, MD: Review and Herald Publishing Association.

Coles, L.B. 1855. *The Philosophy of Health: Natural Principles of Health and Cure, or Health and Cure Without Drugs: Also, the Moral Bearings of Erroneous Appetites.* Battle Creek, MI.

Collins, A.Y., Ed. 1986. Introduction: Early Christian Apocalypticism. *Semeia 36: Early Christian Apocalypticism: Genre and Social Setting.* Atlanta, GA: The Society of Biblical Literature.

Dunbar, S. 2008. *Agape, Special Relations, and the Global Care Crisis: Challenging a "Two-Track" Understanding of the Obligations of Christian Love.* Available at http://divinity.uchicago.edu/martycenter/publications/webforum/012008/.

Finney, C.G. 1878. *Finney's Lectures on Systematic Theology.* Grand Rapids, MI: Eerdmans Publishing Company.

———. 1986. *Principles of Sanctification.* Grand Rapids, MI: Bethany House Publishers.

Fraser, G.E. 2003. *Diet, Life Expectancy, and Chronic Disease: Studies of Seventh-day Adventists and Other Vegetarians.* New York: Oxford University Press.

Fried, C. 1974. *Medical Experimentation: Personal Integrity and Social Policy.* Amsterdam: North-Holland Publishing Co.

General Conference of Seventh-day Adventists. 1984. Fundamental Beliefs of Seventh-day Adventists. *Seventh-day Adventist Church Manual 34.*

Gober, C. 2009. *Analysis of the Wholeness Definition and Its Relation to Assessment* (case study prepared for Loma Linda University's accreditation report to the Western Association of Schools and Colleges). Loma Linda, CA: School of Religion, Loma Linda University.

Hall, D.P. 1854. *Man Not Immortal: The Only Shield Against the Seduction of Modern Spiritualism.* Southfield, MI: Steam Press.

Haloviak, B. 1983. *From Righteousness to Holy Flesh: Disunity and the Perversion of the 1888 Message* (A Documentary Study of the Transition from Righteousness by Faith to Holy Flesh Theology). Unpublished manuscript.

Holifield, E.B. 1986. *Health and Medicine in the Methodist Tradition.* New York: Crossroads.

International Congress on Vegetarian Nutrition. 2002. Available at http://www.Vegetariannutrition.org.

Jeske, D. 2008. Special Obligations. In E. Zalta, Ed., *The Stanford Encyclopedia of Philosophy (Fall 2008 Edition).* Available at http://plato.stanford.edu/archives/fall2008/entries/special-obligations.

Knight, G. 2004. *Joseph Bates: The Real Founder of Seventh-day Adventism.* Hagerstown, MD: Review and Herald Publishing Association.

Land, G., Ed. 1986. *Adventism in America.* Grand Rapids, MI: Eerdmans Publishing.

Loma Linda University. 2008. *Capacity and Preparatory Review.* Western Association of Schools and Colleges for Reaffirmation of Accreditation, 12–13, 22–29.

The LLUSM Physician's Oath—Our Own. 1996. *Alumni Journal* (Jul.-Aug.): 32.

Moore, R.S. 1961. *China Doctor: The Life Story of Harry Willis Miller.* Nampa, ID: Pacific Press Publishing Company.

———. 1986. *Religious Outsiders and the Making of Americans.* New York: Oxford University Press.

Morgan, D. 2001. *Adventism and the American Republic: The Public Involvement of a Major Apocalyptic Movement.* Knoxville, TN: University of Tennessee Press.

Neff, M.L. 1964. *Invincible Irishman: A Biography of Percy T. Magan.* Nampa, ID: Pacific Press Publishing Association.

Numbers, R.L. 1976. *Prophetess of Health: A Study of Ellen G. White.* New York: Harper & Row, Chap. 3–4.

Office of Archives and Statistics SDA. Available at http://www.adventistdirectory.org/default.aspx?&&&&&&page=searchresults&&EntityType=MH&Radius=30&SortBy=0&PageIndex=7.

Provonsha, J.W. [No date.] *The Philosophical Roots of a Wholistic Understanding of Man.* Unpublished manuscript. From the Provonsha File in Thompson Library. Lomo Linda, CA: Loma Linda University Center for Christian Bioethics.

Reid, G.W. 1982. *A Sound of Trumpets: Americans, Adventists, and Health Reform.* Hagerstown, MD: Review and Herald Publishing Association.

Rice, R. 1970. Adventist and Welfare Work: A Comparative Study. *Spectrum* 2 (1):52–63.

Schwarz, R.W. 1964. *John Harvey Kellogg: American Health Reformer.* PhD dissertation, University of Michigan.

———. 1979. *Light Bearers to the Remnant.* Nampa, ID: Pacific Press Publishing Association.

———. 1986. The Perils of Growth, 1886–1905. In G. Land, Ed., *Adventism in America* (pp. 106–9). Grand Rapids, MI: Eerdmans Publishing.

Shurtleff, W. 1981. Dr. Harry Miller: Taking Soymilk Around the world. *Soyfoods* (Winter) 4:28–36.

U.S. Department of Health, Education and Welfare, Smoking and Health. 1964. *Report of the Advisory Committee to the Surgeon General of the Public Health Service.* Washington, DC: U.S. Government Printing Office.

White, E.G. 1851. *Letter,* Dec. 14. White Estate: B-5–1851.

———. 1854. Vision of Feb. 12. Brookfield, NY: Ms. 1.

———. 1860. *Spiritual Gifts, Vol. 2.* Battle Creek, MI: James White. Reprint: 1944. Washington, DC: Review and Herald Publishing Association, 42–45, 84, 118, 135.

———. 1864. *Spiritual Gifts: Important Facts of Faith, Laws of Health, and Testimonies No. 1–10.* Battle Creek, MI: SDA Publishing Association.

———. 1867. *Writing Out the Light on Health Reform.* White Estate: MS-7–1867.

———. 1882. Temperance and the License Law. *Adventist Review and Sabbath Herald* 59 (April 11):289–90.

———. 1944. *Spiritual Gifts, Vol. 2.* Hagerstown, MD: Review and Herald Publishing Association.

———. 1953. *The Adventist Home.* Nashville, TN: Southern Publishing Association.

———. 1964. *Spirit of Prophecy Counsels Relating to Church-State Relations.* Silver Springs, MD: Ellen G. White Estate.

Prevention vs. Treatment in Hong Kong

Constrained Utilitarianism with a Chinese Character

HO MUN CHAN, PhD ∎

INTRODUCTION

"Prevention is better than cure" (預防勝於治療) is a common saying about health in many cultures, particularly Chinese. In traditional Chinese medicine good health is considered a reflection of harmony of the body: between the organs, mind and emotions, and the environment, and great emphasis is placed on prevention of disease and promotion of health (O'Brien and Xue 2003). Chapter *Suwen* of the *Huangdi Neijing* (皇帝內經 - 素問) defines the fundamental approach to health management in Chinese medicine as "try[ing] to live according to the rhythm of nature and avoid getting sick in the first place"—in other words, preventive medicine. Staying healthy rather than curing disease is indeed a good part of Chinese medicine. The *Huangdi Neijing* states that "Good physicians can treat the disease before it appears" (Kong 2010, 5–6). Nourishment of life by exercise, massage, meditation, and traditions of eating is regarded as a primary way of disease prevention and health promotion.

However, in the health care settings of modern Hong Kong with its distinctive background of integrating the cultures of Chinese and Western medicine, prevention came to no longer hold priority when compared to curative treatment. Gérvas et al. (2008) argued that striking the right balance between prevention and treatment is a great challenge. The main challenges include the fact that prevention can cause harm, and that predicting prevention activities can be difficult because many preventive interventions still lack significant evidence of effectiveness. Prevention may be of different value to different individuals, and whether to take a proactive or a reactive approach to health greatly depends on individual beliefs and various government policies. The difficulties also raise doubts—is it always true that prevention is better than cure? Not all preventive interventions have the same health-benefit value, and we know this using standard methodologies to assess prevention activities (Gérvas et al. 2008).

The aim of this chapter is to describe the Hong Kong government's policy, individuals' alternatives on prevention and treatment, and the dilemmas faced in the context of Hong Kong. Another aim is to give a Chinese account of the tension between allocating resources to prevention and treatment. Vaccination as a primary prevention and drug screening as a secondary prevention will be discussed as illustrations of the issues examined in this chapter. Though underemphasized in modern practice, prevention has recently attracted more focus and resources in the health care system of Hong Kong. This trend can be explained in part by a traditional emphasis on prevention that still survives in Hong Kong and other Chinese communities. The traditional relationship between prevention and treatment in Chinese medicine is significantly shaped, though not entirely dictated by a version of utilitarian considerations under the influence of the Chinese ethos. Though in terms of economic level Hong Kong is on par with many wealthy and developed societies in Europe and North America, because of its distinct culture rooted in the Chinese tradition, the response to the tension between allocating resources to prevention and treatment has taken on a very different shape.

POLICIES ON PREVENTION AND TREATMENT IN HONG KONG

As in many other developed countries, Hong Kong's health system focuses mainly on hospital-based curative services, which are mainly provided by the Hospital Authority and substantially subsidized by the government. A wide range of health prevention and promotion services including maternal and child health, student health, elderly health, and port health[1] is provided by the Department of Health (WHO 2008). The Hong Kong government has indicated that "every resident should have access to reasonable quality and affordable health care" (The Harvard Team 1999). However, Hong Kong's health care system is also at a crossroads, and due to aging of the population and advancing

---

1. "Port health" refers to environmental and health protection activities in ports, taken in light of the often unique health needs of ports. The phrase is especially common in Hong Kong, the United Kingdom, and European countries.

technology, financing for health care has become a major problem. Since the 1990s, various consultation documents have been written on health care reform and changes in health policy in Hong Kong. As criticized by the The Harvard Team (1999), health care in Hong Kong is highly compartmentalized, threatening the system's sustainability, quality, and efficiency. The health care delivery system overemphasizes hospital-based services and medical specialization. Preventive care is being neglected and is not adequately resourced (The Harvard Team 1999), and hospitals are considered as Meccas for curing ailments (Leong 1999, 315).

Arguably, the emphasis on treatment rather than prevention that developed in the latter half of the twentieth century began to shift with the pandemic of avian influenza in 1997 and Severe Acute Respiratory Syndrome (SARS) in 2003. Both provided the impetus for greater attention to disease prevention. It appears from mass media coverage that more health education and promotion efforts such as hand washing and cleanliness of the immediate environment are being introduced to the general public. In addition, over many years Hong Kong has successfully promoted a smoke-free culture; since July 2009, a smoking ban includes all indoor areas of restaurants, bars, workplaces, and public areas such as beaches and parks. The Hong Kong government also imposes import controls on the food supply for the protection of public health. In response to the first local human infection of avian influenza in 1997, Hong Kong has developed strategies to prevent, detect, and deal with any future outbreaks: separating people from poultry; worldwide outbreak intelligence gathering; vaccination for all imported and local chickens; stepped-up inspection and hygiene regulation of live poultry retail outlets, wholesale markets, and farms; banning live poultry stocking at retail outlets overnight; and a buyout scheme. Hong Kong gained valuable practical experience in quarantine, infection control, and other public health measures from the outbreak of SARS in 2003. In 2004, a Centre for Health Protection (CHP) was set up under the Department of Health to protect the community from communicable diseases through real-time surveillance, rapid intervention, and responsive risk communication (Hong Kong Themes 2008).

In the following several sections, three examples of primary and secondary prevention in the sociocultural context of Hong Kong will be described in some detail.

PRIMARY PREVENTION—FOOD AND DIETARY PRACTICE IN CHINESE MEDICINE AND SOCIETY

In *The Yellow Emperor's Classic of Medicine,* the *Neijing Suwen* (黃帝內經-素問), considerable mention is made of disease prevention—and by implication, its priority over treatment. In the old days the sages treated disease by preventing illness before it began, just as a good government or emperor was able to take the necessary steps to avert war. "The sages do not wait for the disease to occur, they treat the body so that disease will not occur. By the same token, the sages do not wait till a revolt breaks out, they rule wisely so that people are not rebellious. To administer medicine after a disease has occurred is tantamount to start digging a well when one feels thirsty, or to manufacture weapons when the battle has begun. Is it not a little late by then?" (Kong 2010, 14). ("聖人不治已病治未病, 夫病已成而後藥之, 亂已成而後治之, 譬猶渴而穿井, 鬥而鑄兵, 不亦晚乎?") This implies that prevention should come first in priority. In Chinese medicine, good health is achieved by maintaining harmony within the body, the balance of *Yin* and *Yang* in the body, and the consequent harmonious functioning of the *zang-fu* (organs). Treatment aims at correcting imbalance within the body, just as preventive practice in Chinese medicine aims to detect and address the imbalances in the body before they become serious problems. This is achieved by prophylactic use of herbal medicine, acupuncture, massage, meditation, etc. (O'Brien and Xue 2003, 82). For example, many herbs have been widely used for centuries to prevent diseases by modulating immunofunctions or serving as antioxidants (Cheng 2003). Other factors such as emotions, sufficient sleep, and physical exercises such as *Taichi* and *Qigong* can aid in the relaxation of mind and body and strengthen health (O'Brien and Xue 2003, 82).

Dietary practices and manipulation in particular serve to complement Western medicine both in preventing specific ailments and in treating multiple stages of the disease process. Food plays an important role in fueling a kind of battery of essential bodily energies. In the traditional conception, body homeostasis is maintained through avoiding excess "hot"/"cold" or "wet"/"dry" extremes of body energy, disturbances in energy flow, or inadequate energy levels. Various health problems are classified as being due to imbalances of energy. Excess "hot"/"cold" or "wet"/"dry" ailments were dealt with by increased consumption of foods of the opposite character; those due to disturbance of the normal flow of energy were avoided by the reduced intake of "poisonous" (毒), "irritating" (發), or "stimulating" (刺激) foods; and various tonics were believed to raise the amount of energy flow in the body. For example, "poisonous" energy tends to be manifested as allergic reactions and skin eruption (e.g., measles) and are frequently synonymous with "wet-hot" or "wet-poisonous" foods such as shellfish. "Irritating" foods disturb the proper circulation of body energy by causing it to flow too much or too quickly in some parts of the body and too little or too slow in others. "Stimulating" foods encourage the foods expenditure of body energy, resulting in exhaustion of the body's resources. A rich knowledge of complex dietary rules was prevalent among the lay public because the traditional rules filled explanatory and behavioral niches left open in Western medicine (Koo 1989a, 221–22, 1989b).

This does not mean that people under the influence of Chinese culture will in general reject the Western approach to prevention. On the contrary, given that there is a general acceptance of all kinds of Western medicine as coexisting with a local tradition that puts an emphasis on prevention, it is not surprising that the Western approach to prevention has been taken seriously. This point will be elaborated by the examples of vaccination as a primary prevention and drug screening as a secondary prevention.

PRIMARY PREVENTION—INFLUENZA VACCINATION

Preventive vaccination such as that for influenza artificially stimulates the immune system to fight against viral infections. Influenza is one of the most common infectious diseases, possesses high epidemic and pandemic potential, and is largely vaccine preventable. Vaccination programs attempt to achieve three objectives: individual protection (e.g., to prevent the disease and its complications in high-risk individuals); prevention of institutional outbreaks of the disease, which may in turn affect high-risk patients and staff (e.g., immunization of health care workers and residents of long-term care facilities); and reduction of the burden of disease in the community setting as a public health measure (e.g., vaccination of young children). In Hong Kong, the target groups for influenza vaccination include the elderly and disabled living in residential care homes, the elderly aged 65 or above, those with underlying medical conditions such as chronic illness, health care workers, children aged 6 to 23 months, and poultry workers. Although influenza vaccination is effective in the prevention of infection, it is argued that routine yearly vaccination of all healthy adults has not been deemed to be cost-effective. Moreover, there is always a limitation in the supply of vaccine. Also, some studies have shown that a mass vaccination approach does not demonstrate significant reductions in disease spread, economic loss, morbidity, and hospitalization. It has been reported by WHO that the uptake of influenza vaccination in the general public and among health care workers is suboptimal (Wong and Yuen 2005, 388).

It is generally accepted that vaccinating health care workers against influenza reduces the transmission of the virus in health care settings, decreases staff illness and absenteeism, and indirectly benefits patients by decreasing the chance of being infected. However, it raises the ethical principles of nonmaleficence and beneficence. The duty to do no harm, or nonmaleficence, means that health care workers have a duty not to place patients at undue risk of harm. Thus, health care workers have an obligation to accept the influenza vaccination to prevent the transmission of the virus and to minimize the risk of harm to patients. The duty of beneficence requires health care workers to act in the best interests of their patients by requiring annual influenza vaccination (Anikeeva et al. 2009, 25).

The Hong Kong Hospital Authority has provided free seasonal flu vaccinations to its staff annually, but only approximately 40% accepted the offer in 2007–2009. The Hong Kong government is planning to provide HK$1 billion for free swine flu (H1N1) vaccines in five high-risk groups including the elderly, chronically ill, young children, health care workers, pig farmers, and slaughterhouse workers. However, some caregivers plan to refuse the swine flu shots because some of them may think that the swine flu infection is still very mild and the side effects of the vaccines are still uncertain. Some of them also had known patients who developed serious complications after taking the seasonal flu inoculation. Some have been warned about the side effects of the new vaccines, such as in 1976, when of the 220 million who were vaccinated against swine flu, 400 developed Guillain-Barré syndrome, a disorder in which the body damages its own nerve cells, resulting in muscle weakness and sometimes paralysis. In the end, 32 people who had been vaccinated died of Guillain-Barré syndrome. Even a university microbiologist said that he would not recommend the new vaccines to anyone until the products were well supported by safety data, adding that "Any decision made without reliable safety data is irrational" (Leung 2009). However, based on their review of the existing scientific data and literature and the information provided by the pharmaceutical industry, experts in the Centre for Health Protection (CHP) maintain that this unfortunate side-effect is a far lower risk than that stemming from swine flu infections, especially for the high-risk groups. With the arrival of 500,000 doses of human swine flu vaccine, the government decided to launch the largest vaccination scheme ever in Hong Kong in December 2009 (China Daily 2009; Hong Kong Government 2009). The larger picture here is what Gérvas et al. (2008) painted in predicting that prevention activities can be difficult because many preventive interventions still lack strong evidence of benefit.

SECONDARY PREVENTION—SCREENING FOR SUBSTANCE ABUSE

Lifestyle can be a source of ill-health. Risky discrete behaviors include tobacco and alcohol use, poor diet and weight control, exercise patterns, stress, driving behavior, sexual activity, sleep patterns, and medication use (Lupton 1995, 142). According to the WHO, tobacco, alcohol abuse, and illicit drugs are among the top 20 risk factors for ill health (World Health Organization 2002).

Substance abuse with psychoactive drugs often causes physical or psychological harm, impaired judgment, and other dysfunctional behavior and dependent syndromes. It can involve brain damage and is associated with crime to support the habit, AIDS and other sexually transmitted diseases, imprisonment, social ostracism, and even death. The WHO estimates that 100,000 deaths occur from overdosage annually, many of them adolescents. The abuse involves all levels of society in developed and developing countries (Tulchinsky and Varavikova 2009, 266). Substance abuse in youth is a rising trend. Preventive measures such as control of drug trade and screening adolescents for drug use are believed to be effective. A strong policy aimed at prevention is justified in part because drug addiction involves uncontrollable compulsion to seek drugs. As Faggiano et al. (2005) maintain,

> People may use drugs to seek an effect, to feel accepted by their peers or as a way of dealing with life's problems. Even after undertaking detoxification to reach a drug-free state, many returned to opioid use. *This makes it important to reduce the number of people first using drugs and to prevent transition from experimental use to addiction.* For young people, peers, family and social context are strongly implicated in early drug use. Schools offer the most systematic and efficient way of reaching them. School programs can be designed to provide knowledge about the effect of drugs on the body and psychological effects, as a way of building negative attitudes towards drugs; to build individual self-esteem and self-awareness, working on psychological factors that may place people at risk of use; to teach refusal and social life skills; and to encourage alternative activities to drug use, which instill control abilities. (Faggiano et al. 2005).

Drug abuse in Hong Kong has become more serious in the past few years, particularly in the youth population. According to the Central Registry of Drug Abuse (CRDA), the total number of reported drug abusers increased 7% from 2006 to 2008. Young drug abusers increased an even greater 33% during this period, and among them, 26.3% were students. In 2008, nearly all reported young drug abusers (99%) used psychotropic substances such as ketamine, MDMA, and triazolam/midazolam/zopiclone. The major reasons for youth drug abuse include peer influence and the need to identify with peers, and curiosity and relief of boredom/depression/anxiety. Hence, the Hong Kong government decided to introduce different strategies to tackle the drug abuse problems, including drug testing in school sectors, preventive education and publicity, treatment and rehabilitation, new legislation, and enforcement and cross-boundary cooperation. One of the recommendations is for schools voluntarily to conduct student testing to identify drug abusers for treatment and rehabilitation. Students and their parents will be asked to sign a consent form pursuant to which students may be randomly selected to undergo drug tests; if they test positive, students may be requested to attend follow-up counseling or treatment. The test scheme pilot started in December 2009 in one local region in Hong Kong. School principals and teachers in the regional schools conducted briefings with students and parents concerning the drug test. In case of students' withdrawal of consent, parents will be notified and schools and social workers will follow-up with those students. If the test is positive, a second screening will be performed. A case manager will follow-up those confirmed cases without police participation. Students' positive tests will not be prosecuted unless they are involved in drug trafficking and possession (Lau 2009).

There may be strong resistance from schools and parents, and maintaining a reasonable level of compliance among parents and students will be very complex in local school settings. In addition, the administration of the tests by schools also may lead to a number of complex social, ethical, and technical issues as well as an extra workload to the schools. It may also likely to be difficult to obtain parental consent for the tests (Legislative Council Secretariat 2009). Drug screening indeed raises some important ethical issues, such as obtaining informed consent, who should consent, protecting privacy and confidentiality, balancing risks and potential benefits, and other considerations related to costs and allocation of limited resources for mass screening (Coughlin 2008). When the Hong Kong government first introduced the recommendation of drug testing in schools, the Privacy Commissioner, Roderick Woo, raised concerns about privacy issues and stated that students' parents or guardians had no authority to consent to testing on behalf of a minor (Sun et al. 2009). Even if a student is allowed to refuse, his or her autonomy and privacy may be compromised because of school, peer, and societal pressure.

Weddle and Kokotailo (2002) argued that adolescents lack sufficient intellectual capacity to make decisions about their health behaviors and care. There are four important requirements in obtaining informed consent in biomedical ethics: (1) competence to understand and decide, (2) disclosure of material information, (3) voluntariness, and (4) consent. The levels of competency of adolescents for making decision about their health care have great variations and are difficult to determine. In addition, decision making in health care ethics is guided by the principles of respect for autonomy, beneficence, nonmaleficence, and justice. For decision making about health care for a young child, beneficence and nonmaleficence are the guiding principles. Very often, respect for a child's autonomy is not the compelling principle, as parents have to make decisions for their child. Adolescents fall in a spectrum between the adult model and the pediatric model. However, as Elizabeth, Reppucci, and Woolard (1995) argue, even if adolescents have the competence to make informed consent, it does not follow that they have the maturity to exercise it, and their maturity may vary across different decisional contexts. Adolescents are less willing to risk the disfiguring side effects of medical treatment. They engage more commonly than adults in sex without contraceptives, reckless driving, and substance abuse because of peer pressure, curiosity, and relief of boredom/depression/anxiety. So some paternalistic measure may be justified in the case of drug abuse. According to some surveys done in Hong Kong, in fact, despite many reservations, around 70–80% of school teachers and students supported the school-based drug test scheme proposed by the government (Anonymous 2009a, 2009b; Siu 2009). Indeed, both the general public and the government recognized the importance of introducing reasonably strong preventive measures to tackle the problems of adolescent drug abuse.

TAKING UTILITARIAN CONSIDERATIONS SERIOUSLY, THOUGH NOT EXCLUSIVELY

The above examples show that the perceived cost-effectiveness of prevention is a recognized value in Hong Kong. Cost-effectiveness is one of the important utilitarian considerations in health care decision making. Faust and Menzel's thought experiment (Chapter 1 of this volume) will lead many to conclude that when all utilitarian differences—particularly benefit achieved and expense required—are *removed*, people will tend to prioritize treatment over prevention. It follows that even if a preventive measure surpasses a competing treatment to a certain extent in cost-effectiveness, people may still opt for the treatment. However, if the difference in cost-effectiveness is *significant*, it does not follow that the same people will give no priority to the preventive measures in the greater-difference case, unless they ignore the value of cost-effectiveness entirely. Preferences for prevention in such cases do not contradict the general result of the thought experiment. How great a difference in cost-effectiveness will be counted as significant depends on how much weight is assigned to the value of cost-effectiveness. Then this possibility distinctly emerges: that people in different cultures may assign a different value to cost-effectiveness. It seems from the factual considerations previously described that people in Chinese societies assign greater weight to such a value than their Western counterparts. This claim can be supported further by examining the moral ethos of Chinese society and the results of some relevant empirical studies.

The moral ethos in Chinese societies has been shaped by Confucianism over 2000 years. It is a complicated and sophisticated system of thought. Many comparative philosophers have tried to classify Confucianism in terms of categories developed in the West. Some regard it as a virtue-based theory (Bretzke 1995; Cua 1998; Nivison 1996; Wilson 1995; Yearley 1990), whereas others interpret it to be a form of utilitarianism (Hansen 1992; Im 1997; Munro 2005, 2008). Such classifications are oversimplifications. They give distorted pictures of Confucian ethics, which, I argue, should be regarded as a *pluralistic* theory with different levels of moral considerations. Confucianism draws a distinction between private (personal) and public (political) moralities (Munro 2005, 2008), which is akin to the one drawn by Max Weber in his "Politics as a Vocation" (Weber 1946).

According to Weber, political morality should be largely dictated by an ethics of responsibility (*Gesinnungethik*) that focuses exclusively on the outcome of political actions, whereas the ethics of conviction should largely be confined to private lives. Weber believes that the ethics of responsibility may sometimes require a public official, in order to secure a desirable outcome, not to act in accordance with some moral principle of his or her conviction. In the Weberian view, public decision making, if it is entirely dictated by the ethics of conviction, may lead to fanaticism, and the consequences could be disastrous.

In regard to personal morality, Confucianism emphasizes the importance of character formation in moral education and the cultivation of various virtues, including benevolence, filial piety, loyalty, and courage. The ultimate goal of moral education is to become an ethically ideal person (the so-called *junzi*, or "noble person") (Li 2004, 55–57). Having said that it does not mean that utilitarian considerations are entirely out of the picture in private morality, especially in cases in which the stake of the outcome is exceptionally high. In *Analects*, Confucius says that *bi* (strictness) and *gu* (inflexibility) should be avoided (Confucius 1999, 9.4). Although the virtue of filial piety is fundamental in Confucianism, Confucius said that if your father's punishment is unfair, you, as a filial child, should still accept it if he beats you with a small rod, but you should run away if the rod is big (Confucius 1992: 15.10).

The role of utilitarian considerations will loom much larger in so far as public morality is concerned. In Ancient China, the ideal of a sage is even morally higher than *junzi* (Li 2004). Yet, according to Confucius, a ruler can reach such a higher state by conferring extensive benefits to the multitude of common people. His view was expressed in the following dialogue with his student Zigong in the *Analects*:

> Zigong said, "If a ruler not only conferred wide benefits upon the common people, but also compassed the salvation of the whole state, what would you say of him. Surely, you would call him Good?" The Master said, "It would no longer be a matter of 'Good.' He would without doubt a Divine Sage." (Confucius 1999, 6.30).

Mencius, also, believes that if people concern themselves only with *li* (their own interests), society will run into chaos, and he advises rulers to act from *ren* (benevolence) and *yi* (propriety) by appealing to the consequence of social stability (Mencius 1999, 1.1 and 12.4).

Having said that, it does not follow that Confucians accept public officials dirtying their hands too easily and readily in order to secure desirable social or political outcomes (Chan 2009). Nor will they accept sacrificing the fundamental interests of some individual or social group, especially the worse off, for the sake of promoting the greatest social benefits for all. Confucians are not utilitarian through and through, and their utilitarian considerations are constrained by other moral considerations, such as the claims of the worse off. According to Mencius, human beings have an inborn compassion for the suffering. This innate compassion is regarded as the root of benevolence (Mencius 1999, 3.6). He believes that the ruler should act from benevolence and has the special responsibility to help the victim of natural disasters, the poor, and the elderly, especially those who are widows, widowers, childless, and orphans (Mencius 1999, 2.5). Yet this does not lead to the advocacy of egalitarianism or a strongly welfare program-oriented state. Mencius strongly opposes high taxation and too much government intervention in the economy and people's livelihoods, taxation and intervention that he believes will hinder the prosperity of a society.

The Confucian model of constrained utilitarianism has significantly shaped social policy making in many Chinese societies, manifesting an ethos rooted in the Confucian tradition. According to a survey in Beijing, Taipei, and Hong Kong (Chan 2004, 2005), an overwhelming majority of the subjects accepted the following Floor Constraint Principle for the distribution of income:

The most just distribution of income is that which maximizes the average income in the society only after a certain specified minimum income is guaranteed to everyone.

Both the principle of maximization of utility (without constraints) and Rawls' difference principle were extremely unpopular choices. Though most of the subjects supported maximization as an ideal, they maintained that it should be constrained by a concern for the worse off in society. So the results of the survey suggest that some form of constrained utilitarianism is commonly accepted in Chinese societies.

Further evidence for such a hypothesis is available in some surveys on people's attitude toward the allocation of health care resources in Chinese cities. One survey repeated in Hong Kong, Guangzhou, Shanghai, and Beijing the work done by Peter Ubel and George Loewenstein in the United States

(1996a, 1996b). Subjects were told that there were 100 usable livers to be allocated between the following two groups of patients who were waiting to undergo liver transplant (Chan 2006)[2]:

> Group 1: 100 children with a higher surviving rate of 80%
> Group 2: 100 children with a lower surviving rate of 70%

Subjects were then asked to decide how many livers should be allocated to each group of children. The above was one version of the simulated scenario. In other versions, the prognoses of the two groups were said to be 80% and 50%, 80% and 20%, 40% and 25%, and 40% and 10%. The most popular choice in Ubel and Lowenstein's study conducted in Pittsburgh was to divide the 100 livers for transplant equally between the two groups, but the most popular choice in Hong Kong and other Chinese cities was to give 51–75 livers to the group with higher surviving rates. This provides evidence for the claim that utilitarian considerations play a more significant role for subjects in Chinese societies. Yet it does not follow that their moral considerations were entirely dictated by utilitarianism. Many subjects still chose to give some—though a relatively small fraction—of livers to the group with lower surviving rates because of their concern about the well-being of the worst-off. Yet transplanting any of the 100 livers to the lower prognosis group violated the principle of maximization in the strict sense.

Another study that Ubel (2000) conducted in Philadelphia was also repeated in the above four Chinese cities (Chan 2006).[3] Subjects were asked to prioritize

2. The survey, using the method of face-to-face structure interview, was conducted in Hong Kong, Guangzhou, Beijing, and Shanghai at the selected households' home. In Hong Kong, a sample list of 2000 household addresses—a list of addresses of permanent quarters in build-up areas—covering 18 geographic districts in Hong Kong was drawn by the Census and Statistical Department from the Register of Quarters. The Department applied systematic replicated sampling with a fixed interval in sample unit selection. For Guangzhou, Beijing, and Shanghai, the method of systematic sampling, stratified sampling, and interval sampling was adopted. Each district is regarded as a "stratum." The samples were assigned to each district according to the population distribution in the Statistics Yearbook. In Hong Kong, 18 geographic district areas were sampled and a total of 1072 households were visited during the research period, 281 interviews were successfully achieved, and the response rate was 26.2%. In Beijing, 8 administrative districts were sampled and a total of 3654 households was visited, 1050 interviews were achieved, and the response rate was 29.2%. In Shanghai, 10 administrative districts were sampled and a total of 4717 households was visited, 1050 successful interviews were achieved, and the response rate was 23.4%. In Guangzhou, 6 Administrative districts were sampled and a total of 922 households was visited, 837 interviews were achieved, and the response rate was 90.8%.

3. This study was conducted on the same sample used in the previous survey.

the treatments for the following two illnesses that they were told had an equal chance of developing:

Illness A: seriously ill patients who can improve slightly with treatment
Illness B: moderately ill patients who can improve significantly with treatment

In Philadelphia, the most popular choice was to divide resources for the two groups of patients equally, but a majority of Chinese subjects gave priority to patients with illness B, though they wished to reserve some resources for illness A. Also, to be sure, some preferred giving priority to patients with illness A or dividing the resources equally.

In the above empirical studies, subjects were not asked to choose between preventive and curative interventions. A reason for favoring curative interventions is that those who need treatments are suffering diseases. It may be argued that they are worse off—at least at the time we are acting—and so their claims should have priority over those who need preventive interventions but whose health conditions are better. However, as we have seen, people in Chinese societies do not assign a great priority to the claims of worse off, though such claims will not be ignored entirely. On the contrary, their attitudes are more forward looking in the sense of putting more emphasis on the overall outcome attained by different interventions. That is particularly clear in the transplant prognosis study, in which the results harbored in a better prognosis may not be known for a considerable length of time, nor do we know at the time of allocation either precisely which individuals in the better prognosis group will in fact survive or who in the poorer prognosis group will not survive. To be sure, it is often difficult to ascertain whose condition is really worse off, but even if it can be discerned who has—or will have—severe as distinct from moderate illness, it seems very clear that Chinese subjects put more emphasis on the health care outcome. Therefore, it is plausible to predict that if Chinese subjects are asked to choose between preventive and curative interventions, more Chinese subjects will assign a relatively high priority to prevention than subjects in some Western societies likely do. This will be reflected in preference for prevention over treatment not when cost-effectiveness is equal, but only when the overall cost-effectiveness of the prevention is significantly greater than that of the treatment.

Of course, more empirical studies are needed to verify the above prediction. Nevertheless, there are numerous available examples that show that utilitarian considerations do loom large, though not exclusively, in health care policy making in Chinese societies. The design of the standard drug formulary for public hospitals and clinics introduced in July 2005 in Hong Kong is a very good example. According to the formulary, for drugs with preliminary evidence or marginal benefits over available alternatives but at significantly higher costs, the principle of cost-effectiveness was followed and their use would no longer be subsidized. Drugs proven to have significant benefits but that were extremely expensive for public hospitals and clinics were also excluded from the standard formulary. The following justification was provided for the exclusion, which had the implication that greater priority was given to secondary prevention for illness arising from simple hypertension or diabetes.

> An example of this type of drug is imatinib (Glivec) for the treatment of gastrointestinal stromal tumor (GIST). The existing standard treatment is surgery and supportive care. For patients with unresectable GIST, the prognosis is poor, with few patients, if any, surviving beyond 5 years. For patients who have been put on Glivec, the overall survival estimates will be around 70% at 2 years, as compared with 20% for patients under conventional treatment. The annual cost of this drug for one patient is HK$180,000 to HK$270,000.
>
> The opportunity cost for treating a patient with drugs proven to be of significant benefits but extremely expensive (see the above example) will mean forgoing treatment for a much larger number of patients with other effective means. For example, the annual cost of putting one patient on Glivec is equivalent to the annual costs of treating a few hundred to a thousand patients with simple hypertension or diabetes. As there is an overriding need for rational use of finite public resources and competing needs to maximize health benefits ... patients ... [who require] such expensive treatment and can afford to pay should pay under the targeted subsidy principle. These non-standard drugs are therefore not covered under the standard fees and charges of public hospital clinics. (Hospital Authority 2005)

Having said that, it does not mean that the drug policy entirely ignores the well-being of those who suffer from high cost illness. Partial or full subsidy for extremely expensive drugs will still be provided for patients who pass the means test, although no such test is needed for drugs in the standard formulary. So the design of the formulary is not entirely dictated by utilitarian considerations because there is still some concern about the well-being of the worse off.

CONCLUSIONS

The development of preventive care in Hong Kong, as my review of some relevant cases has shown, faces problems, dilemmas, and challenges similar to those faced in many other societies. There is no simple resolution of the tension between allocating resources to prevention as compared to treatment that is universally applicable to all kinds of cases within a society. Chinese medicine has a long and distinct tradition of putting an emphasis on prevention, and the moral culture of Chinese communities is deeply shaped, though not entirely dictated, by a constrained utilitarianism present in Confucian tradition. Thus, the development of preventive care in Hong Kong, and perhaps in other Chinese societies as well, arguably reflects a different resolution of the tension than what has evolved in many other societies.

ACKNOWLEDGMENTS

I am greatly indebted to Germaine Cheung for her help in drafting this chapter. Thanks are also due to Gary Wong and C.K. Chui for their research support. The preparation of this chapter and the research reported have been funded by the Governance in Asia Research Centre, City University of Hong Kong.

REFERENCES

Anikeeva, O., Braunack_Mayer, A., & Rogers, W. 2009. Health Policy and Ethics: Requiring Influenza Vaccination for Health Care Workers. *American Journal of Public Health* 99(1): 24–29.

Anonymous. 2009a. Nov. 28. 大埔學生支持驗毒 大公報.

Anonymous. 2009b. Nov. 2. 觀塘初中生 80 percent 贊同驗毒. 文匯報.

Bretzke, J.T. 1995. The Tao of Confucian Virtue Ethics. *International Philosophical Quarterly* 35 (1):25 41.

Chan, H.M. 2004. The Ethics of Care and Political Practices in Hong Kong. In B.H. Chua, Ed., *Communitarian Politics in Asia* (pp. 102–21). London: Routledge and Kegan Paul.

———. 2005. Rawls' Theory of Justice: A Naturalistic Evaluation. *Journal of Medicine and Philosophy* 29 (5):449–65.

———. 2006. *How to Strike a Balance between Efficiency and Fairness in Public Health Care Reform?* Unpublished paper presented at the Workshop on Comparative Policy in Hong Kong and Shanghai, East China Normal University, Shanghai, December 15–17.

———. 2009. Whose Responsibility? Marginalization of Personal Responsibility and Moral Character. In L.C. Li, Ed., *Towards Responsible Government in East Asia: Trajectories, Intentions and Meanings* (pp. 101–11). London and New York: Routledge and Kegan Paul.

Cheng, Y.C. 2003. Globalisation of Chinese Medicine. In P.C. Leung, C.C. Xue, and C.M. Cheng, Eds., *A Comprehensive Guide to Chinese Medicine* (pp. 215–44). Singapore: World Scientific Publishing Co. Ltd.

China Daily. 2009. *China Daily* (Hong Kong edition), December 1.

Confucius. 1992. Kongzi Jiayu (The School Sayings of Confucius). In D. C. Lau, Ed., *A Concordance to the Kongzi Jiayu* (pp. 1–91). Hong Kong: The Commercial Press Limited.

———. 1999. *The Analects*. Hunan: Hunan People's Publishing House.

Coughlin, S.S. 2008. Ethics of Screening. In K. Heggenhougen, Ed., *International Encyclopedia of Public Health* (pp. 503–08). Atlanta: Elsevier.

Cua, A. S. 1998. Basic Concepts of Confucian Ethics. In A. S. Cua, Ed., *Moral Vision and Tradition: Essays in Chinese Ethics* (pp. 267–302). Washington D C: The Catholic University of American Press.

Elizabeth, S. S. Reppucci, N. D., and Woolard, J. L. 1995. Evaluating Adolescent Decision Making in Legal Contexts. Law and Human Behavior, 19(3), 221–44.

Faggiano, F., Vigna-Taglianti, F., Versino, E., Zambon, A., Borraccino, A., and Lemmma, P. 2005. School-based Prevention for Illicit Drugs' Use. Cochrane Database of Systematic Review 2.

Gérvas, J., Starfield B., and Heath, I. 2008. Is Clinical Prevention Better than Cure? The Lancet 372: 1997–99.

Hansen, C. 1992. *A Daoist of Chinese Thought: A Philosophical Interpretation*. New York: Oxford University Press.

Harvard Team. 1999. *Improving Hong Kong's Health Care System: Why and For Whom?* Hong Kong: Health and Welfare Bureau

Hong Kong Government. 2009. *Swine Flu Shot Programme to Launch*, Dec 21. Available at http://news.gov.hk/en/category/healthandcommunity/091130/html/091130en050 10.htm.

Hong Kong Themes. 2008. *Health Protection and Pandemic Prevention*. Available at http://www.investhk.gov.hk/UploadFile/IPA_health_protection_eng.pdf.

Hospital Authority. 2005. *HA Drug Formulary*. Available at http://www.ha.org.hk/hadf/en_welcome.html.

Im, M. 1997. *Emotion and Ethical Theory in Mencius*. Ann Arbor: The University of Michigan Press.

Kong, Y.C. 2010. *Huangdi Neijing: A Synopsis with Commentaries*. Hong Kong: The Chinese University of Hong Kong Press.

Koo, L.C. 1989a. Ethnonutrition in Hong Kong: Traditional Dietary Methods of Treating and Preventing Disease. *The Hong Kong Practitioner* 11 (5):221–31.

———. 1989b. A Journey into the Cultural Aspects of Health and Ill-Health in Chinese Society in Hong Kong—the Importance of Health and Preventive Medicine in Chinese Society. *The Hong Kong Practitioner* 11 (2):51–58.

Lau, N. 2009. $11m Tagged for School Drug Testing. *The Standard*, October 29.

Legislative Council Secretariat. 2009. *The Youth Drug Abuse Problem in Hong Kong* (No. IN12/08–09). Hong Kong: Research and Library Services Division.

Leong, C.H. 1999. Primary Health Care Policy in Hong Kong. *Hong Kong Practitioner* 21 (7):312–16.

Leung, K.L. 2009. Health Care Workers Wary of Flu Vaccine. *South China Morning Post*, June 13.

Li, Y. 2004. *The Unity of Rule and Virtue*. Singapore: Eastern Universities Press.

Lupton, D. 1995. *The Imperative of Health*. London: SAGE.

Mencius. 1999. *Mencius.* Hunan China: Hunan People's Publishing House.

Munro, D.J. 2005. *A Chinese Ethics for the New Century.* Hong Kong: The Chinese University Press.

———. 2008. *Ethics in Action: Workable Guidelines for Private and Public Choice.* Hong Kong: The Chinese University Press.

Nivison, D.S. 1996. *The Ways of Confucianism.* Chicago: Open Court.

O'Brien, K.A., and Xue, C.C. 2003. Theoretical Framework of Chinese Medicine. In P.C. Leung, C.C. Xue, and Y.C. Cheng, Eds., *A Comprehensive Guide to Chinese Medicine* (pp. 47–84). Singapore: World Scientific Publishing Co. Ltd.

Siu, B. 2009. Student Concern over Drug-Test Discrimination. *Hong Kong Standard,* November 2.

Sun, C., Lam, A., and Lo, C. 2009. Doctor Questions City's Readiness for Drug Tests. *South China Morning Post.* Hong Kong, August 13.

The Harvard Team. 1999. *Improving Hong Kong's Health Care System: Why and For Whom?* Hong Kong: Health and Welfare Bureau.

Tulchinsky, T.H., and Varavikova, E.A. 2009. *The New Public Health,* 2nd ed. London: Elsevier.

Ubel, P.A. 2000. *Pricing Life: Why It's Time for Health Care Rationing.* Cambridge, MA: The MIT Press.

Ubel, P.A., and Loewenstein, G. 1996a. Public Perceptions of the Importance of Prognosis in Allocating Transplantable Livers to Children. *Medical Decision Making* 16:234–41.

———. 1996b. Distributing Scarce Livers: The Moral Reasoning of the General Public. *Social Science and Medicine* 42:1049–55.

Weber, M. 1946. *From Max Weber: Essays in Sociology.* In H.H. Gerth and C. Wright Mills, Eds., trans. London: Routledge and Kegan Paul.

Weddle, M., and Kokotailo, P. 2002. Adolescent Substance Abuse Confidentiality and Consent. *The Pediatric Clinics of North America* 49:301–15.

Wilson, S.A. 1995. Conformity, Individuality, and the Nature of Virtue. *Journal of Religious Ethics* 23 (2):263–87.

Wong, Y.Y.S., and Yuen, K.Y. 2005. Influenza Vaccination: Options and Issues. *Hong Kong Medical Journal* 11:381–90.

World Health Organization (WHO). 2002. *The World Health Report 2002: Reducing Risks, Promoting Healthy Life.* Geneva: WHO.

———. 2008. *Country Health Information Profile*: Hong Kong (China). Available at http://www.wpro.who.int/NR/rdonlyres/0FA1B5CA-B81D-40BF-A26B-F9680 DF1FFC9/0/14HongKong08.pdf.

Yearley, L.H. 1990. *Mencius and Aquinas: Theories of Virtue and Conceptions of Courage.* New York: State University of New York Press.

Printed in the USA/Agawam, MA
December 27, 2011

563171.009